Ophthalmic Tumours

MONOGRAPHS IN OPHTHALMOLOGY

P.C. Maudgal and L. Missotten (eds.), Superficial Keratitis. 1981.
ISBN 90-6193-801-5.

P.F.J. Hoyng, Pharmacological Denervation and Glaucoma. A Clinical Trial Report with Guanethidine and Adrenaline in One Eye Drop. 1981.
ISBN 90-6193-802-3.

N.W.H.M. Dekkers, The Cornea in Measles. 1981. ISBN 90-6193-803-1.

P. Leonard and J. Rommel, Lens Implantation – 30 years of progress. 1982.
ISBN 90-6193-804-X.

C.E. van Nouhuys, Dominant Exudative Vitreoretinopathy and Other Vascular Developmental Disorders of the Peripheral Retina. 1982. ISBN 90-6193-805-8.

L. Evens (ed.), Convergent Strabismus. 1982. ISBN 90-6193-806-6.

A. Neetens, A. Löwenthal and J.J. Martin (eds.), The Visual System in Myelin Disorders. 1984. ISBN 90-6193-807-4.

H.J.M. Völker-Dieben, The Effect of Immunological and Non-Immunological Factors on Corneal Graft Survival. 1984. ISBN 90-6193-808-2.

J.A. Oosterhuis, Ophthalmic Tumours. 1985. ISBN 90-6193-528-8.

Ophthalmic Tumours

Including lectures presented at the Boerhaave Course on "Ophthalmic Tumours" of the Leiden Medical Faculty, held in Leiden, The Netherlands, on February 2–3, 1984

edited by

Jendo A. Oosterhuis

1985 **DR W. JUNK PUBLISHERS**
a member of the KLUWER ACADEMIC PUBLISHERS GROUP
DORDRECHT / BOSTON / LANCASTER

Distributors

for the United States and Canada: Kluwer Academic Publishers, 190 Old Derby Street, Hingham, MA 02043, USA
for the UK and Ireland: Kluwer Academic Publishers, MTP Press Limited, Falcon House, Queen Square, Lancaster LA1 1RN, UK
for all other countries: Kluwer Academic Publishers Group, Distribution Center, P.O. Box 322, 3300 AH Dordrecht, The Netherlands

Library of Congress Cataloging in Publication Data

Boerhaave Course on "Ophthalmic Tumours" (1984 :
Leiden, Netherlands)
Ophthalmic tumours.

(Monographs in ophthalmology ; 9)
1. Eye--Tumors--Congresses. 2. Eye-sockets--Tumors--
Congresses. 3. Adnexa oculi--Tumors--Congresses.
I. Oosterhuis, J. A. II. Rijksuniversiteit te Leiden.
Faculteit der Geneeskunde. III. Title. IV. Series.
[DNLM: 1. Eye Neoplasms--congresses. W1 MO568D v.9 /
WW 149 B672o 1984]
RC280.E9B64 1984 616.99'284 85-5605
ISBN 90-6193-528-8

ISBN 90-6193-528-8 (this volume)

PRINTED IN THE NETHERLANDS

CONTENTS

Note to the reader:

The figures on the dust jacket are colour reproductions of the figures found on page 95 of this book.

INTRODUCTORY REMARKS

Tumours of the eye, orbit and adnexa are fields in ophthalmology which in recent years have shown rapid advances both in diagnostics and in treatment. This volume deals with many questions, such as

- which is the survival rate in choroidal melanoma in relation to its clinical and histopathological characteristics?
- what treatment modalities alternative to enucleation are currently being used, which of them have been abandoned, and which of them show promise for the future?
- what irradiation techniques are currently being used to treat choroidal and ciliary body melanomas and which are their indications, results and rate of complications?
- how can one differentiate non-pigmented tumours in the ocular fundus?
- to what extent has the survival rate in retinoblastoma patients improved over the years and what irradiation technique offers minimal risk of side effects?
- which are the rates of metastasis and survival in conjuntival melanomas?
- which are the general principles in oncological surgery and how are they to be applied in the management of orbital tumours?
- how do ENT tumours affect the orbit?
- which are the features of pseudo-tumours, vascular tumours, and benign tumours of the orbit?
- which is the significance of cytostatic or irradiation treatment in tumours of the orbit and adnexa?
- how does one diagnose and how does one treat adnexal tumours?
- which is the significance of cryotherapy in the treatment of adnexal tumours?

If you know the answers to these questions you do not need to buy this volume.

If you do not know the answers to these questions, you will find them in this volume, together with a lot of other information on tumours of the eye, orbit and adnexa.

This volume includes lectures presented at a "Boerhaave Course" of the Leiden University by experts in the various fields.

I would especially like to thank Professor G.M. Bleeker, the mentor of the wellknown Orbita Team of the Amsterdam University Hospital, and his collaborators for their contributions on the orbit, and Miss I.G. Jeltes for her editorial assistance.

Jendo A. Oosterhuis

DIFFERENTIAL DIAGNOSIS OF VERY SMALL MELANOMAS AND NAEVI OF THE CHOROID

J.A. Oosterhuis and D. de Wolff-Rouendaal

Diagnosis of large choroidal melanomas usually does not present special problems, especially when the tumour is very prominent and shows the characteristic features of a choroidal melanoma. The ophthalmologist must be familiar with the various ophthalmologic aspects of the pigmented as well as the amelanotic type of melanoma; the latter develops especially when the tumour has perforated through Bruch's membrane. The diagnosis can be confirmed by means of fluorescein angiography and ultrasonography. When the diagnosis remains doubtful the phosphor 32 test is a very reliable examination method in the differential diagnosis.

In small melanocytic choroidal tumours situated near the posterior pole clinical differentiation between choroidal naevus and malignant melanoma can be very difficult. Nowadays, when most of these tumours are not treated any longer by enucleation of the eye but by irradiation, a reliable assessment of the diagnosis is more important than ever as we have no histopathological confirmation of the diagnosis any more. Irradiation mistakenly performed in benign tumours may endanger vision because of irradiation side effects and make statistic calculation of the results unreliable.

We have studied the eyes of 41 patients with a small choroidal pigmented lesion which on ophthalmoscopy did not show the typical characteristics of a naevus or a melanoma but had an aspect which could be associated with both types of tumour.

Oosterhuis, A. (ed.), Ophthalmic tumors.

ISBN 90-6193-528-8. Printed in the Netherlands.

Clinical examination

As parameters for differentiation we used: prominence of the tumour, P32 uptake test, fluorescence angiography, perimetry, and presence or absence of visual complaints.

Ophthalmoscopy is valuable in cases characteristic of melanoma (Gass, 1974) or naevus (Oosterhuis & von Winning, 1979), but the fundus aspect of a naevus associated with pigment-epithelial degeneration and subretinal leakage may be difficult to differentiate from that of a small, flat melanoma. We used ophthalmoscopy to determine the maximum diameter and prominence of the tumour, the presence or absence of drusen, orange pigment, and pigment-epithelial degeneration. Subretinal exudation was looked for by means of binocular ophthalmoscopy, with slitlamp and Goldmann contact lens. The degree of prominence of the tumour is important, because the vast majority of naevi is flat or shows a prominence of only 0.5-1.0 dioptre, in exceptional cases 1-2 dioptres (Naumann, 1970); thus, a prominence of more than 2 dioptres may indicate the tumour to be a melanoma.

The phosphor 32 (P32) uptake test was carried out in all our patients. A conjunctival incision was always required and in some of the patients also a rectus muscle had to be detached to give the probe access to the macular area. A difference of more than 60% between tumour and control site found 48 hours after administration of the P32 was considered to be suggestive of malignancy, a difference of more than 100% as a very strong indication of malignancy. The P32 isotope examination is the most reliable ancillary test currently available for the diagnosis of choroidal melanocytic tumours.

In our series of 194 eyes with histopathologically proven malignant melanoma the P32 test results were positive in 192 cases (99%) (Oosterhuis et al., 1980), which agrees with the results of Shields (1978), who found a positive P32 test result in 213 out of 226 melanoma eyes (98.7%). All our P32 test values of more than +100% were associated, like those of Shields (1978), with malignant tumours, but in the range between +60% and +100% we had 2 false-positive results among 60 benign lesions, one in a histopathologically proven choroidal haemangioma (Oosterhuis et al., 1980) and one in a tumour clinically presumed to be naevus. Shields (1978) too obtained a positive P32 test result in 2 out of 20 haemangiomas, but none among 23 clinically assessed choroidal naevi.

Accurate performance of the P32 test in small tumours requires perfect localisation of the tumour, which we performed with the aid of a fibre optic localisator of own design, and great experience in this seemingly simple technique (Ruiz, 1977; Shields, 1978). It has been suggested that a lesion smaller than 7 mm in diameter can not always be tested accurately (Shields, 1978), but all our melanomas with a diameter as small as 3-7 mm in the histologic sections had given a positive P32 test result.

Fluorescein angiography is a helpful adjunct in the evaluation of suspect intraocular tumours (Gass, 1974; Hayreh, 1974; Oosterhuis & van Waveren, 1968). Choroidal naevi with only the typical slate-gray appearance, with or without signs of drusen, and with the characteristic fluorescein-angiographic pattern (Oosterhuis & von Winning, 1979) but without pigment-epithelial lesions or accumulation of subretinal fluid, were not included in the present study, because in these cases there is no doubt as to the diagnosis and therefore the P32 test was considered to be superfluous.

A typical choroidal melanoma pattern seen on fluorescein angiography, especially one showing a circular zone of pinpoint hyperfluorescence due to damaged pigment epithelium surrounded by a non-fluorescent zone, strongly supports malignancy (Oosterhuis & Scheffer, 1976). In naevi, a reticular structure in the choroidal filling phase corresponding with the architecture of the choriocapillaris is a sign of benignity (Oosterhuis & von Winning, 1979); this was found in 3 out of 18 naevi. The fluorescence angiogram may become non-specific when subretinal fluid blurs the fluorescence pattern of the tumour.

Kinetic perimetry was carried out with the Goldmann perimeter, using isoptres I:1-4 and V:4, and the Friedmann visual field analyser; when relative scotomas were found or visual field defects were absent, static perimetry was performed with the Tübinger perimeter.

Perimetry has been neglected as an aid in differentiation between naevus and melanoma. In our opinion, however, it is a valuable aid in the differential diagnosis, because the non-toxic naevus cells do not interfere with the choroidal function or do so only slightly over the years leading to the deposition of drusen material in Bruch's membrane and incidentally to pigment-epithelial leakage but rarely to damage of the outer segments of the sensory cells, as has been shown on histopathological examination (Karickhoff, 1967; Naumann et al., 1966). Therefore, in choroidal naevi visual field defects are absent (Aulhorn, 1966) or there is only a relative scotoma, the latter having been found in 7.5-30% on kinetic perimetry (van Dijk, 1978; Naumann et al., 1966 & 1971; Tamler, 1970; Tamler & Maumenee, 1959). The relative visual field defects have been clinically associated with 1-2 D elevation of the tumour, usually with drusen or focal pigment-epithelial atrophy (Naumann et al., 1971). Subretinal fluid only rarely develops; it has been found in only 3 out of 102 naevi (Naumann et al., 1966)and in 2.1% of 933 naevi (Pro et al., 1978).

Melanoma cells exert a toxic effect; on histopathology secondary retinal degeneration is far more severe in malignant melanoma than in naevus (Karickhoff, 1967). Therefore, the finding of a normal visual field in malignant melanoma is quite exceptional (Shields et al., 1975). Several studies performed in up to 600 melanoma patients (Aulhorn, 1966; van Dijk, 1978; Karickhoff, 1967) showed a visual field defect in all patients and an absolute defect in 58%

(Aulhorn, 1966) and 86% (van Dijk, 1978).

Perimetry studies have shown that a relative scotoma can be associated with either naevus or melanoma, but that the absence of a scotoma is strongly indicative of a naevus and that the presence of an absolute scotoma is strongly indicative of a melanoma. In our series of 18 clinical naevi scotomas were absent in 10 patients, a relative scotoma was found on kinetic and/or static perimetry in 6 patients and an absolute scotoma in 2 patients. Perimetry performed in 22 of our 23 patients with a very small choroidal melanoma revealed an absolute scotoma in 21 and a relative scotoma in only 1 patient.

Visual complaints can be expected more readily in a melanoma, being an expanding tumour, than in a naevus. In naevi, visual loss is usually related to subretinal fluid in the macular area, but it is an uncommon complication (Naumann et al., 1966; Pro et al., 1978). Only 3 of our 18 patients with clinical naevi but 21 of our 23 patients with very small melanomas had visual complaints.

From our study we conclude that none of the examination methods used in our study was in itself totally reliable and therefore complete dependence on any of the tests is not justified.

Out of the 18 patients with a clinical naevus, one had a positive P32 test result, one showed a fluorescence pattern simulating that of a melanoma, two patients with subretinal leakage had an absolute scotoma, and two had a prominence of the tumour of 2½ dioptres; however, in each of these 18 only one test result was suggestive of a melanoma. As the results of all other functional tests were inconclusive or negative, we decided to consider these tumours as benign; in fact, none of them did show clinical growth during the follow-up period averaging 5½ years.

On the other hand, 20 out of the 23 patients with a very small melanoma each showed three or even four examination results strongly indicative of malignancy: a P32 test result of more than 100%, an absolute scotoma, a characteristic melanoma pattern on fluorescein angiography, a tumour prominence of more than 2 dioptres. In the other 3 patients only two test results pointed toward malignancy: in two of them the P32 test result was higher than +100% and the fluorogram was characteristic; the third patient had a typical fluorogram and an absolute scotoma but the P32 test result of +75% was only suspect.

In view of the present results the importance of taking into account all information obtained by a multifunctional examination before starting treatment of pigmented choroidal lesions can not be overstressed.

Histopathological examination (cell type)

Thirteen of the 23 melanoma eyes (57%) contained pure spindle cell melanomas, three (13%) pure epithelioid cell tumours and seven (30%) mixed cell melanomas with varying amounts of spindle cells and epithelioid cells. Thus, ten melanomas (43%) harboured epithelioid cells. Ten eyes (43%) showed no or only slight infiltration of tumour tissue into the innermost scleral layers. Nine eyes (39%) showed deep infiltration up to 1/2-3/4 of the scleral thickness, mainly around blood vessels and nerve penetrating the sclera. In three eyes (13%) melanoma cells had reached the scleral surface but without episcleral tumour formation. Penetration through Bruch's membrane was found in 22%.

Thus, we found a high incidence (43%) of epithelioid cells in our series of very small melanomas with a diameter of up to 7 mm and elevation of up to 2 mm. In series of melanomas of up to 10 mm diameter and 3 mm elevation the incidence of epithelioid cells found by others was 22% (Davidorf & Lang, 1975), 33% (Curtin, 1977; Zimmerman & McLean, 1975) and 62% (Hagler et al., 1977). The high incidence of epithelioid cells and the high degree of scleral ingrowth of 52% in our series of very small melanomas indicate that in case of growth they will lead to a poor prognosis with respect to life expectancy (Manschot & van Peperzeel, 1980).

References

Aulhorn, E.: Funktionsstörungen im Bereich von Aderhauttumoren. Ophthalmologica Additamentum ad vol. 151: 647-653, 1966.

Curtin, V.T.: Malignant melanoma management. In: Controversy in Ophthalmology, ed. R.J. Brockhurst et al. W.B. Saunders Co., Philadelphia, 1977, pp 635-640.

Davidorf, F.H. and Lang, J.R.: The natural course of malignant melanoma of the choroid: small vs large tumors. Trans. AAOO 79: OP.310-OP.320, 1975.

Dijk, R.A. van: The 32P-test and other methods in the diagnosis of intraocular tumours. Thesis. Dr.W.Junk Publ., The Hague, 1978.

Gass, J.D.M.: Differential diagnosis of intraocular tumors. C.V. Mosby, St. Louis, 1974.

Hagler, S.W., Jarett II, W.H. and Killian, J.H.: The use of the 32P test in the management of malignant melanoma of the choroid: A five-year follow-up study. Trans. AAOO 83: OP.49-OP.60, 1977.

Hayreh, S.S.: Choroidal tumors: role of fluorescein fundus angiography in their diagnosis. Current Concepts in Ophthalmology IV: 168-201, 1974.

Karickhoff, J.R.: Loss of visual function and visual cells in 600 cases of malignant melanoma. Amer.J.Ophthal. 64: 268-273, 1967.

Manschot, W.A. and van Peperzeel, H.A.: Choroidal melanoma. Enucleation or observation? A new approach. Arch.Ophthal. 98: 71-77, 1980.

Naumann, G.: Pigmentierte Naevi der Aderhaut und des Ciliarkörpers. Adv.Ophthal. 23: 187-272, 1970.

Naumann, G.O.H., Hellner, K. and Naumann, L.R.: Pigmented nevi of the choroid. Clinical study of secondary changes in the overlying tissues. Trans. AAOO 75: 110-122, 1971.

Naumann, G., Zimmerman, L.E. and Yanoff, M.: Visual field defect associated with choroidal nevus. Amer.J.Ophthal. 62: 914-917, 1966.

Oosterhuis, J.A., Pauwels, E.K.J., de Wolff-Rouendaal, D. and Jeltes, I.G.: 32P Phosphorus uptake test in choroidal melanomas, naevi and haemangiomas. Docum.Ophthal. 50: 9-19, 1980.

Oosterhuis, J.A. and Scheffer, C.H.: Choroidal naevus and melanoma. Docum.Ophthal.Proc.Series 9 ISFA, ed. J.J. de Laey. Dr. W.Junk Publ., The Hague, 1976, pp 263-267.

Oosterhuis, J.A. and van Waveren, Ch.W.: Fluorescein photography in malignant melanoma. Ophthalmologica 156: 101-116, 1968.

Oosterhuis, J.A. and von Winning, C.H.O.M.: Naevus of the choroid. Ophthalmologica 178: 156-165, 1979.

Pro, M., Shields, J.A. and Tomer, T.L.: Serous detachment of the macula associated with presumed choroidal nevi. Arch. Ophthal. 96: 1374-1377, 1978.

Ruiz, R.S.: Early treatment in malignant melanomas of the choroid. In: Controversy in Ophthalmology, ed. R.J. Brockhurst et al. W.B. Saunders Co., Philadelphia, 1977, pp 604-610.

Shields, J.A.: Accuracy and limitations of the 32P test in the diagnosis of ocular tumors: an analysis of 500 cases. Ophthalmology 85: 950-966, 1978.

Shields, J.A., Annesley Jr., W.H. and Totino, J.A.: Non-fluorescent malignant melanomas of the choroid diagnosed with the radioactive phosphorus uptake test. Amer.J. Ophthal. 79: 634-640, 1975.

Tamler, E.: A clinical study of choroidal nevi. A follow-up report. Arch.Ophthal. 84: 29-32, 1970.

Tamler, E. and Maumenee, A.E.: A clinical study of choroidal nevi. Arch.Ophthal. 62: 196-202, 1959.

Zimmerman, L.E. and McLean, I.W.: Changing concepts of the prognosis and management of small malignant melanomas of the choroid. Montgomery Lecture 1975. Trans.Ophthal.Soc. U.K. 95: 487-494, 1975.

FIVE-YEAR FOLLOW-UP STUDY OF CHOROIDAL AND CILIARY BODY MELANOMAS AFTER ENUCLEATION*

H.M. Kakebeeke-Kemme, J.A. Oosterhuis and D. de Wolff-Rouendaal

Since 1973 326 patients with a uveal melanoma have been examined in the Leiden University Eye Clinic. Three hundred and five eyes of 304 patients were enucleated because of a choroidal or ciliary body melanoma; one patient with the dysplastic naevus or familial atypical multiple mole melanoma (FAMMM) syndrome had a choroidal melanoma in both eyes. In 4 patients local resection of ciliary body melanoma was performed. Three rather old patients were successfully treated by photocoagulation in view of their age; all died from non-tumour-related causes. Eight patients were not treated for various reasons; one had clinical signs of metastasis at the time of diagnosis, the other 7 have been carefully observed up till now. Seven patients have been treated with local irradiation by ruthenium-106 or cobalt-60 applicators.

As new conservative ways of treatment have been introduced and are successfully being carried out nowadays, it is important to have complete data and good statistics on all kinds of treatment of uveal melanomas. Numerous studies have been published on the survival rate of patients who underwent enucleation because of a uveal melanoma. Unfortunately, many of these studies do not have a follow-up period comparable to our own study. We feel dat data can only be compared when similar periods of survival are taken into account, for instance 5-year periods as in general oncology, as has been done by Jensen (1982), Thomas et al. (1979),

* This study was supported by a grant from the "Koningin Wilhelmina Fonds"

Oosterhuis, A. (ed.), Ophthalmic tumors.

ISBN 90-6193-528-8. Printed in the Netherlands.

Davidorf and Lang (1975), Packard (1980), Shammas and Blodi (1977), Seddon et al. (1983) and McLean et al. (1977).

Material and Method

Between January 1973 and June 1978 enucleation was performed in 176 patients because of a choroidal (170) or ciliary body (6) melanoma. In all patients examination included ophthalmoscopy, fundus drawings, perimetry, photography, fluorescein angiography, P32-uptake test, and in part of them also ultrasonography. In all eyes the diagnosis malignant melanoma was confirmed on histopathologic examination by one of us (DdW-R).

After enucleation the whole tumour was examined. Slides were prepared according to the nitrocellulose technique. The degree of pigmentation of the histologic specimens was coded according to four carefully chosen examples of absent, slight, moderate, and intense pigmentation, respectively. The mitotic activity was counted per 15 high power fields (HPF). In order to compare the size of the tumours they were divided into groups according to the largest diameter and height of the tumour conform to the TNM classification for uveal melanomas of the Union Internationale contre le Cancer (UICC) to be published in the near future (table 1). Survival data were gathered in cooperation with the Oncologic Documentation Centre of the Cancer Registration Department of our hospital by contacting civil registries, general practitioners, and referring ophthalmologists. The X^2 test was used for the statistical studies.

Results

The age of the patients ranged from 15 to 93 years with an average of 54 years. More than 50% of them were between 50 and 70 years of age (fig. 1). The sex distribution was 34 males and 82 females. There was no difference in age distribution between males and females.

TNM classif.	Diameter in mm	Elevation in mm	Number of eyes	Own classif.
pT1a	⩽ 7	⩽ 2	21 (12%)	small
pT1b	> 7 and ⩽10	> 2 and ⩽3	36 (25%)	medium
pT2	>10 and ⩽15	>3 and ⩽5	43 (24%)	large
pT3	>15	>5	76 (44%)	

TABLE 1. Distribution of our 176 tumours according to the TNM classification of the UICC and to our own classification.

Location	Number of eyes	%
ciliary body	6	3.4
peripheral fundus	40	22.7
between equator and posterior pole	86	48.9
posterior pole	29	16.5
adjacent to optic disc	5	2.8
impossible to assess (whole eye filled with tumour)	10	5.7
total	176	100.0

TABLE 2. Tumour location according to the location of the greater part of the tumour.

Tumour size	Number of eyes	Mean age	S.D.
small	21	50.5 years	14.78
medium	35	53.7 years	15.68
large	120	54.4 years	17.20
total	176	53.8 years	16.59

TABLE 3. Relation of tumour size to mean age. (Analysis of variance: P = 0.61).

Clinical observations

In 16 cases the melanoma had been detected on routine examination; in all of them the localisation was posterior to the equator; the tumours were small or of medium size, and flat. The 160 other melanomas had caused visual complaints because of, for instance, a retinal detachment (91x), vitreous haemorrhages (6x), cataract (10x), glaucoma (6x).

In 14 patients the eye was enucleated more than 1 year, up to 12 years, after discovery of the lesion. In 6 of them initially a different diagnosis had been made, such as disciform macular degeneration, vitreous haemorrhage e.c.i., central serous detachment. To 2 patients the ophthalmologist had recommended enucleation of the tumour-containing eye, but they had refused this until growth was observed, and in 6 patients with a small melanoma the ophthalmologist had preferred observation until growth was established; in these 8 patients the tumours were of medium (6x) and large (2x) size at the time of enucleation.

The majority of the melanomas was localized near the equator (table 2); 84% of the large tumours was localized very peripherally or near the equator. Peripheral tumours may become large before giving visual complaints. In 10 patients the eye was so much filled with partly necrotic tumour tissue that the primary site of the tumour could not be assessed.

On perimetry an absolute scotoma (I_4 on the Goldmann perimeter) was found in all but three of the choroidal melanomas. Only a relative scotoma (I_3 on the Goldmann perimeter) was found in 3 small, flat melanomas that were localized in or near the posterior pole.

We feel that in the differential diagnosis between naevus and melanoma perimetry is not sufficiently appreciated as an important diagnostic aid (Oosterhuis and de Wolff-Rouendaal, 1981).

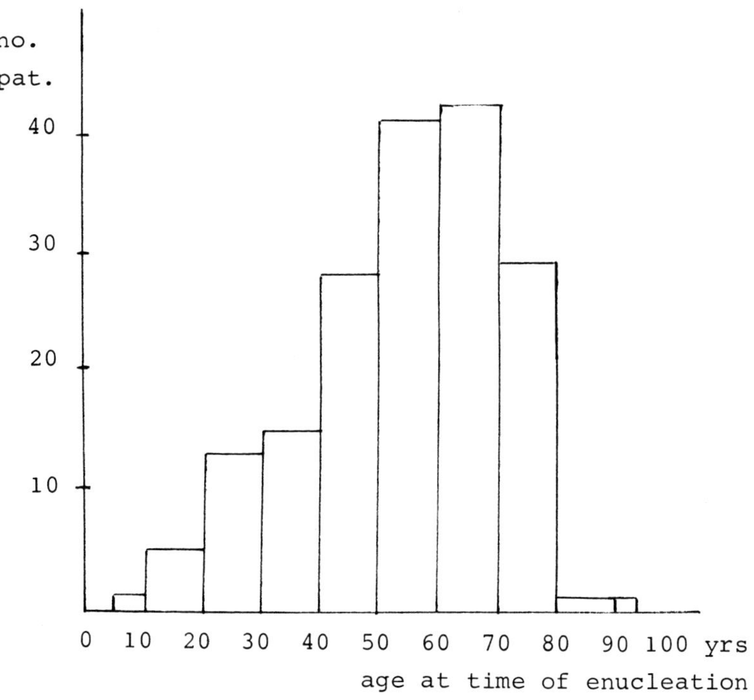

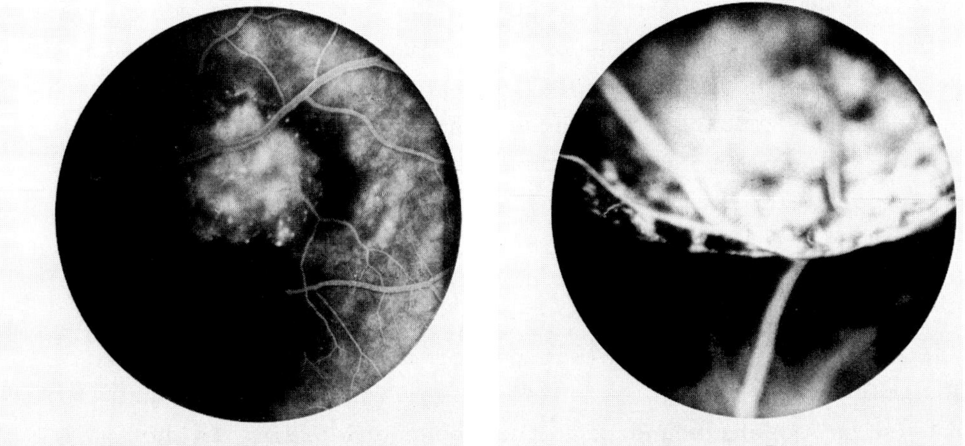

Fig. 2 Typical fluorescence pattern of a choroidal melanoma.

Fig. 3 Fluorescence pattern of a serous retinal detachment over a large choroidal melanoma.

Fluorescein angiography proved to be a reliable diagnostic tool, especially in small and medium-sized tumours without a prominent retinal detachment. Characteristic features are the pin-point hyperfluorescent lesions along the margin of the tumour surrounded by a zone of hypofluorescence, and hyperfluorescent areas of leakage in the central part of the tumour (fig. 2). Large tumours mostly show only widespread irregular, diffuse, subretinal leakage, especially when a retinal detachment is present (Oosterhuis and van Waveren, 1968) (fig. 3).

Ultrasonography has only been regularly used as a diagnostic aid in our department since 1978; only 42 patients were investigated by ultrasound. In 30 cases (71%) the ultrasonic pattern was highly suggestive of the presence of a melanoma. In 10 cases the pattern was not typical and in 2 cases the tumours were too flat for obtaining useful ultrasonographic information.

The P32 isotope uptake test was carried out in 173 patients as part of a special study (van Dijk, 1978). In one eye with a totally necrotic tumour the test result was negative. In 11 eyes the outcome was positive between +60% and +100%, and in 161 eyes (93%) it was more than +100%. The P32 test values tended to be higher in epithelioid cell and large tumours, but these findings were not statistically significant. The tumour-containing eyes were enucleated directly after the P32 test. The test is not carried out routinely any more but we still consider it to be of great value in case of doubtful diagnosis. The test has no prognostic value.

General examination was performed in all patients; it included X-rays of the chest, liver function tests and, in case of doubt, scans of liver, bone and brain. In our series signs of metastatic disease were not found before enucleation.

Histopathological findings

Tumour size

The tumours were grouped according to the TNM classification of the UICC as follows: pT1a 21 tumours (12%), pT1b 36 tumours (20%), pT2 43 tumours (24%) and pT3 76 tumours (44%) (table 1). In our series no statistically significant correlation between age and tumour size which might indicate that uveal melanomas grow at a slow rate could be found (table 3).

Cell type

Ninety-nine tumours (56%) were of the spindle cell, 54 (30%) of the mixed cell, and 20 (11%) of the epithelioid cell type. Three tumours (2%) were too necrotic for determination of the cell type. Foci of necrosis were found in 27 (16%) out of the 176 tumours. This occurred only in medium sized tumours, but was not related to cell type.

The correlation between tumour size and cell type is shown in table 4; 10% of the small (pT1a) and 13% of the large (pT3) melanomas was of the epithelioid cell type. The correlation was not statistically significant.

Bruch's membrane

The membrane was ruptured in 98 cases (59%); it was ruptured in 50 to 60% of all cell type groups. A statistically significant correlation with tumour size was found (table 5).

Intravascular ingrowth

This was found in 35 eyes (20%). For the spindle, mixed and epithelioid cell type groups this was 30%, 40% and 35%, respectively ($P > 0.5$). The correlation according to tumour size was statistically highly significant (table 6).

Scleral ingrowth

This was not found in 13 eyes (8%), it was less than half the scleral thickness in 100 eyes (58%), more than half in 34 eyes (20%), reaching the outer layers of the sclera in 8 eyes (5%), and extending extrasclerally in 16

Cell type	Tumour size				Number of eyes
	pT1a	pT1b	pT2	pT3	
spindle	76%	63%	59%	46%	99
mixed	14%	29%	30%	37%	54
epithelioid	10%	8%	11%	13%	20
necrosis	-	-	-	4%	3
number of eyes	21	35	44	76	176

TABLE 4. Relation of tumour size to cell type.
(X^2 = 10.94; df = 9; P = 0.27).

Bruch's membrane	Tumour size				Number of eyes
	pT1a	pT1b	pT2	pT3	
ruptured	24%	34%	58%	85%	98
intact	76%	62%	32%	10%	56
condition could not be assessed	-	4%	10%	5%	8
number of eyes	21	32	40	69	162

TABLE 5. Relation of tumour size to condition of Bruch's membrane.
(X^2 = 43.94; df = 3; P = $<$0.001).

Intravascular ingrowth	Tumour size				Number of eyes
	pT1a	pT1b	pT2	pT3	
ingrowth	10%	15%	33%	49%	55
no ingrowth	90%	85%	67%	51%	111
number of eyes	21	33	42	70	166

TABLE 6. Relation of tumour size to presence or absence of intravascular ingrowth.
(X^2 = 17.63; df = 3; P = $<$0.001).

eyes (9%). Only in 3 cases was the extrascleral extension found on clinical examination or on surgery. No statistically significant relationship was found betwen the degree of scleral ingrowth and cell type or tumour size. In the group of 21 small tumours 17 showed scleral ingrowth, 2 of them even showing extrascleral extension on histopathological examination. No local orbital recurrence was observed.

P i g m e n t a t i o n

In the first 136 cases of our series the degree of pigmentation has been coded. Fifteen tumours (12%) contained no pigment, 54 (45%) showed only slight pigmentation, 41 (33%) were moderately pigmented, 14 (10%) were intensely pigmented. Small tumours tended to be less pigmented than large ones and epithelioid cell tumours tended to be the most heavily pigmented ones, but the correlation between pigmentation and size or cell type of the tumour was not statistically significant.

M i t o t i c a c t i v i t y

In the first 123 cases of our series mitotic figures per 15 HPF were counted. More mitotic figures were counted in the epithelioid cell type tumours (27% had more than 20 mitotic figures) than in the spindle cell type tumours (7% had more than 20 mitotic figures) but the difference was not statistically significant (P=0.2). However, the correlation between the number of mitotic figures and tumour size was statistically significant (table 7).

In relatives of 2 patients melanomas had been found; one of these 2 patients had the dysplastic naevus or familial atypical multiple mole-melanoma (FAMMM) syndrome (Lynch et al., 1981; Oosterhuis et al., 1982). Twenty-one patients (12%) developed one or more primary malignancies elsewhere in the body; the incidence of multiple primary malignancies in the oncologic patients of the Leiden University Hospital over the period of our investigation was 10%.

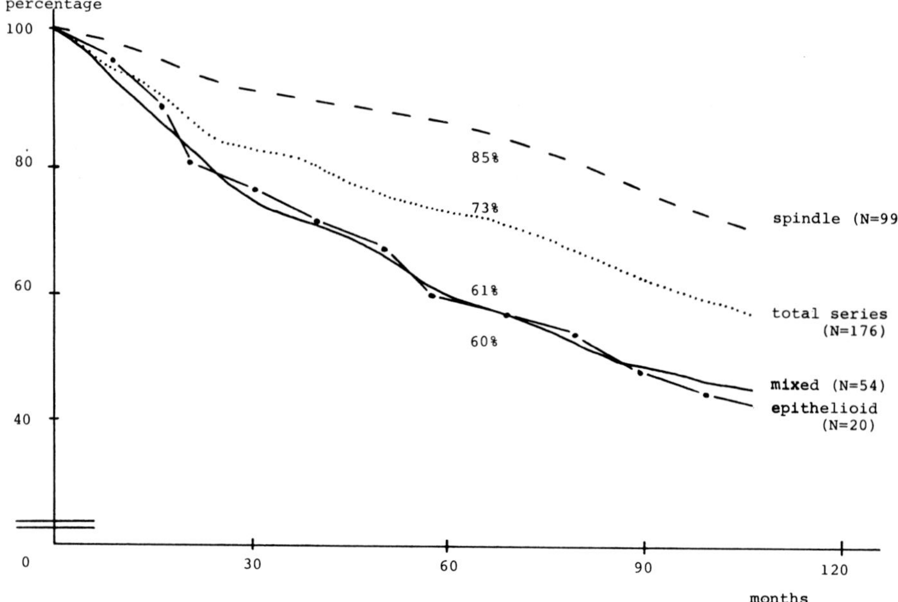

Fig. 4 Survival rates according to cell type.

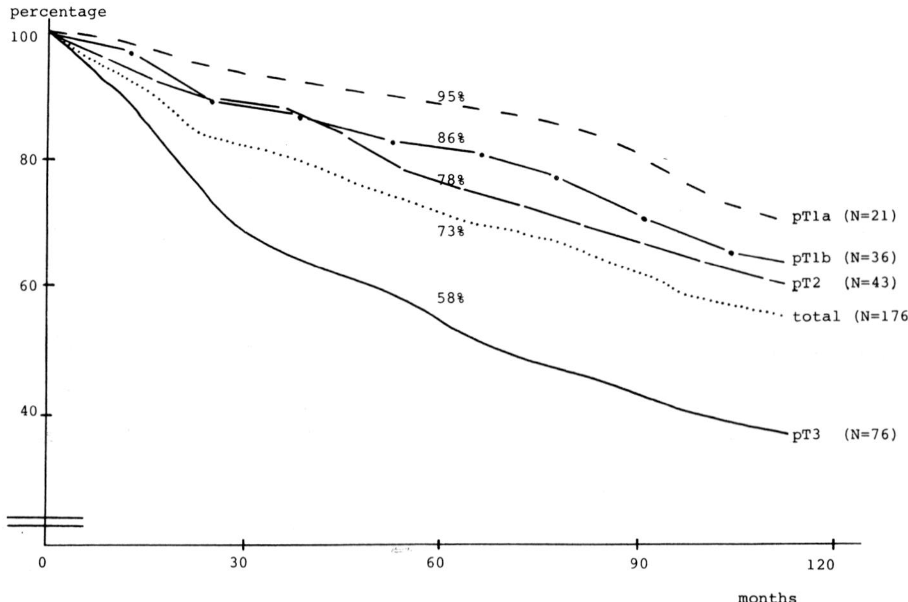

Fig. 5 Survival rates according to tumour size.

Number of mitotic figures per 15 HPF	Tumour size				Number of eyes
	pT1a	pT1b	pT2	pT3	
0 - 9	94%	88%	65%	51%	84
10 - 19	6%	8%	25%	29%	25
20 or more	-	4%	10%	20%	14
number of eyes	17	26	29	51	123

TABLE 7. Relation of number of mitotic figures per 15 HPF to tumour size.
(X^2 = 15.61; df = 4; P = $<$0.01).

	Number of metastatic deaths	
1st year	4	
2nd year	10	
3rd year	5	31
4th year	7	
5th year	5	

TABLE 8. Number of metastatic deaths per year after enucleation

Cell type	Tumour size				Number of eyes
	pT1a	pT1b	pT2	pT3	
spindle	-	-	2	6	8 (26%)
mixed	1	3	1	11	16 (51%)
epithelioid	-	-	2	4	6 (20%)
necrosis	-	-	-	1	1 (3%)
number of eyes	1(3%)	3(10%)	5(16%)	22(71%)	31(100%)

TABLE 9. Relation of tumour size to cell type in the patients who died of metastasis.

	Metastatic death	Survival or non-metastatic death
mixed + epithelioid cell type	71%	36%
large tumours (pT3)	71%	37%
scleral ingrowth	100%	82%
minimal episcleral extension	4%	3%
episcleral tumour tissue	10%	6%
ruptured Bruch's membrane	76%	55%
intravascular ingrowth	48%	29%
20 or more mitotic fig./15 HPF	47%	6%

TABLE 10. Comparison of the melanomas of patients who died of metastatic disease within 5 years after enucleation and those who survived or died of non-tumour-related causes.

	Number of patients	5 Years survival
no scleral extension	13	92%
less than one half scl.extension	100	79%
more than one half scl.extension	42	64%
episcleral extension	16	62%

TABLE 11. Relation of scleral extension to survival rate.

	5 Years survival	5 Years mortality (tumour deaths only)
Davidorf & Lang, 1975		6.1% (small tumours)
McLean et al., 1977	75%	
Thomas et al., 1979		35.8% (large tumours) 5.4% (small tumours)
Jensen, 1982	60-65%	
Seddon et al., 1983	74%	
own study	73%	17.6%

TABLE 12. Survival and mortality rates of various authors.

Metastatic deaths

Thirty-one patients (17.6% of our series) died from metastatic disease within 5 years after enucleation of the tumour-containing eye (table 8). In 3 more patients metastasis of the melanoma was the most likely cause of death.

Complaints due to metastatic disease always occurred at a very late stage; the median survival after metastasis had been diagnosed was 3.5 months (ranging from 0-46 months). In 28 of the 31 patients who died within 5 years after enucleation metastasis of the liver was found. Nine patients had metastasis of the lung, in 6 of them associated with metastasis of the liver, 5 times metastasis of the bone was found, 6 times of the central brain, and 5 times of the skin. The mean age of the patients who died of metastasis was 57 years (18-78 years).

Tumour size and cell type are shown in table 9. Seventy-one per cent of the tumours leading to metastatic death contained epithelioid cells against 42% of the whole series (table 4), and 71% were large tumours against 43% of the whole series (table 4) but even so two patients with a very small tumour died of metastatic disease. All tumours leading to metastatic death showed scleral ingrowth; in 10% of them episcleral tumour tissue was found on surgery and/or on histopathological examination. Bruch's membrane was ruptured in 76% of the patients who died of metastatic disease; in 48% intravascular ingrowth was found (table 10).

Survival rates after 5 years

The 5 year follow-up for the whole group was 73% (fig. 4). According to cell type the prognosis for the spindle cell type was significantly better than for the mixed and epithelioid cell type. In the group of patients with large tumours 58% was still alive after 5 years as against 95% in the group of small tumours (fig. 5).

The survival rate was 91% when Bruch's membrane was intact but 66% when it was ruptured (fig. 6). On subdivision

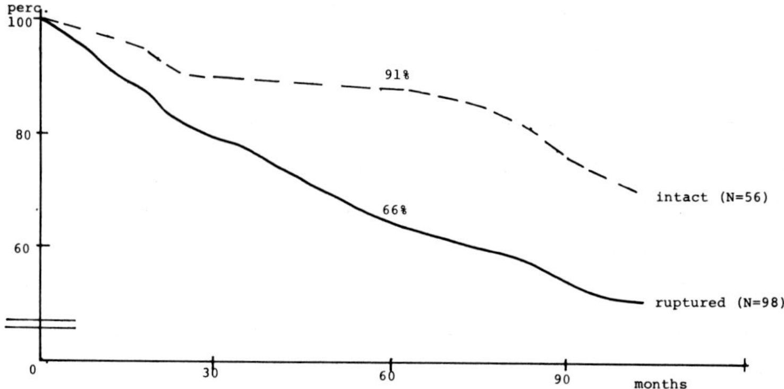

Fig. 6 Survival rates according to condition of Bruch's membrane.

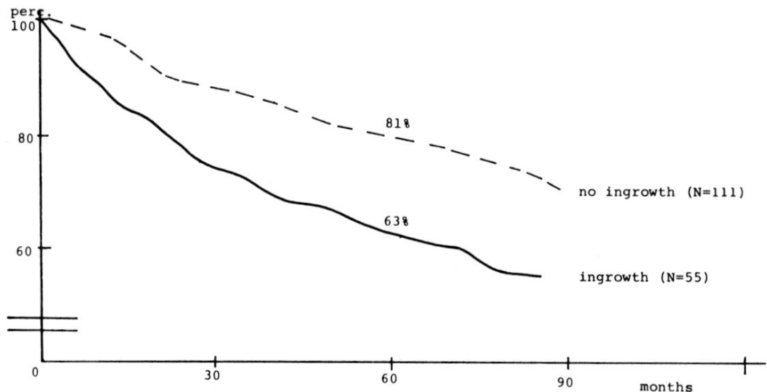

Fig. 7 Survival rates according to absence or presence of intravascular ingrowth.

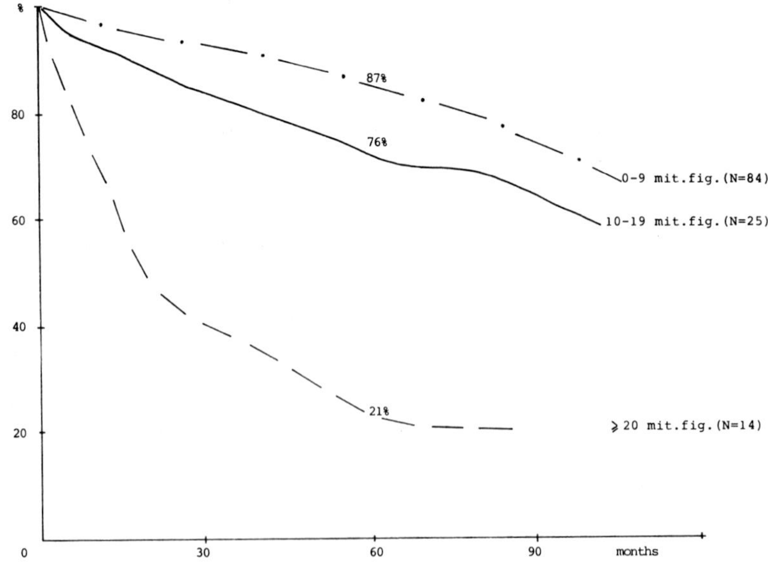

Fig. 8 Survival rates according to mitotic activity.

according to tumour size the difference remained statistically significant.

Without intravascular ingrowth 81% of the patients was alive after 5 years as against 63% when intravascular ingrowth was present (fig. 7). This difference was not related to tumour size. The survival rate decreased from 92% when the tumour had not extended into the sclera to 62% when episcleral extension was present macro- or microscopically (table 11).

The influence of the degree of pigmentation on the survival rate was not statistically significant but its relationship with the mitotic activity was statistically highly significant ($P < 0.01$); the survival rate decreased from 87% when up to 9 mitotic figures per 15 HPF were counted, to 21% when 20 or more mitotic figures were counted (fig. 8).

The location of the tumour did indirectly influence the prognosis, since the larger tumours having the worst prognosis were mostly located peripherally.

Discussion

We have studied 176 uveal melanomas. The survival rate after 5 years for the whole series was 73%. The tumour-related mortality rate after 5 years was 17.6%. Tumour diameter and mitotic activity were found to be the most important prognostic factors. Cell type, rupture of Bruch's membrane, and intravascular ingrowth also influenced the prognosis statistically significantly. Scleral invasion only influenced the prognosis when it was deep or episcleral. Location of the tumour influenced the onset of visual disturbance which made the patient visit the ophthalmologist, and consequently the size of the tumour. The P32 test is a very reliable test in cases of doubt as to the malignancy of a lesion, but it has no prognostic value. It was performed in almost all our patients as part of a study on the P32 test; the procedure of the P32 measurements did not influence the prognosis, since our survival rate is not lower than those mentioned in other studies (table 12). The 5 years' mortality rate in the group of small tumours, i.e. diameter 10 mm or less and elevation 3 mm or less (pT1a + pT1b), was 2.3% as compared to 6.1% in the study of Davidorf et al. (1975) and 5.4% in the study of Thomas et al. (1979).

Jensen (1982) found tumour size, cell type, and extra-scleral extension to be the most important prognostic factors. Shammas and Blodi (1977) found tumour diameter to be the most important factor besides elevation, cell type, rupture of Bruch's membrane, location of the tumour, and pigmentation. Also Seddon et al. (1983), Packard (1980), McLean et al. (1977) and Davidorf and Lang (1975) mentioned tumour size as being highly important to the prognosis.

Davidorf and Lang (1975) found in their series of small tumours 22% mixed or epithelioid tumours. They found no tumour deaths in the group of very small tumours (pT1a), neither did McLean et al. (1977), nor Thomas et al. (1979) who even found 56% mixed cell type tumours in their small melanoma group. In all three studies a number of small tumours showed deep scleral and even episcleral extension and intravascular ingrowth.

We were able to confirm these findings in our study, but we also found that very small tumours (pT1a) may cause metastatic disease. One patient with a pT1a tumour died two years after enucleation owing to metastasis; the tumour was a mixed cell type one, located in the posterior pole, with a diameter of only 7 mm and an elevation of only 1.5 mm but with ruptured Bruch's membrane and deep scleral invasion.

Like Seddon et al. (1983), Shammas and Blodi (1977) and McLean et al. (1977), we found a difference in prognosis related to location of the tumour, but this parameter was highly influenced by the tumour size. Intense pigmentation had no statistically significant influence on the prognosis in our study. Shammas and Blodi (1977) found this parameter to be linked with rupture of Bruch's membrane because melanomas perforating Bruch's membrane usually are of the amelanotic type. McLean et al. (1977), Jensen (1982), and Shammas and Blodi (1977) considered pigmentation to be of importance. This difference in outcome is probably influenced by differences in follow-up time and number of cases.

The number of mitotic figures/HPF have only been mentioned by Seddon et al. (1983) and McLean et al. (1977). The former found that it was related to cell type, the epithelioid cell type having the highest number of mitotic figures. We however did not find a significant correlation between mitotic activity and cell type, but we did find a correlation between mitotic activity and tumour size; however, even irrespective of tumour size a high number of mitotic figures was a bad prognostic sign.

We have reviewed all our data exactly five years after enucleation. The possibility to compare data of various authors is rather restricted as not all authors evaluate their data after periods of 5 years as is the custom in oncology, or if they do evaluate survival after fixed periods, they are not all equally strict with their clinical and histopathological parameters. Moreover, classifications and parameters differ, some investigators using diameter and elevation separately, others using tumour volumes.

Since surgical and various conservative treatment are currently being used in the treatment of uveal melanomas, it is important to have comparable parameters and to evaluate data every 5 years. As tumour size is the only parameter that can be assessed clinically and is an important prognostic feature, it is necessary to use a uniform classification of the tumours. Fortunately, the International Union against Cancer has now developed such a classification for ophthalmic tumours.

Acknowledgements

We are greatly indebted to Mrs. E. Begemann-Groesbeek for her secretarial help and to the Leiden University Computing Centre for the statistical analysis of our data.

References

Davidorf, F.H. and Lang, J.R.: The natural history of malignant melanoma of the choroid: small vs large tumors. Trans.Amer.Acad.Ophthal.Otolaryngol. 79: 310-320, 1975.

Dijk, R.A. van: The 32P test and other methods in the diagnosis of intraocular tumours. Thesis, Dr. W. Junk Publ., The Hague, 1978.

Jensen, O.A.: Malignant melanomas of the human uvea: 25-year follow-up of cases in Denmark, 1943-1952. Acta Ophthal. 60: 161-182, 1982.

Lynch, H.T., Fusaro, R.M., Pester, J., Oosterhuis, J.A., Went, L.N., Rumke, P., Neering, H. and Lynch, J.F.: Tumour spectrum in the FAMMM syndrome. Brit.J.Cancer 44: 553-560, 1981.

McLean, M.I.W., Foster, W.D., and Zimmerman, L.E.: Prognostic factors in small malignant melanomas of choroid and ciliary body. Arch.Ophthal. 95: 48-58, 1977.

Oosterhuis, J.A. and van Waveren, Ch.W.: Fluorescein photography in malignant melanoma. Ophthalmologica 156: 101-116, 1968.

Oosterhuis, J.A. and de Wolff-Rouendaal, D.: Differential diagnosis of small pigmented choroidal tumours. Docum. Ophthal. 50: 299-301, 1981.

Oosterhuis, J.A., Went, L.N. and Lynch, H.T.: Primary choroidal and cutaneous melanomas, bilateral choroidal melanomas, and familial occurence of melanomas. Brit.J. Ophthal. 66: 230-233, 1982.

Packard, R.B.S.: Pattern of mortality in choroidal malignant melanoma. Brit.J.Ophthal. 64: 565-575, 1980.

Seddon, J.M., Albert, D.M., Lavin, P.T. and Robinson, N.: A prognostic factor study of disease-free interval and survival following enucleation for uveal melanoma. Arch.Ophthal. 101, 1894-1899, 1983.

Shammas, H.F. and Blodi, F.C.: Prognostic factors in choroidal and ciliary body melanomas. Arch.Ophthal. 95: 63-69, 1977.

Thomas, J.F., Green, W.R. and Maumenee, A.E.: Small choroidal melanomas. Arch.Ophthal. 97: 861-864, 1979.

CONSERVATIVE TREATMENT MODALITIES OF CHOROIDAL MELANOMAS

J.A. Oosterhuis

For a long time enucleation of the eye has been the usual treatment for choroidal melanomas as surgical excision of the tumour was only possible by removing the whole eye, which was carried out as soon as the diagnosis had been established. Treatment was only omitted in old or ill patients with a limited life span or when the tumour was located in the only useful eye of the patient.

Losing an eye with sometimes good vision and even the loss of a blind eye cause more stress than most patients show, which is often not properly acknowledged by the ophthalmologist. Both are a heavy psychological burden to the patient and give the ophthalmic surgeon a feeling of incompetence.

Hence for many years various alternative methods have been tried out for management of choroidal melanomas in an attempt to save the eye and its vision. Some treatment modalities have not gained acceptance as an alternative to enucleation, some are currently carried out and some are still in an experimental stage and may or may not develop into the stage of clinical use.

Diathermy

Melchers[1] reviewed the results of diathermy treatment carried out by Weve[2,3] between 1935 and 1953 in 17 out of 80 eyes with uveal melanomas. Surface diathermy was combined with perforating diathermy in melanomas with an elevation of more than 2 mm. Most of the patients were treated only once.

Oosterhuis, A. (ed.), Ophthalmic tumors.

ISBN 90-6193-528-8. Printed in the Netherlands.

In 3 eyes with large tumours postoperative complications such as glaucoma, iridocyclitis and retinal detachment necessitated enucleation; in 2 of the eyes, enucleated 10 days after diathermy treatment, remnants of viable melanoma tissue were found on histopathologic examination; in the third eye, enucleated 3 years after diathermy, the tumour had been totally destroyed. It is remarkable that in none of the other 14 eyes a recidive of the melanoma developed during the postoperative control period of 1 to 14 years. Two of the 17 patients died, one from prostate cancer and one from acute rheumatoid fever, but presumably none of the patients from melanoma metastasis.

Diathermy as treatment for uveal melanoma has not gained acceptance. Only Dunphy[4] and Davidorf[5] reported on 1 and 4 cases, respectively, all of them successfully treated with diathermy.

Cryotherapy

Only few results of cryotreatment of melanomas have been reported in literature. Lincoff et al.[6] treated 2 patients with a choroidal melanoma. In one patient a subretinal bleeding developed and persisted for 6 days after the treatment; a total retinal detachment developed. On histopathologic examination of the eyes of this patient, who had a bilateral melanoma of the choroid, the structure of the treated tumour was undistinguishable from that of the untreated one. The melanoma in the other patient was treated twice. After the second treatment a massive exudative response occurred; the vitreous became cloudy, vitreous retraction and organization caused a total retinal detachment. After enucleation of this eye examination showed most of the tumour cells to be still viable.

After these disappointing results this modality has not been tried again until recently by Buschmann and Linnert[7]. They attributed their favourable results of cryotherapy in two patients with choroidal melanoma to the use of an apparatus equipped with liquid nitrogen, enabling rapid and intense freezing, which was twice repeated; moreover, they combined cryotreatment with photocoagulation. Haemorrhages originating from the tumour did not extend beyond the tumour area. Necrosis of the tumour caused a transient exudative retinal detachment and clouding of the vitreous.

Bleckmann[8] successfully treated 5 patients with small choroidal melanomas with cryo at -80°C, in all but one more than once, in all of them combined with repeated argon laser photocoagulation. His preliminary results seem to be encouraging but results of larger series are needed for assessment of the value of cryotherapy in choroidal melanoma.

Histopathologic examination of an eye with a melanoma of the ciliary body and the choroid treated with cryopexy showed an area of cell destruction corresponding with the cold-treated area[9].

Local excision

Surgical removal of the tumour by local excision is fundamentally an ideal treatment modality for choroidal melanoma, as it spares the healthy tissue surrounding the tumour. However, because of their anatomical localization choroidal melanomas are more difficult to remove by surgical excision than melanomas of the iris and ciliary body. The technique most commonly used is based on the experimental and clinical work of Peyman and co-workers[10,11]. Even tumours as large as 10 mm[12] to 15 mm in diameter and within 2-3 mm from the optic disc[13] have been excised successfully. Beneath a lamellar scleral dissection overlying the tumour the choroidal tumour is excised; the retina overlying the tumour is left intact[13] or is removed with the tumour[11].

Foulds[14] performed approximately 120 local resections for choroidal tumours, about half of which also involved the ciliary body. Surprisingly, large tumours and those with an accompanying retinal detachment were easier to deal with than small flat tumours. He successfully operated on tumours within 2-3 mm of the optic disc. About 40% of his patients retained a visual acuity of 6/18 to 6/6 and some 56% 6/60 or better. In 91% of the patients the result was cosmetically satisfactory. After local choroidectomy 7 out of 58 eyes had to be enucleated, 2 of them for recurrent tumours. Only 3 (17%) of 17 patients with a postoperative control of more than 5 years died.

Resection is especially indicated in tumours of 8-15 mm diameter. Foulds[14] advocates enucleation of large tumours over 15 mm in diameter; for small tumours up to 8 mm in diameter observation or other conservative treatment modalities have to be considered as well.

Peyman et al.[11] performed sclerochorioretinal resection in 28 patients with suspected melanoma of the choroid. The tumour proved to be totally resected in 24 eyes; in 2 cases the resected specimens showed tumour cells at their margins and the eyes were enucleated, 2 patients in whom the resected specimen showed dubious margins are being observed. There were no signs of local or systemic metastasis in 24 patients with histologically proven melanoma after an average follow-up of 55 months. Surgical treatment permitted retention of 18 eyes; 8 of them have a visual acuity of more than 2/10. The cosmetic results are excellent.

Naumann[15] performed block excision of melanomas of ciliary body and choroid in 15 patients. Three eyes were enucleated because histology was indicative of incomplete removal but no tumour was found in the enucleated eyes. Visual function was retained in 12 eyes, in 4 visual acuity was 0.1-0.6.

Shields and Augsburger[16] performed 13 local excisions for choroidal melanoma. The integrity of the eye was better than the visual outcome because of complications such as cystoid macula oedema, vitreous haemorrhages and retinal detachment.

Kara[12] performed excision of 12 melanomas located in the choroid, 5 of them associated with a ciliary body melanoma and 5 associated with a melanoma of the ciliary body and iris. The results in 6 tumours of less than 10 mm diameter were favourable, only one eye becoming blind, but out of 5 eyes with melanoma of iris, ciliary body and choroid measuring 10-15 mm in diameter 4 became blind and one was enucleated. Five years after the excision there had been only one tumour death.

In the Soviet Union local excision of choroidal melanoma has been performed by Brovkina[17], Linnic[18] and Volkov[19]. In the 24 patients operated by Volkov secondary enucleation was performed in 12, mostly because transparency of the ocular media was insufficient for proper control; two patients died soon after enucleation owing to metastatic disease. Linnic performed 28 choroidectomies and cyclochoroidectomies; the tumour proved to be completely excised in all eyes. Only in the initial stage vitreous loss was a serious complication.

Local excision of choroidal melanomas requires great surgical skill and is demanding for the anaesthesiologist because of a controlled arterial hypotension being imperative to avoid bleeding. One may assume that when removing the melanoma out of the eye one leaves behind melanoma cells which are attached to the retina or have invaded the superficial layer of the sclera covering the area of excision. It is therefore quite remarkable that this does not lead to tumour recurrence, which was not observed even after a relatively long postoperative observation period of up to 8 years[11] and 13 years[13].

Photocoagulation

In 1952 Meyer-Schwickerath started to use xenon photocoagulation to destroy choroidal melanomas. Results of photocoagulation treatment in large series of patients have only been published from two centres: Essen[20,21,22] and Ghent[23,24]

Only relatively small tumours of 5-6 disc diameters and with a prominence of up to 5 dioptres are suitable for photocoagulation treatment. There should not be a retinal detachment and it must be technically possible to surround the tumour completely with photocoagulation burns.

In 79 eyes of 134 patients (59%) with a mean follow-up of more than 9 years growth of the tumour could be arrested and these eyes could be saved[22]. Seventy-six patients are either still alive or have died from not tumour-related causes. Three patients may have died from metastatic disease but this was confirmed in only one. In 55 patients (41%) the eye was enucleated because of complications: recurrences, new vessel formation, retinal detachment, loss of fundus visibility, but the main reason for enucleation was fear in patients and referring physicians. In 17 eyes no vital tumour cells were found on histologic examination; 6 eyes showed extrascleral outgrowth. It is remarkable that after enucleation 11 of 55 patients (20%) died from metastatic disease as against only 1, possibly 3, of 79 patients without enucleation.

François[23,24] observed 100 patients with choroidal melanoma for more than 5 years after photocoagulation. Usually 3-7 photocoagulation sessions were needed. Sixty-two patients (62%) could be considered cured; the cure rate was related to the size of the tumour: 13 of 14 patients (93%) with a tumour of less than 2 disc diameters and an elevation of less than 2 dioptres, 35 of 49 patients (71%) with a tumour of 2-5 disc diameters and an elevation of 2-6 dioptres, and only 13 of 33 patients (39%) with a tumour larger than 5 disc diameters and an elevation of more than 6 dioptres were cured. Most recurrences occurred after 6-9 years, generally at the margin of the coagulation scar.

Twenty-five of the 100 eyes were enucleated, 10 because of recurrence of the tumour, in two of them associated with extraocular outgrowth.

Thirteen of the 100 patients developed metastatic disease: 7 (9%) of the 75 patients without enucleation and 6 (24%) of the 25 patients after enucleation. François recommends a very careful follow-up as extrascleral outgrowth may occur in cases that seem to be locally cured and recurrences may appear even 10 to 15 years after treatment.

Even after 30 years of photocoagulation in choroidal melanoma this modality of treatment has not been generally accepted, as its indications are very restricted and control of extraocular outgrowth is not possible. It seems to be mostly used nowadays in combination with other modalities such as radioactive applicators.

Radiotherapy

Irradiation treatment in choroidal melanoma has only gradually developed over a period of many decades. Clinical trials are usually carried out in a limited number of patients, as in case of failure endangering the life expectancy of the patient enucleation has still to be performed. For assessment of recurrences and metastatic rate a period of many years is required. This explains why most therapeutical alternatives to enucleation have first been tried out for a long period in a few centres only, before gaining acceptance on a wider scale.

The development of irradiation treatment has been hampered by the long standing assumption of radioresistance of melanoma cells. More recent studies, however, showed that melanoma cells as such do not differ in radiosensitivity or radioresistance from cells of other types of tumour[25,26,27,28,29]. The clinical radioresistance that exists may be partly explained by the high fraction of up to 85% hypoxic cells in melanomas, which is among the highest found in malignant tumours[27,30].

The first results of irradiation treatment such as those obtained by Stallard[31,32] were not uniformly promising and were regarded with scepticism rather than enthusiasm[33]. A revival of the treatment with radioactive applicators is largely based on the work of Lommatzsch[34], who in 1962 had started to treat choroidal melanomas with ruthenium-106.

Irradiation of melanomas of the ciliary body and choroid can be performed in two different ways, firstly by external beam irradiation by means of charged particles or linear accelerator, secondly by suturing applicators containing radio-isotopes onto the sclera.

External beam irradiation

Most clinical experience has been obtained by proton beam irradiation of melanomas of the choroid and the ciliary body. High energy proton beams offer multiple advantages for the irradiation of intraocular tumours, because they provide highly attractive depth dose distribution patterns. Protons travel through matter in nearly straight lines and with minimal scatter. The protons deliver maximum intensity of ionisation at the end of the path, the so-called Bragg peak; at the end of the beam the terminal 90% to 50% dose fall off is approximately 2 mm. An advantage of charged particle irradiation is that a uniform dosage can be given throughout the tumour and the adjacent 1.5 mm for adequate coverage of the melanoma borders. The sharp lateral dose fall off results in a lower risk of radiation retinopathy in the adjacent areas, which makes this technique exquisitely suitable for irradiation of choroidal and ciliary body melanomas[35,36,37,38,39].

For careful focussing the head of the patient is immobilized by an adjustable head holder. The proton beam is adjusted with the help of radiopaque tantalum rings, sutured onto the sclera around the base of the tumour, which serve as reference markers for radiographic alignment of the tumour with the proton beam. A dose equivalent to 70 cobalt Gy is given, delivered in 5 treatments during 8 to 10 days.

The results of Gragoudas et al.[39] of proton beam irradiation in 241 uveal melanomas over the past 7½ years are favourable. Their material comprises 12 (5%) small melanomas (up to 10 mm in diameter and 2 mm in height), 99 (41%) medium-sized melanomas (10-15 mm in diameter and 2-5 mm in height), 103 (43%) large melanomas (15-20 mm in diameter and 5-10 mm in height) and 27 (11%) extra large melanomas (more than 20 mm in diameter and more than 10 mm in height).

The mean follow-up was 21 months.

Ninety-four per cent of the irradiated eyes with a follow-up of more than 2 years showed regression of the tumour. The most recent visual acuity was 0.5 or better in 47% and 0.2 or better in 66%. Visual acuity improved in 13%, remained unchanged in 53% and deteriorated in 34%. Post-treatment visual acuity was associated with the size of the tumour; it was lower in large tumours than in medium-sized tumours and was lowest in extra large melanomas.

Complications of irradiation of minor importance were lid epitheliitis, epilation and epiphora from punctum occlusion when the eyelids had to be included in the irradiation field. Epithelial keratopathy developed in a small number of cases. Cataract developed in 22 patients after irradiation of large choroidal or ciliary body melanomas, in 5 necessitating cataract extraction. The most serious complication was rubeosis iridis and neovascular glaucoma observed in 8 patients with large or extra large tumours, possibly caused by a vasoproliferative substance originating from the necrotic tumour or retina. Vitreous haemorrhage was observed in 8 eyes with large or extra large melanomas but cleared in 6 of them. Twenty-nine eyes (12%) developed radiation retinopathy involving the fovea.

Ten eyes were enucleated, 9 because of complications such as secondary glaucoma and retinal detachment, 1 because of continued tumour growth. The only other eye which showed post-irradiation tumour growth was successfully treated with argon laser coagulation.

Histopathologic examination of enucleated eyes after proton beam irradiation indicated that in addition to a direct cytotoxic effect on tumour cells damage to the tumour was also achieved indirectly by irradiation vasculopathy of the tumour, as marked vascular changes were found and necrotic areas and degenerated cells were observed in the vicinity of these abnormal vessels[40].

Only 13 patients (5.4%) developed metastases, 12 with large or extra large melanomas and one with a medium-sized melanoma, which suggests that proton irradiation does not promote metastasis.

The regression pattern after proton beam irradiation consists of a rather slow shrinkage; the earliest onset of decrease in height was one month, the latest 2 years, in the majority of the patients between 4 months and one year, after irradiation. After an initial regression the tumour continued to regress at a lower rate after the first post-irradiation year but continuous regression has been observed even 4 years after treatment[39,41]. Disappearance of the tumour or formation of a flat scar was observed in a small number of eyes; in the other eyes the residual tumours seemed to have lost their capacity for reproduction as they did not grow again after shrinkage.

After proton beam irradiation of 60 eyes with choroidal melanomas 3 mm or less from the fovea visual acuity remained the same in 47%, improved in 20%, and deteriorated in 33%[42]. In 58% of the treated eyes visual acuity was 0.2 or more. The most common cause of decrease in visual acuity was macular oedema as a result of macular vasculopathy which developed in 13 eyes (22%), resulting in loss of visual acuity in 8 eyes. Macular oedema was not related to the distance of the tumour from the fovea but it was observed twice as often in eyes with large melanomas (diameter more than 15 mm and height more than 5 mm) as in eyes with medium size tumours (diameter 10-15 mm, height 2-5 mm). Improvement of visual acuity resulted from resolution of subfoveal serous detachment. Some maculae tolerated the total irradiation dosage without damage but all four diabetic patients developed marked vascular changes from radiation even in the absence of diabetic retinopathy. As radiation retinopathy may occur many years after irradiation and the follow-up averaged 18 months (2-82 months) some increase of the number of eyes with radiation vasculopathy has to be expected.

Char et al.[43,44] reported on irradiation of 40 patients with choroidal melanomas with helium ion charged particles. Four eyes were enucleated because of continued growth; in 2 of them the melanoma seemed to be radioresistent, in the other 2 it seemed that the lesion was not entirely within the irradiation field. The mean reduction of tumour height measured by echography in 17 patients followed for at least 1 year after therapy was approximately 40%(17-76%). The interval between therapy and detectable shrinkage was 6 months (1-23 months). Fifteen of the 40 eyes contained large tumours, more than 15 mm in diameter and more than 5 mm in height. Approximately 200 patients have been treated up till now[45]. Over 95% of the patients have retained their eyes and in the follow-up of less than 7 years the mortality rate is 5%.

In the Soviet Union Brovkina and Zarubey[46] have successfully treated patients with choroidal melanomas with proton beam irradiation.

The results of heavy particle irradiation show that this is a useful treatment as an alternative to enucleation and so far the only conservative treatment modality for the management of large uveal melanomas and tumours adjacent to the optic disc. Until recently, the expensive and technically complicated equipment for proton beam irradiation was in Europe only available in Moscow but recently the SIN (Swiss Institute for Nuclear research) has started this modality of treatment in cooperation with the University Eye Clinic in Lausanne, Switzerland (Professor Gailloud and Dr Zografos).

Bornfeld et al.[47] reported on preliminary results of irradiation of 20 choroidal melanomas with a linear accelerator using a tumour dose of 50 Gy delivered in a 5 weeks' period by a single lateral field. After a mean follow-up period of 15 months the tumour showed regression or arrest of growth in all but one patient. One eye was enucleated because of a haemorrhagic glaucoma complicating total tumour necrosis. Most patients developed radiation retinopathy. The period of control is too short for assessment of the degree of usefulness of this irradiation technique.

Applicators containing radio-isotopes

Quite a few studies have been performed on the method to destroy choroidal and ciliary body melanomas by suturing an applicator containing radio-isotopes onto the sclera and leaving it there for a period of time corresponding with the dosage of radiation to be delivered to the tumour. The rationale of using applicators is to deliver a sufficiently high dose for destruction of the tumour but to restrict radiation damage of the healthy structures of the eye. Experience has been gained with applicators containing the β-ray emitting isotope ruthenium-106 and the γ-emitting cobalt-60 and iodine-125. For the physical characteristics of cobalt-60 and ruthenium-106 see Hallermann, table 2, elsewhere in this volume.

C o b a l t - 60

The results of cobalt plaque treatment are summarized in the table.

Stallard[31] published results on 100 choroidal melanomas treated with cobalt applicators between 1939 and 1964. The radiation dosage varied greatly: on the summit of the tumours 70-420 Gy, in most cases 100-140 Gy; on the base 200-1200 Gy, in most cases 300-400 Gy. Most of the successes were obtained by a single application at a dosage of about 70-140 Gy at the top and 180-360 Gy at the base of the tumour, and in tumours up to 8 mm in diameter.

MacFaul[33] reviewed the results of cobalt plaque treatment in 130 patients treated between 1960 and 1975. Out of 107 patients for whom the clinical reports are complete 29 died, 12 (11%) from metastatic disease. In 27 patients (20%) the treated eye had to be removed because of failure to control the tumour or because of radiation complications. In 20 of the remaining 51 patients (39%) a useful vision of 6/18 to 6/6 was preserved. In the patients with poor visual outcome the tumour was close to the optic disc or macula and irradiation resulted in circinate retinopathy, vascular occlusion

	Stallard 1966/1968	MacFaul & Morgan 1977 MacFaul 1977	Shields et al. 1982	Migdal 1983	Zygulska-Mach et al. 1983	Zografos & Gailloud*
Number of patients	107	107	100	99	93	104
Period of investig.	1939-1964	17 yrs	7 yrs	1954-1978	1968-1980	1969-1982
Observation period		2.5 - 17 yrs	1 - 5 yrs	≥ 5 yrs	3 - >10 yrs	mean 4.6 yrs
Tumour dosis (Gy) (t = top, b = base)	t 70- 420 b 180-1080	t 80 b ± 500	t 80 b ± 450	t ± 80 b ± 400	t 110-200	t 90 b ± 350
Regression tumour	78% (82)	48%	96% (96)		62.4%	
Enucleation	16.8% (18)	25% (27)		23%	24%	21.2%
Metastatic death	9.3% (10)	11% (12)	3% (3)	5%	18.3%	5.8% (6)
5 yrs mortality	4.7% (5)	14%			18%	8.3%
Radiation retinopathy	20% (22)		30% (30)	16%	56%	
Vitr.haemorrhage	2.8% (3)		11% (11)	6%	26%	11.5% (12)
Radiation cataract	9.3% (10)		7% (7)	29%	65%	10.6% (11)
Scleral necrosis	1.9% (2)		2% (2)			
Secondary glaucoma	2.8% (3)				13%	

* see elsewhere in this volume

Table. Results of cobalt-60 irradiation treatment.

and optic nerve atrophy. MacFaul advocates to restrict cobalt plaque treatment to small tumours under 10 mm in diameter and 3-4 mm in height and not located near the optic disc and macula. Regression of the tumours took 1½-2 years; this was considered suggestive of ischaemia resulting from progressive vascular changes in the tumour as a factor in addition to the direct radiation damage of the cells[48].

On pathologic examination of 17 out of 23 eyes removed after cobalt plaque treatment for melanoma of the choroid no evidence of tumour necrosis was found although radiation changes were present in the adjacent tissues; necrosis was found in 6 eyes but was a prominent feature in only 2. Enucleation was performed on average at about 32 months after treatment because of continued growth or complications leading to a painful blind eye[49].

Zografos and Gailloud[50] have treated 100 choroidal melanomas with cobalt-60 applicators at a dosage of 90 Gy at the top of the tumour. They have controlled 57 patients for 5 years or more. Recurrence of the tumour was found in 5 eyes, in 1 eye 2 years and in the other 4 eyes 7-9 years after irradiation. In 13 eyes (22.8%) visual acuity had diminished, in 21 eyes (36.9%) it was unchanged or had even improved. Xenon photocoagulation of the surface of the tumour prior to irradiation considerably reduced the risk of haemorrhages. The 5 year metastatic rate was only 7%. For details of their results see their paper elsewhere in this volume.

Migdal[51] reported on 99 patients treated with cobalt plaques and followed for at least 5 years. On average 80 Gy was delivered at the top of the tumour. Twenty-three eyes (23%) were enucleated because of loss of vison or growth of the tumour. After 5 years in 45 patients (45%) visual acuity was unchanged or had improved, in 15 patients (15%) the visual acuity had decreased by more than one line on the Snellen chart, and in 23 patients (23%) the visual acuity was less than 6/60. Five patients died of metastatic disease, remarkably all of them with tumours 10 mm or less in diameter. Radiation retinopathy was a frequent complication, which even developed many years after cobalt therapy. Therefore only long term studies will reveal the exact incidence of complications and recurrences of the tumour.

A short term study has been performed by Shields et al.[52]. One hundred patients with choroidal melanomas were treated with cobalt plaque therapy; the average radiation dose delivered to the top of the tumour was 85 Gy. The follow-up ranged from one to 5 years with an average of two years. Prior to the treatment visual acuity was 6/16 or less in 37 eyes; at the final follow-up examination 50 eyes were in this visual acuity range. About 40% of the patients developed complications: radiation retinopathy and/or maculopathy in 30%, intravitreal haemorrhage in 11%, and radiation cataract in 7%. In 23 patients visual acuity was impaired because radiation retinopathy involved perifoveal retinal blood vessels. The tumour decreased in size in 96 of the 100 patients.

Zygulska-Mach et al.[53] reported on cobalt plaque therapy in 93 patients with choroidal melanomas with an observation period of 3 to more than 10 years. Tumours up to 14 mm in diameter and up to 6 mm in height were treated. The radiation dose at the top of the tumour ranged from 110 to 200 Gy. Complications were numerous: cataract 65%, glaucoma 33%, radiation retinopathy 56%, retinal haemorrhage 25%. Twenty-two eyes (24%) were enucleated, 7 of which because of a recurrence of the tumour and 14 because of a secondary glaucoma. In 31% a good or useful visual acuity was retained.

Smaller series of 32 and 47 patients published by Rotman et al.[54] and Ellsworth[55], respectively, showed similar results as those described above.

Ruthenium-106

Irradiation of choroidal melanomas with ruthenium-106 applicators has been performed by Lommatzsch[34] for more than 20 years. For the characteristics of ruthenium-106 see Hallermann, table 1, elsewhere in this volume. Ruthenium-106 emits mainly beta rays; in tissue it has a 50% isodose curve at a distance of 3 mm from the applicator surface[56]. A 1 mm silver layer at the back of the applicator absorbs the electrons completely. The halflife is 1 year.

A total of 205 choroidal melanomas with a diameter up to 15 mm and a height not exceeding 5 mm was irradiated[34]. A dose of 80-100 Gy at the top of the tumour was given in 8-14 days. Treatment was successful in 132 patients (64.4%): the tumour had changed into a flat scar or to a grey or black mass which remained unchanged for more than a year. The development into a flat pigmented scar depended primarily on the size of the tumour, as all small tumours developed into small scars. A visual acuity of 0.5-1.5 was retained in 35 (25.8%) of the successfully treated patients. The visual outcome depended on the distance between melanoma and macula or optic disc as visual loss was caused by radiogenic side effects on those structures. Radiation retinopathy was observed in 55 patients with a melanoma located at a distance of 1-2 disc diameters from the foveola. In these cases the scarring around the tumour necessarily involved the macula. A second treatment was performed in 14 patients because of a recurrence of the tumour. Additional photocoagulation treatment was performed in 18 eyes. In 36 patients (18%) the eye was enucleated, in 26 of them because of tumour growth, in the other 10 because of loss of visual function. The survival rate of 85.1% after 5 years and 71.9% after 10 years was better than in a comparable group of small melanomas after primary enucleation.

Lommatzsch does not advocate ruthenium treatment for ciliary body melanomas but Foerster et al.[57] successfully treated 26 eyes with a ciliary body melanoma with 50 Gy at 5 mm tumour depth. Two eyes failed to respond and had to be enucleated; one eye was re-treated because of recurrence.

Regression of the tumour after irradiation may take many months. After irradiation of 95 choroidal melanomas with a prominence of up to 6 mm Hallermann and Guthoff[58] observed a 50% reduction of the prominence after 9 months in male and 5 months in female patients. The gradual regression of the tumour may well be related to an expanding necrosis due to a gradually developing vasculopathy in the tumour which Wessing et al.[59] found on fluorescein angiography 6-12 months after irradiation; even complete non-perfusion in the whole tumour area was observed.

The beta irradiation of ruthenium-106 with its lower photon energy than that of the gamma-emitting cobalt-60 might be less damaging to the normal structures adjacent to the tumour, resulting in less side-effects and complications[34]. Wessing et al.[59] feel that radiation dosage should not primarily be calculated from the peak dose in relation to the prominence of the tumour; in their opinion the dose at the scleral surface must be enough Gy to create an occlusive vasculopathy in the tumour and in the feeder vessels in the choroid. In those parts of the tumour where cells are not destroyed by a direct radiation effect cell necrosis will occur later on, when the tumour vessels and choroidal feeder vessels become occluded. Reviewing the regression of 267 melanomas in relation to the irradiation dosage Bornfeld et al.[60] found that the best results were obtained when 700-1000 Gy was delivered to the basis of the tumour; at the top at least 100 Gy should be delivered.

Elsewhere in this volume Hallermann gives details of his own results and a review of the results of others of ruthenium plaque treatment and Wessing et al. describe their results on ruthenium plaque treatment of choroidal and ciliary body melanomas. The first results of Busse and Müller[61] are in accordance with those described above.

I o d i n e - 1 2 5

The use of applicators containing iodine-125 is advocated by Packer and Rotman[62] and Rotman et al.[63]. They consider the radiation characteristics of iodine-125 to be ideal for the treatment of intraocular tumours as the half-value layer of 20 mm allows for use in larger intraocular tumours. When comparing the radiation effect of iodine-125 and cobalt-60 applicators in the Greene melanoma in the posterior segment of rabbit eyes Packer et al.[64] found iodine-125 to be superior to cobalt-60. At a similar apex dose of 80 Gy the melanoma in the eye irradiated by iodine-125 showed complete necrosis on histopathologic examination, whereas cobalt-60 irradiation resulted in an uneven effect of partly necrotic areas and areas with viable tumour cells. Radiation damage of the retina adjacent to the tumour was clearly visible with cobalt-60 but only minimal with iodine-125. A disadvantage is that regularly new iodine-125 containing seeds have to be glued onto the applicator as the halflife of the isotope is only 60.2 days. So far only results of a short-time follow-up of 21 patients after treatment with a dose of 73-110 Gy to the top of the tumour are known[63]. In large tumours with a diameter of 11 mm or more and an elevation of 6 mm or more the one year disease-free survival was 69%; for the patients with smaller tumours the one year disease-free survival rate was 78%. Irradiation-induced complications were infrequent; the major complication after irradiation of large choroidal melanomas was rubeosis iridis.

For assessment of the therapeutic effectivity of the iodine-125 treatment we have to await information on larger series of patients with a longer follow-up period.

Radon and aureum-198 seeds

Radon seeds have been used as early as 1930[65] and 1949[66] in the treatment of choroidal melanoma. After irradiation with radon seeds in 18 patients Ehlers et al.[67] observed post-irradiation complications such as vitreous haemorrhages, retinal detachment, progressive loss of vision, in half of the patients regardless of tumour control; in 6 eyes the tumour activity necessitated enucleation. After implantation of radioactive radon rings in 22 patients Davidorf[5] observed tumour regression in 14 eyes; the irradiation dose was 80-100 Gy to the top and 200-250 Gy to the base of the tumour.

Eight eyes were enucleated because of inadequate tumour response, one because of scleral atrophy and rupture of the globe; 5 patients developed intraocular haemorrhages. The high energy and short halflife of 3.8 days necessitate delivery of the total dose at a very high dose rate, which may promote complications[62].

There are only two reports on the use of aureum-198. Boniuk and Cohen[68] treated patients with choroidal melanoma with plaques covered with radioactive gold seeds which emit gamma rays. The dosage was 70-240 Gy in 48-96 hours at the top of the tumour. Out of the 40 patients treated 35 (88%) retained their eye; of these 35 patients 65% retained a visual acuity of 20/50 or more. The major complications of the treatment were cystoid macular oedema (45%) followed by radiation retinopathy and vitreous haemorrhages, each observed in 12.5%, and cataract in 10%.

Menapace et al.[69] reported on a patient who, after telecobalt irradiation with 60 Gy, was locally treated with radio-active gold seeds for an additional delivery of 25 Gy, resulting in a good regression of the tumour in one year.

The lack of publications on serial studies since 1978 may indicate that the use of radon and aureum-198 seeds has been abandoned in the treatment of melanoma.

Critical assessment and future prospects

Conservative treatment of choroidal melanomas is in a stage of rapid development. Modalities such as diathermy and cryotreatment either did not survive or did not develop into the phase of widespread clinical use. Photocoagulation treatment is performed on a limited scale and is restricted to flat tumours. Irradiation modalities, both by heavy particles and by radioactive applicators, are rapidly developing, the latter now being carried out in an increasing number of tumour centres.

It is to be hoped that treatment results will give answers to the as yet unanswered questions and will give solutions to the as yet unsolved problems. Heavy particle irradiation apparently gives the best results as regards regression of the tumour and saving visual function of the eye, and has the advantage of being applicable in large tumours. However, this treatment modality requires a cyclotron and highly sophisticated technical facilities, which at the moment are only available in two centres in the U.S.A. and two centres in Europe.

Treatment by radioactive applicators saves a large part of the melanoma-containing eyes but a number of them does not respond sufficiently and requires additional photocoagulation treatment, 15-25% even so requiring enucleation in the end. Complications, mainly radiation retinopathy, are far from negligible and may necessitate enucleation when proper control of the tumour is not possible any more, for instance in case of vitreous haemorrhages.

It is not yet known which of the radiopharmaceuticals gives the best results: cobalt-60, ruthenium-106 or iodine-125. The beta radiation of the ruthenium applicators is the most sparing one to the healthy ocular structures but this modality is not applicable in very prominent tumours. For the more elevated tumours gamma irradiation by cobalt-60 is required. Thus size and especially prominence of the tumour may be indicative as to the type of radioactive agent needed.

Another unsolved problem is the optimal irradiation dosage. There is no uniformity in the dosage used by the various investigators. It is not known which dosage is the most important one, the one to the top or the one to the base of the tumour. At the top of the tumour the dosage seems to be related to the cell-killing effect, whereas at the base the radiation vasculopathy of the tumour vessels and the feeder vessels in the choroid surrounding the tumour may be of major importance.

It is not known why regression in size of the tumour does not start until 6 to 12 months or even longer after treatment. It seems that the melanoma cells are devitalized by the radiation but that shrinkage of the tumour largely depends on irradiation-induced vascular occlusion, which only occurs after a certain lapse of time. Neither is it known how long one is justified to wait before installing further treatment when the tumour does not show any signs of regression. The tumour cells may be permanently devitalized and the tumour may show no tendency to grow any more, but on the other hand neither may it show any tendency to shrink, which might mistakenly be explained as insufficient radiation effect.

Histopathologic examination of melanomas as a means of assessing the degree of viability of the tumour may be misleading. Rousseau et al.[70] treated 10 out of 20 patients with a choroidal melanoma with 40 Gy in 20 days prior to enucleation. They found that the tumour cells lost their capacity to grow in tissue culture medium and did not take up thymidine, whereas in the control eyes the melanoma cells did grow and showed an uptake of thymidine. However, the histopathologic aspect of the irradiated melanoma cells did not differ from that of the untreated melanoma cells.

It is to be hoped that in the near future more information on the rate of metastasis after irradiation of melanomas will become available. All investigators state that in their series the rate of metastasis does not appear to be higher than after enucleation, but in most studies, except in the study of Lommatzsch[34], the material is too small and the period of observation too short for a statistical evaluation. Moreover, in relatively small tumours the rate of metastasis is low anyhow.

The prospects for the future as regards treatment of choroidal melanoma are favourable. New treatment modalities such as hyperthermia and haematoporphyrin derivative photoradiation, are currently being investigated; it is to be hoped that they will develop into clinically useful techniques. When they can be applied in combination with the afore described irradiation techniques they may allow reduction of the irradiation dose and of unwanted side-effects and complications.

Recently we have carried out experiments to study the feasibility of the administration of a haematoporphyrin derivative (HpD) followed by photoradiation with red laser light to destroy melanomas implanted into the anterior chamber of rabbit eyes. I discuss this in detail elsewhere in this volume.

Hyperthermia is gaining interest as auxiliary treatment in combination with irradiation. Hyperthermia in the eye can be induced by microwave or ultrasonic heating. Lagendijk[71,72] has developed a microwave system which enables controlled hyperthermia of anterior or posterior segment of the eye. Coleman[73] induced hyperthermia confined to the tumour area by means of an ultrasound probe which is also used for localization of the tumour; his first results with this modality of treatment in combination with irradiation are encouraging.

For a number of years immunologic aspects have been considered of importance in melanoma. On immunologic investigation circulating tumour-associated antibodies have been found in patients with uveal malignant melanoma[74]. Average post-therapy titres remained high after cobalt-60 plaque therapy or photocoagulation but decreased rapidly after enucleation. However, the antibodies were not specific for ocular melanoma[75].

In order to stimulate immunologic response, non-specific treatment with dicarbazine (imidazole carboxamine, or DTIC) and BCG vaccine have been given as treatment of disseminated malignant melanoma but in the absence of a distinct effect this modality of treatment gradually faded into oblivion; in ocular melanoma it has only been used on a limited scale and temporarily[75].

Nevertheless, antibody treatment may have a comeback in the future in the form of monoclonal antibodies against melanoma cells. Research is being done to tag monoclonal antibodies against malignant melanoma with chemotherapeutic or radio-isotopic agents. If this can be achieved, it may be possible to deliver a high dose of toxic material locally to kill malignant cells. At the moment it is not to be foreseen whether this fascinating line of basic research will in the near or more remote future develop into a clinical mode of selective treatment of uveal melanoma in man.

Explorations of the new and promising therapeutic modalities in uveal melanoma indicate that this field in ophthalmology is very much on the move, rousing high expectations for improving treatment results to the benefit of the patients.

References

1. Melchers, M.J.: Diathermy treatment of intraocular tumours. Thesis. Schotanus & Jens, Utrecht, 1953.
2. Weve, H.J.M.: Ueber operative Behandlung von intraokularen Tumoren mit Erhaltung des Bulbus. Arch.f.Augenheilk. 110: 482-491, 1936.
3. Weve, H.J.M.: Traitement chirurgical des tumeurs intraoculaires. L'Annẽe Thẽrapeutique en Ophtalmologie 1953: 345-358, 1953.
4. Dunphy, E.B.: Management of intraocular malignancy. Amer. J.Ophthal. 44: 313-322, 1957.
5. Davidorf, F.H.: Radiotherapy and diathermy of malignant melanoma of the choroid. In: Peyman, G.A., Apple, D.J. and Sanders, D.R.: Intraocular Tumors. Appleton, New York, 1977, pp 135-153.
6. Lincoff, H., McLean, J. and Long, R.: The cryosurgical treatment of intraocular tumors. Amer.J.Ophthal. 63: 389-399, 1967.
7. Buschmann, W. and Linnert, D.: Zur Kryotherapie von Tumoren. Ber.Dtsch.Ophthal.Ges. 77: 305-311, 1980.
8. Bleckmann, H.: Laser- und Kryokoagulation zur Behandlung "kleiner" Aderhaut-Melanome. Fortschr.Ophthal. 80: 309-311, 1983.
9. Abramson, D.H. and Lisman , R.D.: Cryopexy of a choroidal melanoma. Ann.Ophthal. 11: 1418-1421, 1979.

10. Peyman, G.A. and Raichand, M.: Full-thickness eye wall resection of choroidal neoplasms. Ophthalmology 86: 1024-1036, 1979.
11. Peyman, G.A., Raichand, M. and Green, J.: The management of uveal neoplasm with local excision. In: P.K. Lommatzsch and F.C. Blodi: Intraocular Tumors. Fortschritte der Onkologie, Band 9. Akademie-Verlag, Berlin, 1983, pp. 396-403.
12. Kara, G.B.: Excision of uveal melanomas: A 15-year experience. Ophthalmology 86: 997-1023, 1979.
13. Foulds, W.S.: Current options in the management of choroidal melanoma. Trans.Ophthal.Soc.U.K. 103: 28-34, 1983.
14. Foulds, W.S.: Personal communication, 1984.
15. Naumann, G.O.H.: Blockexcision of tumors of the ciliary body and choroid. In: P.K. Lommatzsch and F.C. Blodi: Intraocular Tumors. Fortschritte der Onkologie, Band 9. Akademie-Verlag, Berlin, 1983, pp 386-396.
16. Shields, J.A. and Augsburger, J.J.: Changing attitudes toward the management of posterior uveal melanomas. In: P.K. Lommatzsch and F.C. Blodi: Intraocular Tumors. Fortschritte der Onkologie, Band 9. Akademie-Verlag, Berlin, 1983, pp 367-373.
17. Brovkina, A.F.: Surgical treatment of tumors of the anterior uvea. In: P.K. Lommatzsch and F.C. Blodi: Intraocular Tumors. Fortschritte der Onkologie, Band 9. Akademie-Verlag, Berlin, 1983, pp 404-408.
18. Linnic, L.F. Surgical treatment of melanomas of the iris, ciliary body and choroid. In: P.K. Lommatzsch and F.C. Blodi: Intraocular Tumors. Fortschritte der Onkologie, Band 9. Akademie-Verlag, Berlin, 1983, pp 409-416.
19. Volkov, V.V.: Indications, technique and results of the surgical treatment of intraocular melanomas. In: P.K. Lommatzsch and F.C. Blodi: Intraocular Tumors. Fortschritte der Onkologie, Band 9. Akademie-Verlag, Berlin, 1983, pp 378-385.
20. Vogel, M.H.: Treatment of malignant choroidal melanomas with photocoagulation. Amer.J.Ophthal. 74: 1-11, 1972.
21. Meyer-Schwickerath, G.: Photocoagulation of choroidal melanomas. Docum.Ophthal.Proc.Series 24: 57-61, 1980.
22. Meyer-Schwickerath, G. and Bornfeld, N.: Photocoagulation of choroidal melanomas - Thirty years experience -. In: P.K. Lommatzsch and F.C. Blodi: Intraocular Tumors. Fortschritte der Onkologie, Band 9. Akademie-Verlag, Berlin, 1983, pp 269-276.
23. François, J.: Treatment of malignant choroidal melanomas by photocoagulation. Ophthalmologica 184: 121-130, 1982.
24. François, J.: Treatment of malignant choroidal melanomas by xenon photocoagulation. In: P.K. Lommatzsch and F.C. Blodi: Intraocular Tumors. Fortschritte der Onkologie, Band 9. Akademie-Verlag, Berlin, 1983, pp 277-285.
25. Trott, K.R., Kummermehr, J., Hug, O., Lukacs, S. and Braun-Falco, O.: Die Strahlenempfindlichkeit des amelanotischen Hamstermelanoms in vitro und in vivo. Strahlentherapie 154: 571-577, 1978.

26. Trott, K.R., Von Lieven, H., Kummermehr, J., Skopal, D., Lukacs, S. and Braun-Falco, O.: The radiosensitivity of malignant melanomas part I: Experimental studies. Int.J. Radiation Oncology Biol.Phys. 7: 9-13, 1981.
27. Chavaudra, N., Guichard, M. and Malaise, E.-P.: Hypoxic fraction and repair of potentially lethal radiation damage in two human melanomas transplanted into nude mice. Radiation Research 88: 56-68, 1981.
28. Thomson, L.F., Smith, A.R. and Humphrey, R.M.: The response of a human malignant melanoma cell line to high LET radiation. Radiology 117: 155-158, 1975.
29. Kummermehr, J.C.: Kurabilität des Harding-Passey-Melanoms durch Einzeitbestrahlung. Strahlentherapie 154: 578-581, 1978.
30. Guichard, M., Gosse, C. and Malaise, E.-P.: Survival curve of a human melanoma in nude mice. J.Natl.Cancer Inst.58: 1665-1669, 1977.
31. Stallard, H.B.: Radiotherapy for malignant melanoma of the choroid. Brit.J.Ophthal. 50: 147-155, 1966.
32. Stallard, H.B.: Malignant melanoblastoma of the choroid. Mod.Probl.Ophthal. 7: 16-38, 1968.
33. MacFaul, P.A.: Local radiotherapy in the treatment of malignant melanoma of the choroid. Trans.Ophthal.Soc. U.K. 97: 421-427, 1977.
34. Lommatzsch, P.K.: β-Irradiation of choroidal melanoma with ^{106}Ru/^{106}Rh applicators. 16 Years' experience. Arch.Ophthal. 101: 713- 717, 1983
35. Gragoudas, E.S., Goitein, M., Koehler, A.M., Verhey, L., Tepper, J., Suit, H.D., Brockhurst, R. and Constable, I.J.: Proton irradiation of small choroidal malignant melanomas. Amer.J.Ophthal. 83: 665-673, 1977.
36. Gragoudas, E.S., Goitein, M., Koehler, A., Constable, I.J., Wagner, M.S., Verhey, L., Tepper, J., Suit, H.D., Brockhurst, R.J., Schneider, R.J., and Johnson, K.N.: Proton irradiation of choroidal melanomas. Preliminary results. Arch.Ophthal. 96: 1583-1591, 1978,.
37. Gragoudas, E.S., Goitein, M., Verhey, L., Munzenreider, J., Urie, M., Suit, H. and Koehler, A.: Proton beam irradiation of uveal melanomas. Results of 5½-year study. Arch.Ophthal. 100: 928-934, 1982.
38. Gragoudas, E.S.: Proton beam irradiation of uveal melanomas: An alternative of enucleation. In: P.K. Lommatzsch and F.C. Blodi: Intraocular Tumors. Fortschritte der Onkologie, Band 9. Akademie-Verlag, Berlin, 1983, pp 347-354.
39. Gragoudas, E.S., Seddon, J., Goitein, M., Verhey, L., Munzenrider, J., Urie, M., Suit, H.D., Blitzer, P. and Koehler, A.: Current results of proton beam irradiation of uveal melanomas. Presented at the 88th Ann.Meeting Amer.Acad.Ophthal., Chicago-Ill., Oct.30-Nov.3, 1983. To be published.
40. Seddon, J.M., Gragoudas, E.S. and Albert, D.M.: Ciliary body and choroidal melanomas treated by proton beam irradiation. Histopathologic study of eyes. Arch.Ophthal. 101: 1402-1408, 1983

41. Wilkes, S.R. and Gragoudas, E.S.: Regression patterns of uveal melanomas after proton beam irradiation. Ophthalmology 87: 840-844, 1982.
42. Gragoudas, E.S., Goitein, M., Seddon, J., Verhey, L., Munzenrider, J., Urie, M., Suit, H.D., Blitzer, P., Johnson, K.N. and Koehler, A.: Preliminary results of proton beam irradiation of macular and paramacular melanomas. Brit.J.Ophthal. 68: 479-485, 1984.
43. Char, D.H. and Castro, J.R.: Helium ion therapy for choroidal melanoma. Arch.Ophthal. 100: 935-938, 1982.
44. Char, D.H., Brooks Crawford, J., Castro, J.R. and Woodruff, K.H.: Failure of choroidal melanoma to respond to helium ion therapy. Arch.Ophthal. 101: 236-241, 1983.
45. Char, D.H.: Personal communication, 1984.
46. Brovkina, A.F. and Zarubey, G.D.: Proton-therapy for eye-preserving treatment of choroidal tumors. Presented at the Symposium Diagnosis and Management of Intraocular Tumors, Moscow USSR Oct.30-Nov.1, 1984. To be published.
47. Bornfeld, N., Alberti, W., Foerster, M.H., Gerke, E., Wessing, A. and Meyer-Schwickerath, G.: External beam therapy of choroidal melanomata. Preliminary report. Trans.Ophthal.Soc.U.K. 103: 68-71, 1983.
48. Bedford, M.A.: The use and abuse of cobalt plaques in the treatment of choroidal malignant melanomata. Trans. Ophthal.Soc.U.K. 93: 139-143, 1973.
49. MacFaul, P.A. and Morgan, G.: Histopathological changes in malignant melanomas of the choroid after cobalt plaque therapy. Brit.J.Ophthal. 61: 221-228, 1977.
50. Zografos, L. and Gailloud, Cl.: Traitement conservateur des mélanomes de la choroïde avec les applicateurs de cobalt 60 radioactifs. Klin.Mbl.f.Augenheilk. 182: 499-501, 1983.
51. Migdal, C.: Choroidal melanoma: The role of conservative therapy. Trans.Ophthal.Soc.U.K. 103: 54-58, 1983.
52. Shields, J.A., Augsburger, J.J., Brady, L.W. and Day, J.L.: Cobalt plaque therapy of posterior uveal melanomas. Ophthalmology 89: 1201-1207, 1982.
53. Zygulska-Mach, H., Maciejewski, Z. and Link, E.: Conservative treatment of choroidal melanomas. Combined use of cobalt plaques and photocoagulation. In: P.K. Lommatzsch and F.C. Blodi: Intraocular Tumors. Fortschritte der Onkologie, Band 9. Akademie-Verlag, Berlin, 1983, pp 417-423.
54. Rotman, M., Long, R.S., Packer, S., Moroson, H., Galin, M.A. and Chan, B.: Radiation therapy of choroidal melanoma. Trans.Ophthal.Soc.U.K. 97: 431-435, 1977.
55. Ellsworth, R.M.: Cobalt plaques for melanoma of the choroid. In: F.A. Jakobiec: Ocular and Adnexal Tumors. Aesculapius Publ.Cy., Birmingham, 1978, pp 76-79.
56. Lommatzsch, P.: Treatment of choroidal melanomas with ^{106}Ru/^{106}Rh beta-ray applicators. Survey Ophthal. 19: 85-100, 1974.
57. Foerster, M.H., Wessing, A. and Meyer-Schwickerath, G.: The treatment of ciliary body melanoma by beta radiation. Trans.Ophthal.Soc.U.K. 103: 64-67, 1983.

58. Hallermann, D. and Guthoff, R.: Retrogression of choroidal melanoma after beta-irradiation with ruthenium-106/rhodium-106. In: P.K. Lommatzsch and F.C. Blodi: Intraocular Tumors. Fortschritte der Onkologie, Band 9. Akademie-Verlag, Berlin, 1983, pp 307-315.
59. Wessing, A., Foerster, M. and Fried, M.: Fluorescenz-angiographische Befunde nach Ruthenium-Behandlung maligner Aderhaut-Melanome. Fortschr.Ophthal. 80: 415-417, 1983.
60. Bornfeld, N., Foerster, M.H., Shulz, U. and Wessing, A.: Tumor regression and scleral contact dose in ruthenium therapy of uveal melanomas. Presented at the Symposium Diagnosis and Management of Intraocular Tumors, Moscow USSR Oct. 30-Nov. 1, 1984. To be published.
61. Busse, H. and Müller, R.-P.: Techniques and results of $^{106}Ru/^{106}Rh$ radiation of choroidal tumours. Trans.Ophthal. Soc.U.K. 103: 72-77, 1983.
62. Packer, S. and Rotman, M.: Radiotherapy of choroidal melanoma with iodine-125. Ophthalmology 87: 582-590, 1980.
63. Rotman, M., Packer, S., Long, R., Chiu-Tsao, S.T. and Zaki Sedhom, L.: Ophthalmic plaque irradiation of choroidal melanoma. In: P.K. Lommatzsch and F.C. Blodi: Intraocular Tumors. Fortschritte der Onkologie, Band 9. Akademie-Verlag, Berlin, 1983, pp 341-346.
64. Packer, S., Rotman, M., Fairchild, R.G., Albert, D.M., Atkins, H.L. and Chan, B.: Irradiation of choroidal melanoma with iodine 125 ophthalmic plaque. Arch.Ophthal. 98: 1453-1457, 1980.
65. Foster Moore, R.: Choroidal sarcoma treated by the intraocular insertion of radon seeds. Brit.J.Ophthal. 14: 145-152, 1930.
66. Stallard, H.B.: A case of malignant melanoma of the choroid successfully treated by radon seeds. Trans. Ophthal.Soc.U.K. 69: 293-297, 1949.
67. Ehlers, G., Batley, F. and Kartha, M.: Radiotherapeutic management of malignant melanoma of the eye. Amer.J. Roentgen. 123: 486-491, 1975.
68. Boniuk, M. and Cohen, J.S.: Combined use of radiation plaques and photocoagulation in the treatment of choroidal melanomas. In: F.A. Jakobiec: Ocular and Adnexal Tumors. Aesculapius Publ.Co., Birmingham USA, 1978, pp 80-85.
69. Menapace, R.M., Gnad, H.D. and Heckenthaler, W.: Interstitielle Radiotherapie maligner Aderhautmelanome: Spickung mit dem Goldkorn-Applikator nach Hodt. Klin. Mbl.f.Augenheilk. 182: 560-564, 1983.
70. Rousseau, A., Deschênes, J., Pelletier, G., Boudreault, G., Tremblay, M., Tardif, Y. and Larochelle, M.: Malignant melanoma: An evaluation of pre-enucleation radiotherapy. XIVth Meeting Jules Gonin Club, Lausanne, Sept. 24-28, 1984. To be published.
71. Lagendijk, J.J.W.: A mathematical model to calculate temperature distributions in human and rabbit eyes during hyperthermic treatment. Phys.med.Biol. 27: 1301-1311, 1982.

72. Lagendijk, J.J.W.: A microwave heating technique for the hyperthermic treatment of tumours in the eye. Phys.Med. Biol. 27: 1313-1324, 1982.
73. Coleman, J.: Effects of hyperthermia (ultrasound) on ocular tumours. XIVth Meeting Jules Gonin Club, Lausanne, Sept. 24-28, 1984. To be published.
74. Char, D.H.: Immunological mechanisms in choroidal melanoma. Trans.Ophthal.Soc.U.K. 97: 389-393, 1977.
75. Federman, J.L., Felberg, N.T. and Shields, J.A.: Effects of local treatment on antibody levels in malignant melanoma of the choroid. Trans.Ophthal.Soc.U.K. 97: 436-439, 1977.

TREATMENT OF INTRAOCULAR MELANOMAS BY RUTHENIUM-106 BETA IRRADIATION

D. Hallermann

For 150 years scientific research has been done on the problem of finding a suitable method of treatment for choroidal melanoma. Even today contradictory opinions exist; the causes are many, such as

- insufficient insight into the origin and development of the tumour;
- the so far unexplained function of an immunologic defense mechanism against the tumour;
- the clinically unpredictable development and rate of growth of the tumour;
- insufficient knowledge of the factors leading to a general metastasis,

which together contribute to

- uncertainty in the evaluation of therapeutic measures;
- lack of proof of a decisive extension of life by chemotherapy (cytostatics);
- insufficient proof of an influence of immunotherapy.

When considering the modalities of treatment used at present, we must conclude that opinions vary widely. The theory published by Zimmerman and co-workers (1978, 1979) caused a major controversy. They questioned, even partly rejected enucleation as suitable therapy for melanomas; on the other hand it continued to be advocated as the therapy of choice (Manschot and Van Peperzeel, 1980).

In the intervening territory of these controversial opinions the bulbus-preserving irradiation therapy has lately proved itself as a curative way of treatment with good results and has won acceptance in some centres.

Oosterhuis, A. (ed.), Ophthalmic tumors.

ISBN 90 6193 528 8. Printed in the Netherlands.

General principles of treatment

The principles of today's treatment of melanoma are the following:

- enucleation of the eye in case of larger tumours which do not allow bulbus-preserving treatment any more, sometimes in combination with a pre- or postoperative irradiation;
- xenon or argon laser photocoagulation in smaller choroidal melanomas with an elevation of up to 1-2 mm;
- surgical removal of tumours of ciliary body or iris not extending into the anterior segment (block excision);
- bulbus-preserving irradiation therapy with radiopharmaceuticals (strontium-90, cobalt-60, iodine-125, ruthenium-106) or heavy particle irradiation with linear accelerator or cyclotron (protons, helium ions).

History of the irradiation treatment of choroidal melanoma

Foster Moore (1930) was the first ophthalmologist to succeed in confuting the generally prevailing view held till then that choroidal melanomas are radiation-resistent. He used radium needles shaped for the purpose ("radon seeds") which were introduced transsclerally in the direction of the tumour at various sites of the posterior segment of the bulbus. His pupil Stallard (1966, 1968) subsequently developed this method into the proper applicator technique, first with radium but later with cobalt-60, and reported on 107 patients treated with cobalt-60. He designed a series of differently shaped applicators with loops for suturing the applicators onto the sclera for some days until the pre-calculated dose to destroy the tumour had been delivered.

Others have modified his technique. Fossati (1964) introduced cobalt-containing threads into the sclera overlying the base of the tumour. Rosengreen and Tengroth (1963) developed a spherical cobalt source for irradiation of smaller choroidal melanomas at the posterior pole. Boniuk and Cohen (1978) treated 40 patients with radioactive gold-

198 by gluing gold needles onto a pre-fabricated plastic applicator which had been modelled according to the shape of the tumour base. Packer and Rotman (1980) and Packer et al. (1980) modified the applicator technique by introducing the isotope iodine-125, also a gamma ray emitter, which they considered to be superior to cobalt-60. Brovkina (1983) reported on successful irradiation treatment of choroidal melanomas with the radioisotope strontium-90.

McFaul and Bedford (1970) made a critical review of the ocular complications after irradiation of choroidal melanoma. The gamma irradiation did not only affect the tumour itself but also the anterior parts of the eye. The following serious complications of irradiation were encountered: obliteration of large retinal vessels, both arteries and veins, resulting in an irreversible secondary glaucoma; cataract; a decrease of tear production due to shrinkage of the lacrimal glands, which not seldom caused trophic lesions of the cornea with secondary ulcers.

Shields et al. (1982) mentioned data about noxious side effects of irradiation. They found complications in 40 out of 100 patients treated with cobalt irradiation; in 23 radiation retinopathy resulted in impairment of visual acuity. Zografos and Gailloud (1983, 1984) report on their results of cobalt plaque therapy elsewhere in this issue. Rotman et al. (1977) reported on 32 patients, Zygulska-Mach et al. (1983) reported on 149 patients and Migdal (1983) reported on 99 patients with choroidal melanomas treated with cobalt plaques. Oosterhuis gives a review of the results of cobalt-60 treatment elsewhere in this issue.

Irradiation treatment with ruthenium-106

A decisive turn of events was brought about by Lommatzsch who in 1964 started treatment of intraocular melanomas with the beta ray emitter ruthenium-106, which he considered to be more suitable than cobalt-60 in view of its isodose curve distribution (Table 1). The findings of Lommatzsch (1983) in 205 patients over the past 16 years, especially the complications of irradiation, are summarized in Table 2.

Nuclide	Ru-106	
Daughter		Rh-106
Half life	1 y	30 s
Effective half life		
whole body	7.2 d	
kidney	2.48 d	
bone	15 d	
Beta energy max. (MeV)	0.039 (100%)	3.54 (79%)
		3.6 (8%)
		2.4 (11%)
		2.0 (2%)
Extrapolated range (mg/cm^2)	2.5	1.750
Extrapolated range in water (mm)		20
Half thickness in water (mm)		2.4
Gamma energy (MeV)		0.51 (21%)
		0.62 (11%)

Table 1. Radiophysical properties of $^{106}Ru/^{106}Rh$.

	Strontium	Ruthenium-106		
	Brovkina	Lommatzsch	Hallermann	Wessing et al.*
Number of patients	278	205	215	100
Period of investigation	1972-1983	1964-1980	1975-1983	3 years
Observation period	mean 3 yrs	0.5-16 yrs mean 5.4 yrs	mean 3 yrs	mean 2 yrs
Tumour dosis (Gy)	200	top 80-100 base ⩽1000	top 150-200 base ⩽1500	base 700-800
Regression of tumour		64.4% (132)		85% (85)
Enucleation	3%	17.6% (36)	5%	15% (15)
Metastatic death		10.2% (21)	5%	3% (3)
5-Years mortality	30%	14.9%	20%	
Radiation retinopathy		3.9% (8)	4%	
Vitreous haemorrhage		1.9% (4)	1%	
Optic atrophy		8.8% (18)		
Central ret.vein occl.		1.0% (2)		
Scleral necrosis		0.5% (1)		
Radiation cataract		2.4% (5)		

* see elsewhere in this issue

Table 2. Results of strontium-90 and ruthenium-106 irradiation treatment.

Indications for treatment

Before considering irradiation treatment the diagnosis of choroidal melanoma has to be established, for which we use biomicroscopy, fluorescein angiography, infrared photography, ultrasonography, and incidentally also the P32-test. The decision whether or not to perform irradiation treatment by means of ruthenium-106 applicators depends primarily on the elevation and localization of the tumour. As a rule, all tumours with an elevation of up to 5-7 mm and a diameter at the base of up to 15 mm can be considered for irradiation, but choroidal melanomas with extension into the ciliary body can not be demarcated with precision and for this reason are not suitable for irradiation treatment with applicators.

Prior to treatment the risk of loss of visual function has to be extensively discussed with the patient. There is a distinct relationship between the site of the tumour and the functional loss to be expected. The residual visual acuity after irradiation does indeed depend on the localization and extension of the tumour after irradiation. Irradiation retinopathy and damage to the optic nerve have to be expected when the margin of the tumour is near the posterior pole or the optic disc. Therefore, ruthenium treatment is only indicated when the tumour is located in midperiphery, at a distance of at least 1.5 mm from the optic disc. However, if the melanoma has developed in the only eye with visual function, the indication for irradiation must sometimes be adapted to the individual situation of the patient.

Dosage

It is our experience that for irradiation of choroidal melanomas a dosage of 400-700 rads/h is the most favourable one. The duration of the irradiation depends on the degree of elevation of the tumour; to destroy the tumour a total dosage of 15,000-20,000 rads at the top of the tumour is needed. In order to obtain an optimal protraction effect the irradiation should last about 5-10 days. Tumours with an elevation of more than 3 mm should receive a higher dosage than smaller tumours, in any case more than 15,000 rads delivered at the top of the tumour; for these tumours applicators with a higher radiation output in rads/h should be used (more than 400 rads/h). In order to avoid undesirable radiation side effects the duration of irradiation should not be less than 3 days. On the other hand, when in large tumours irradiation requires more than 2 weeks, an insufficient regression of tumours of more than 5 mm elevation has to be expected. In these cases an applicator has to be selected with a higher radiation delivery per hour (up to 1,000 rads/h) and sometimes irradiation has to be combined with xenon arc photocoagulation or followed by additional irradiation treatment after an interval of 6-9 months.

Special surgical aspects

Irradiation of the eye may be followed by a number of complications, which one has to bear in mind when considering irradiation treatment and its advantages for the patient. The risk of side effects and their influence on vision have to be discussed extensively with the patient. As a rule, patients prefer irradiation treatment when enucleation is the only alternative. However, irradiation treatment should only be given in those cases which strictly conform with the indications for treatment.

General anaesthesia is preferable but treatment can be carried out under local anaesthesia. After perilimbal conjunctival incision the scleral surface is denuded in the tumour area; if necessary, muscles are detached. Then the base of the tumour is marked on the scleral surface under guidance of diaphanoscopy; sometimes this is not possible, especially when the tumour is located at the posterior pole. Careful cauterization of all bleeding vessels must be carried out before the applicator is sutured to the sclera; this is of utmost importance. If the diagnosis is still doubtful, a P32-test is carried out to confirm the diagnosis. When the P32-test is positive, a suitable applicator is selected, which is fastened onto the sclera with 2 suturamid sutures; the applicator has to cover the tumour area completely plus 1 mm extra in all directions, as otherwise a recidive may occur in the area that was not sufficiently covered.

The applicators are stored in the Department of Radiology in containers which absorb all radiation. This department calculates the radiation activity of the applicator on the day on which it is sutured onto the eye. A physicist of the Department of Radiology transports the applicator in a leaden container. In Germany there are strict rules for the use of radiopharmaceuticals. Continuous careful control of the patient can only be carried out in the Department of Radiology, where the patient is transported to when he leaves the recovery room after the applicator has been applied.

After delivery of the precalculated tumour dose the applicator is removed, again preferably under general anaesthesia, and handed over to the physicist. Application time and dosage are calculated and registered.

Clinical course after irradiation

After removal of the applicator the period of clinical observation depends on the degree of irradiation uveitis. In all patients we found an acute exudative anterior and posterior uveitis within the first few days after removal of the applicator. The inflammatory reaction in the anterior segment may lead to synechiae, to a neovascularization on the iris, even to a secondary glaucoma. As a rule, these early exudative complications respond very well to local or subconjunctival steroid treatment (Hallermann and Lommatzsch, 1979).

In ruthenium treatment of uveal melanoma the scleral surface receives up to 100,000 rads without undue reaction. However, the radiogenic load on the much more radiosensitive choroid leads to a considerable disturbance of the chorioretinal circulation and subsequently of the intraocular haemodynamic balance.

Post-irradiation retinal oedema slowly regresses in a few weeks. In the treated area a characteristic pigment shifting gradually develops in concomitance with a regression of the retinal detachment over the tumour and, if present, elsewhere in the fundus. A flattening of the tumour is not to be expected until after about 2-3 months. Its first signs are incipient retinal and choroidal atrophy at the periphery of the tumour area. These alterations in the tumour indicating regression may extend over a period of 1½ to 2 years.

According to the data presently available on long-term results of irradiation of intraocular melanomas with ruthenium-106, irradiation therapy has the advantage over enucleation in that not only the eye itself is preserved for the patient but also the rate of survival after irradiation treatment is distinctly higher (Hallermann and Lommatzsch, 1979; Lommatzsch, 1983).

Own results

Irradiation therapy of choroidal melanoma only has a permanent effect when the malignant tissue formation in the subretinal space is destroyed completely without damage to the non-tumorous part of the eye. From our material of the last 9 years we may conclude that in general this can be accomplished.

Irradiation therapy was given in 215 patients, including 7 in whom the eye concerned was the "last eye" and 21 in whom the visual acuity of the fellow eye was less than of the melanoma-containing eye. In agreement with literature most patients were aged 50 to 70 years; over the last few years there has been a remarkable increase of frequency among younger women of 30 to 50 years.

The effectiveness of the irradiation therapy can not be assessed until 1½ years have elapsed after treatment. An analysis of 142 patients (66%) in this respect is given in Table 3; the mean observation period of these patients was 36.7 months. The irradiation-induced regression of the tumour can be assessed by measuring the decrease of elevat-

Follow-up period	Number of patients	Percentage
18 - 24 months	43	20%
2 - 4 years	71	33%
4 - 6 years	23	11%
6 - 9 years	5	2%
Mean 36.7 months	142	66%

Table 3. Observation periods of 142 patients after ruthenium irradiation treatment.

Visual acuity	Before irradiation		After irradiation	
	number of eyes	percentage	number of eyes	percentage
Light perception to 0.05	19	9%	73	34%
0.06 - 0.1	11	5%	36	17%
0.2 - 0.6	54	25%	50	23%
0.7 - 1.0	131	61%	56	26%

Table 4. Visual acuity before and after ruthenium irradiation treatment in 215 patients.

ion of the tumour or by ultrasonographic measurement of the volume of the tumour (Hallermann and Guthoff, 1983). The effect of ruthenium irradiation on elevation and volume of the tumour may vary greatly, the cause of which has not yet been found. Further studies on radiation dosage and the resulting effect are required. Melanomas with a residual elevation of more than 3 mm should be additionally treated with xenon or argon laser photocoagulation or re-irradiation; it is our experience, however, that the total scleral dosage should not exceed about 150,000 rads.

In accordance with the frequency of larger melanomas at the posterior pole the visual acuity after irradiation was 0.2-1.0 in 49% of our patients (Table 4). In most patients a decrease of vision was due to irradiation damage of the optic nerve. Therefore, in a number of other patients with as yet good vision a decrease of visual acuity is to be expected due to a late development of radiation lesions, which according to our experience may continue for about 1½ to 2 years.

The complications which we have encountered in the patients with a follow-up of 1½ years and longer are summarized in Table 5. In 10 out of 142 patients a recidive developed, in 11 patients a secondary enucleation was necessary, 10 patients died, 8 of them owing to metastatic disease confirmed on histologic examination. In 1/3 of the treated patients regression of the tumour into a flat chorioretinal scar was achieved. In a further 1/3 we are justified in assuming the course will be favourable. In 26 patients the tumour regression was considered to be insufficient and additional irradiation treatment was given. For the latter as well as for the recently treated patients the follow-up period is too short to be of prognostic significance.

<u>Recently advanced techniques (proton, helium ion irradiation)</u>

A review of the present situation in irradiation treatment for intraocular melanomas would be incomplete without mentioning the latest techniques developed in the USA,

Follow-up in years	No. of cases	Initial V.A. restored	Decrease of V.A.	Recurrence	Secondary enucl.	Metastasis	Death	
							meta-stasis	other cause
1.5-2	43	30	13	6	3	1	1	-
2-4	71	50	21	-	5	3	3	-
4-6	23	5	18	3	3	6	4	2
6-9	5	2	3	1	-	-	-	-
mean 3	142	87	55	10	11	10	8	2

Table 5. Results of long term follow-up of 142 patients after ruthenium irradiation.

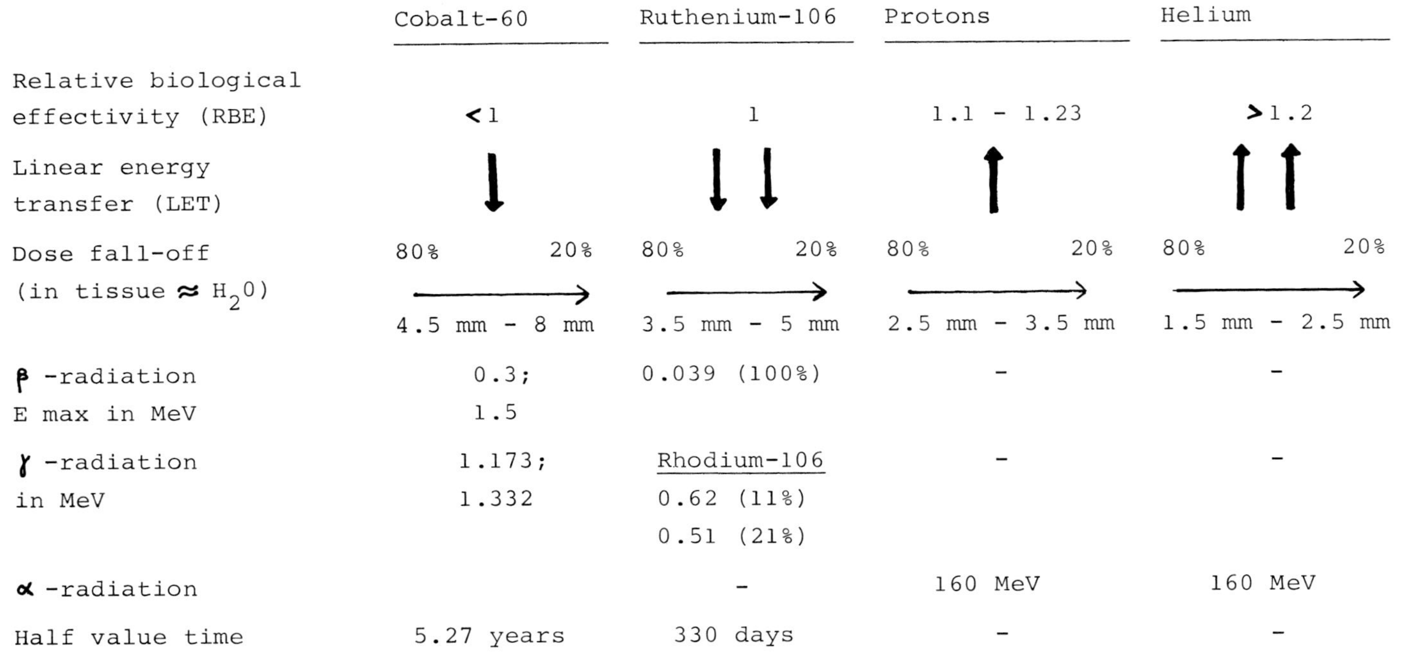

	Cobalt-60	Ruthenium-106	Protons	Helium
Relative biological effectivity (RBE)	< 1	1	1.1 - 1.23	> 1.2
Linear energy transfer (LET)	↓	↓↓	↑	↑↑
Dose fall-off (in tissue ≈ H_2O)	80% → 20% 4.5 mm - 8 mm	80% → 20% 3.5 mm - 5 mm	80% → 20% 2.5 mm - 3.5 mm	80% → 20% 1.5 mm - 2.5 mm
β -radiation E max in MeV	0.3; 1.5	0.039 (100%)	-	-
γ -radiation in MeV	1.173; 1.332	<u>Rhodium-106</u> 0.62 (11%) 0.51 (21%)	-	-
α -radiation		-	160 MeV	160 MeV
Half value time	5.27 years	330 days	-	-

Table 6. Characteristics of various irradiation modalities.

although they have yet to prove their clinical value in the long run. According to the results so far obtained the proton irradiation proposed by Gragoudas et al. (1982), especially for larger tumours, seems to surpass the ruthenium irradiation. The same applies to the helium ion irradiation (Char & Castro, 1982).

In irradiation therapy the relative biological effectivity (RBE) of alpha, beta and gamma rays is usually related to that of cobalt-60 or comparable conventional X-rays of 220 kV. Ruthenium has a smaller RBE than cobalt. Protons and helium ions ionize more densely in the tissues than beta and gamma ray emitters because of their heavier mass. The proton radiation is characterized by the development of its maximum radiobiological effectivity at a defined tissue depth with sparing of the overlying tissues. Helium ions have an even more favourable dose distribution than protons.

Table 6 summarizes the characteristics of cobalt-60, ruthenium-106, protons and helium ions. At the moment proton irradiation seems to be a better technique for our purpose than the conventional applicator techniques, as it apparently delivers a higher concentration of energy at the tumour with less risk for the healthy tissues of the eye.

Protons and helium ions are delivered by a cyclotron, involving an expensive accelerator which requires a whole staff of nuclear physicists and electronic engineers in order to guarantee a safe procedure. In the near future also in Villigen (Switzerland) proton irradiation of intraocular melanomas will be possible under supervision of Professor Gailloud of Lausanne.

References

Boniuk, M. and Cohen, J.S.: Combined use of radiation plaques and photocoagulation in the treatment of choroidal melanomas. In: Ocular and Adnexal Tumors. Ed.: F.A. Jakobiec. Aesculapius Publ.Cy., New York, 1978, pp 80-87.

Brovkina, A.F.: Personal communication, 1983.

Char, D.H. and Castro, J.R.: Helium ion therapy for choroidal melanoma. Arch.Ophthalmol. 100: 935, 1982.

Fossati, F.: Die Behandlung von Retinoblastomen und Melanoblastomen der Uvea mit Implantation radioaktiver Kobaltdrähte. Strahlentherapie 124: 180, 1964.
Foster Moore, R.: Choroidal sarcoma treated by the intraocular insertion of radon seeds. Brit.J.Ophthalmol. 14: 145, 1930.
Gragoudas, E.S., Goitein, M., Verhey, L., Munzenreider, J., Urie, M., Suit, H. and Koehler, A.: Proton beam irradiation of uveal melanomas. Results of 5½-year study. Arch. Ophthalmol. 100: 928, 1982.
Hallermann, D. and Lommatzsch, P.K.: Langzeitbeobachtungen nach Strahlentherapie des malignen Melanoms der Aderhaut mit dem Ru-106/Rh-106-Applikator. Ber.Dtsch.Ophthalmol. Ges. 76: 177, 1979.
Hallermann, D. and Guthoff, R.: Retrogression of choroidal melanoma after beta-irradiation with ruthenium-106/rhodium-106. Internat.Symp. on Intraocular Tumors, Schwerin 1981. Eds. P.K. Lommatzsch and F.C. Blodi. Springer-Verlag Berlin -Heidelberg-New York-Tokyo, 1983, pp 307-315.
Lommatzsch, P.: Beta-irradiation of choroidal melanoma with 106-Ru/106-Rh-applicators. 16 Years' experience. Arch. Ophthalmol. 101: 713-717, 1983.
McFaul, P.A. and Bedford, M.A.: Ocular complications after therapeutic irradiation. Brit.J.Ophthalmol. 54: 237-247, 1970.
Manschot, W.A. and van Peperzeel, H.A.: Choroidal melanoma: enucleation or observation? A new approach. Arch.Ophthalmol. 98: 71-77, 1980.
Migdal, C.: Choroidal melanoma. The role of conservative therapy. Trans.Ophthal.Soc. U.K. 103: 54-58, 1983.
Oosterhuis, J.A.: Conservative treatment modalities of choroidal melanomas. See elsewhere in this volume.
Packer, S. and Rotman, M.: Radiotherapy of choroidal melanoma with iodine-125. Ophthalmology 87: 582-590, 1980.
Packer, S., Rotman, M., Fairchild, R., Albert, D.M., Atkins, H.L. and Chan, B.: Irradiation of choroidal melanoma with iodine-125 ophthalmic plaque. Arch.Ophthalmol. 98: 1453-1457, 1980.
Rosengren, B. and Tengroth, B.: A modified Co-60-applicator for the treatment of the retinoblastoma. Acta Radiol. 1: 305, 1963.
Rotman, M., Long, R.S., Packer, S., Moroson, H., Galin, M.A. and Chan, B.: Radiation therapy of choroidal melanoma. Trans.Ophthal.Soc.U.K. 97: 431-435, 1977.
Shields, J.A., Augsburger, J.J., Brady, L.W. and Day, J.L.: Cobalt plaque therapy of posterior uveal melanomas. Ophthalmology 89: 1201-1207, 1982.
Stallard, H.B.: Radiotherapy for malignant melanoma of the choroid. Brit.J.Ophthalmol. 50: 147-155, 1966.
Stallard, H.B.: Malignant melanoma of the choroid. Mod.Probl. Ophthalmol. 7: 16-38, 1968.
Wessing, A., Foerster, M. and Bornfeld, N.: Ruthenium plaque treatment of malignant choroidal melanomas. See elsewhere in this volume.

Zimmerman, L.E. and McLean, I.W.: An evaluation of enucleation in the management of uveal melanomas. Amer.J.Ophthalmol. 87: 741-760, 1979.

Zimmerman, L.E., McLean, I.W. and Foster, W.P.: Does enucleation of an eye containing a malignant melanoma prevent or accelerate the dissemination of tumor cells? Brit.J.Ophthalmol. 62: 420-425, 1978.

Zografos, L. and Gailloud, Cl.: Conservative treatment of choroidal melanoma by cobalt 60 applicators. Internat. Symp. on Intraocular Tumors, Schwerin 1981. Eds. P.K. Lommatzsch and F.C. Blodi. Springer Verlag, Berlin-Heidelberg-New York-Tokyo, 1983, pp 286-289.

Zografos, L. and Gailloud, Cl.: Cobalt plaque treatment of choroidal melanomas. See elsewhere in this volume.

Zygulska-Mach, H., Maciejewski, Z. and Link, E.: Conservative treatment of choroidal melanomas. Combined use of cobalt plaques and photocoagulation. Internat.Symp. on Intraocular Tumors, Schwerin 1981. Eds. P.K. Lommatzsch and F.C. Blodi. Springer Verlag, Berlin-Heidelberg-New York-Tokyo, 1983, pp 417-423.

RUTHENIUM PLAQUE TREATMENT OF MALIGNANT CHOROIDAL MELANOMAS

A. Wessing, M. Foerster and N. Bornfeld

Conservative treatment of choroidal malignant melanomas has gained interest in recent years and has been caried out in increasing numbers of patients. This is based on new ideas as regards conservative treatment of malignant tumours. In ophthalmology conservative treatment has been stimulated by Zimmerman (1978) who, based on statistical data, stated that enucleation promotes the development of metastatic disease. Based on our own results of photocoagulation treatment and some very favourable results after cobalt-60 plaque treatment in choroidal melanomas we have been performing ruthenium plaque treatment since 1979.

Ruthenium (106 Ru/106 Rh) plaque treatment has been introduced by Lommatzsch in 1964. A review on his results has recently been published by Kiel et al. (1984).

Material and method

According to the size of the tumour 3 different applicators with a diameter of 17, 20 and 25 mm, respectively, can be used. Attachment of the applicator to the eye is a relatively simple procedure. After conjunctival incision the tumour is carefully localized by means of diaphanoscopy. The applicator is sutured onto the eye, covering the tumour in all directions, extending over the surface of the tumour by 2-3 mm. In case the insertion of a muscle must be covered by the applicator, the muscle is detached and temporarily attached next to the applicator. In case of localization of the tumour at the posterior pole, the situation is somewhat more complicated; as a rule resection of both oblique muscles

Oosterhuis, A. (ed.), Ophthalmic tumors.

ISBN 90-6193-528-8. Printed in the Netherlands.

is required. During surgery and during the period of irradiation the localization of the applicator can be checked by means of ultrasonography. Care should be taken that the applicator is in close contact with the sclera without interspace.

When treating tumours of the ciliary body, part of the cornea is covered by the applicator. In these cases sufficient and continuous anaesthesia of the surface of the cornea is required during the period of application. Usually regular application of an anaesthetic ointment is sufficient.

Attachment and removal of the applicator are performed under local anaesthesia; general anaesthesia is only required in exceptional cases.

The irradiation dosage has been changed in the course of the period irradiation treatment has been carried out. We started with a dosage at the top of the tumour of 100 Gy according to the scheme of Lommatzsch (1977). Later on we changed to a tumour dose of 50 Gy to be delivered at the level of 5 mm tumour depth. We now treat all tumours irrespective of their size with a scleral contact dose of 700-800 Gy.

The selection of the tumours for irradiation is performed according to the criteria of Lommatzsch (1977) and Hallermann & Lommatzsch (1979). Tumours with a diameter of up to 10 disc diameters and an elevation of up to 5 mm are suitable for irradiation. In certain cases we have surpassed these limits and treated larger tumours, especially mushroom-shaped ones with a small basis. Contrary to the advice of Lommatzsch, we also treated melanomas of the ciliary body.

Results

The following case histories are typical examples of the irradiation treatment.

Case history 1

A woman aged 58 years presented in 1981 with a large choroidal melanoma in her right eye. The tumour was located superior to the optic disc and macula; it had an elevation of 4 mm and a diameter of 35° (Fig. 1).

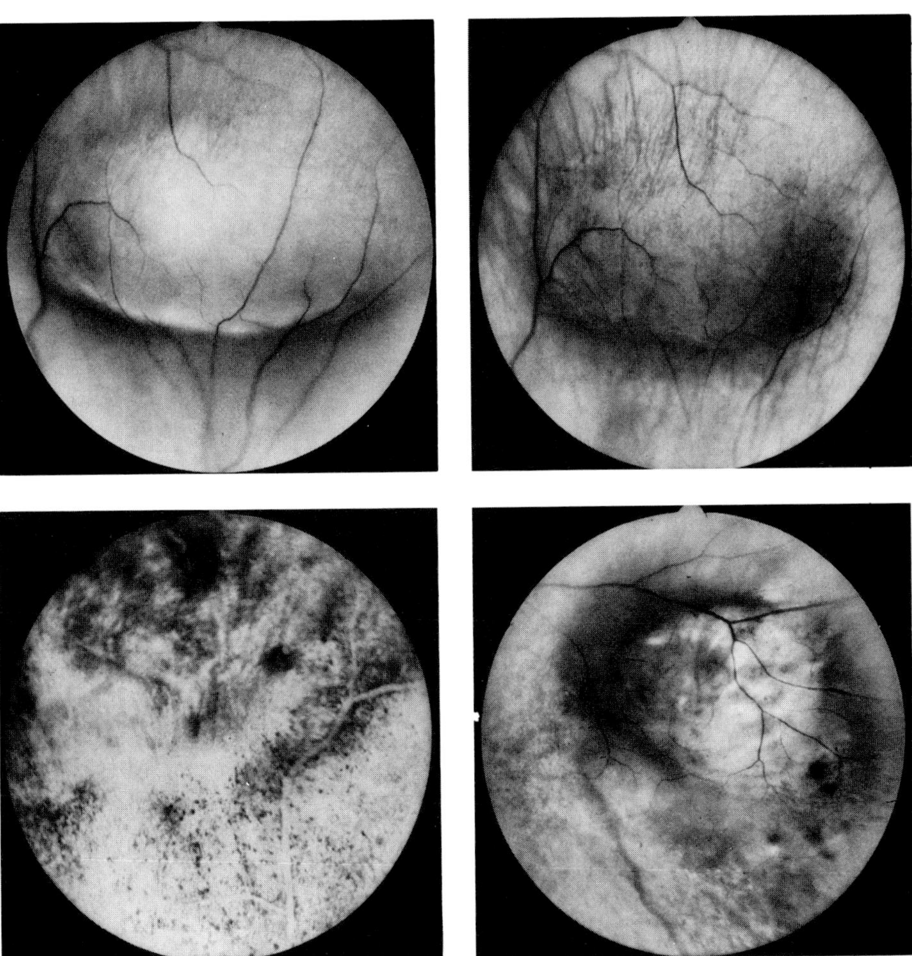

Fig. 1 Malignant melanoma of the choroid before therapy.

Fig. 2 Same tumour as in fig. 1 after ruthenium irradiation showing distinct regression.

Fig. 3 Malignant melanoma of the choroid after intense ruthenium irradiation showing atrophic choroidal scar.

Fig. 4 Malignant melanoma of the choroid after ruthenium irradiation showing residual prominence in the centre.

Irradiation was performed with a 17 mm ruthenium applicator (type CCA). The scleral contact dosage was 300 Gy. Six months after irradiation the choroid had become distinctly atrophic, the tumour had decreased in size and the elevation had decreased from 4 to 2 mm (Fig. 2).

Case history 2

This is an example of the development of very atrophic scars of retina and choroid covering a large fundus area.

A man aged 53 years presented in 1980 with a choroidal melanoma in the far periphery of his left eye. Elevation of the tumour was 4.2 mm, diameter was 45°.

Irradiation treatment was performed with a 17 mm applicator (CCA) and with a more than average scleral contact dosage of 1200 Gy. In the course of 23 weeks elevation of the tumour regressed completely. The tumour changed into a completely flat, atrophic and avascular scar (Fig. 3).

Case history 3

In some cases a smaller or larger part of the tumour will remain as residue.

A man of 65 years presented in 1981 with a tumour of 4.3 mm elevation and 30° diameter in the mid-periphery in the temporal fundus of his left eye.

Irradiation treatment was performed with a 17 mm applicator (CCA) and a contact dosage of 1100 Gy. Six months after irradiation a spherical residual tumour with a prominence of 2 mm was present in an otherwise atrophic scar (fig. 4). The residual tumour has not shown any significant change since then, in particular it has not changed in size and even now its elevation is still 2 mm.

Case history 4

Photocoagulation can be a useful adjunct in the conservative treatment in case of insufficient regression of the tumour after irradiation.

In a woman aged 62 years a melanoma was found in her right eye in 1979; its prominence was 5 mm, its diameter was 35° and it had already perforated the retinal pigment epithelium.

After irradiation with the 20 mm applicator (CCB) and a scleral contact dosage of 700 Gy a distinct regression of the tumour with haemorrhagic infarction was observed. Four months later the residual tumour was treated with photocoagulation twice with an interval of 4 weeks (Fig. 5). Finally the tumour changed into a completely flat scar with irregular pigmentation (Fig. 6).

Up till now we have treated 280 patients with a malignant choroidal melanoma by means of ruthenium applicators. We have the following data on the first 100 eyes thus treated.

In 1979 5 eyes were treated, in 1980 18, in 1981 34 and in 1982 43 eyes. The observation periods ranged from 0.12 to 4.7 years, averaging 2.3 years. Fifty-eight of the 100 eyes were only treated once with a ruthenium applicator, 24 eyes required additional photocoagulation treatment, in 11 eyes ruthenium applicator irradiation was performed twice and 7 eyes needed additional photocoagulation after the second irradiation.

In 32 eyes the tumour was completely destroyed and had developed into a flat irregularly pigmented scar. In 48 eyes a larger or smaller residual tumour remained, but in none of them did a fundus aspect suspicious of recidivation of the tumour develop. Enucleation was performed in 16 patients because of insufficient regression of the tumour or because of serious complications such as vitreous haemorrhages and retinal detachment; the interval between irradiation and enucleation varied from 3.5 months to 4 years 3 months, averaging 1 year 2 months.

The prominence of the 100 melanomas varied from 2.3 to 12.6 mm and averaged 7.48 mm. These values were assessed by ultrasonography and corresponded to 3.0, 16.5 and 9.77 microseconds. The average pre-treatment prominence of the 32 com-

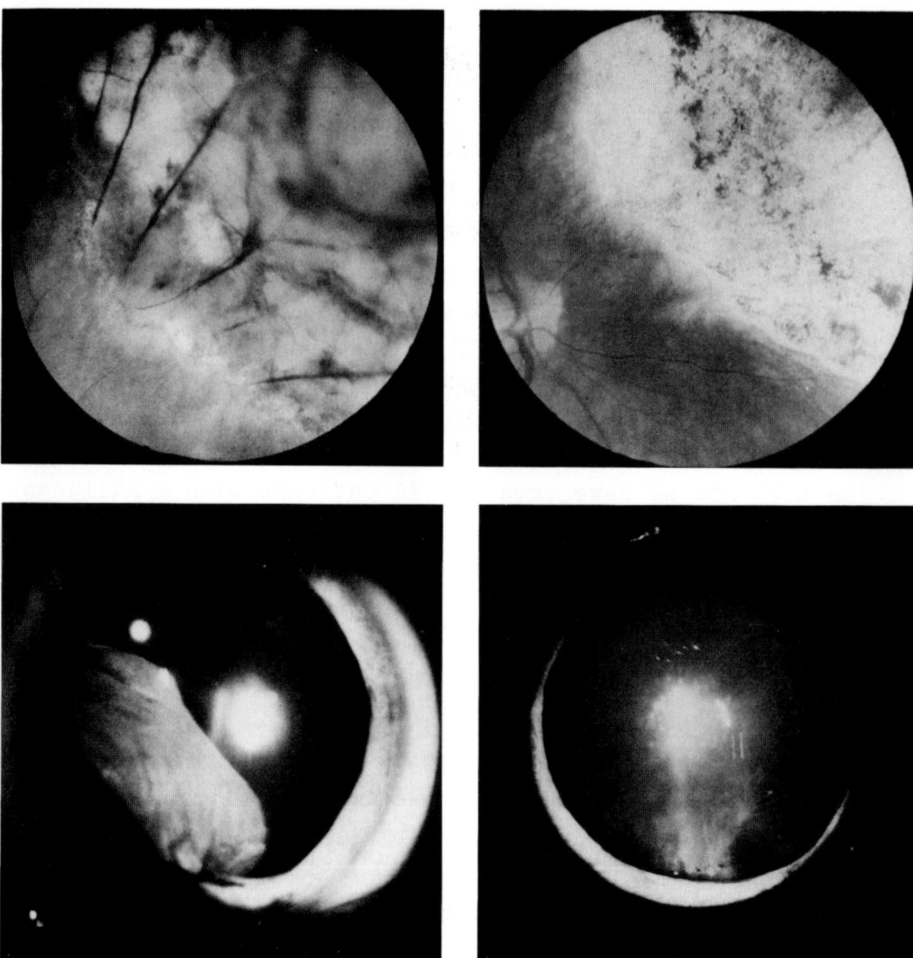

Fig. 5 Malignant melanoma of the choroid after ruthenium irradiation and photocoagulation treatment.

Fig. 6 Same tumour is in fig. 5 in scar stage.

Fig. 7 Melanoma of the ciliary body before therapy.

Fig. 8 Same tumour as in fig. 7 after ruthenium irradiation showing extensive regression.

pletely destroyed tumours was 4.33 mm (= 5.7 micro-sec). The average pre-treatment prominence of the 18 tumours twice treated with ruthenium was 6.33 mm (= 8.34 micro-sec). The average pre-treatment prominence of the tumours in the 16 enucleated eyes was 8.2 mm (= 10.6 micro-sec).

These figures show the limits as regards the size of the tumours suitable for ruthenium irradiation treatment which had already been given by Lommatzsch but which we had surpassed in a number of cases.

Eight of our first 100 patients died during the follow-up period, 3 of them due to metastatic disease, which will be discussed later on.

Malignant melanoma of the ciliary body

According to Lommatzsch, melanomas of the ciliary body are not suitable for ruthenium treatment. However, we have tried this modality in melanomas located far anteriorly and found that also these tumours do as a rule respond to treatment.

After intense irradiation of ciliary body melanomas we found two typical patterns of regression. The first pattern shows a rapid regression of the tumour, which develops into a flat, avascular scar in the course of 4-6 months. The second pattern shows changes at the surface of the tumour indicative of tumour necrosis. The colour changes into grey-white. Retinal folds develop at the surface of the tumour. Fluorescence angiography shows areas of non perfusion in the centre of the tumour. On ultrasonography the internal reflectivity has increased, indicating development of fibrosis in the tumour.

The case history of a female of 34 years is a typical example. In her right eye a melanoma of the ciliary body with a very strong prominence was visible in the temporal inferior quadrant, almost behind the pupillary centre (Fig. 7). Ruthenium irradiation with the 20 mm applicator (CCB) was performed because the patient refused enucleation. The scleral contact dosage was 350 Gy. One and a half years later the tumour had shrunken to 1/3 of its original size. Quite an amount of cellular debris had been dispersed into the vitreous (Fig. 8). About half the cornea had been covered by the applicator but this had not led to complications of any significance; the cornea remained clear. The iris became only slightly atrophic. Lately coarse opacities have developed in part of the lens adjacent to the tumour.

Among the 100 choroidal melanomas treated were 21 melanomas involving the ciliary body, 17 of which could be successfully treated with ruthenium irradiation, the tumour either turning into a flat scar or shrinking to a residual tumour without any tendency to recidivate. In 4 eyes a second ruthenium treatment was carried out. In 4 eyes additional photocoagulation was performed. Four eyes were enucleated because of complications or tumour regrowth. One patient died from unknown cause, one patient is known to have metastatic disease.

Fluorescence angiography

Serial fluorescein-angiographic studies have been performed in a number of our patients. The irradiation effect shows on the angiogram in three ways.

Destruction of the retinal pigment epithelium is the first fluorographic finding. The structure becomes more coarse, large pigmentary aggregations develop. The pigment epithelium may partly become totally destroyed. This type of reaction reaches as far as 2-3 mm beyond the margin of the applicators. It is remarkable that despite complete depigmentation no leakage of fluorescein of any significance develops.

The second finding concerns degenerative changes of the retinal vessels. Retinal capillaries at the surface of the tumour and in the adjacent retina become obliterated about 3-4 months after irradiation. Lesions of the larger vessels develop later on; they show considerable changes in calibre and vascular sheathing. At the margin of the non-perfused retina microaneurysms develop. Sectorial or total loss of vascularity of the optic disc develops in cases where the optic disc has been included in the field of irradiation.

The third and most important finding concerns the choroidal circulation and therefore the feeding vessels of the tumour. After about 3 months areas of hypofluorescence develop in the centre of the tumour, which only in the late phase of the angiogram develops hyperfluorescence, a pattern attributed to foci of necrosis. Tumour vessels, when visible, develop the same calibre changes as the retinal vessels. After intense irradiation avascular choroidal scars may develop, in which no vascular structure at all can be found any more.

The effect after irradiation treatment of melanomas is exerted in two ways. One is the direct irradiation effect on the tumour cells, the other one is indirect by affecting the feeding vessels of the tumour. Irradiation angiopathy is caused at the base of the tumour by the extremely high irradiation dosage at this level. This diminishes the circulation in the tumour, sometimes even to such an extent that the tumour is cut off from all feeding vessels.

Metastasis

Out of the 100 ruthenium-treated patients 8 have died in the period of observation, 3 owing to metastatic disease, 3 owing to proven non tumour-related causes (coronary infarction, bronchial carcinoma, suicide), 2 owing to unknown cause.

The case histories of the 3 patients who died from metastatic disease are as follows.

The first patient was a male aged 68 years with an intensely pigmented tumour in the macular area of 30° diameter and an elevation of 2.7 mm. Irradiation was performed with a 17 mm applicator (CCA) and a scleral contact dose of 675 Gy. The tumour regressed rapidly; after 1 year there was only a residual scar without any prominence at all. Twenty-two months after the irradiation patient died owing to metastatic disease of the liver.

The second patient was a male aged 21 years who had a tumour with 10.5 mm elevation in the temporal periphery of his fundus and a secondary retinal detachment. Irradiation was performed with a 17 mm applicator (CCA); the scleral contact dose was 660 Gy. At first the tumour regressed to some extent. As later on tumour regrowth was observed and the serous retinal detachment increased, the eye was enucleated 16 months after the irradiation. Histopathology showed the tumour to be of the spindle B cell type; tumour cells had infiltrated the retina but the internal limiting membrane was still intact. Scleral ingrowth as far as half the thickness of the sclera was found but there was no extraocular extension. Eighteen months after the irradiation and 2 months after enucleation of the eye patient died owing to liver metastasis.

The third patient was a woman aged 40 years who had a tumour in the macular area of 45° diameter and 4.7 mm elevation. Treatment was performed with a 17 mm applicator (CCA) and a scleral contact dose of 360 Gy. One year after the irradiation the elevation of the tumour had regressed to 0.8 mm. The scar which gradually resulted developed a remarkably intense pigmentation. Thirty months after irradiation patient died owing to liver metastasis.

Complications

The acute complications after beta irradiation are without exception related to a rapidly developing, too intense necrosis of the melanoma tissue. An exudative retinal detachment is often observed, which regresses within 1-2 weeks. Six times we observed a total and irreversible retinal detachment, usually associated with intense signs of inflammation and vitreous clouding. There was a predilection for those patients who already had an exudative retinal detachment prior to the irradiation. However, occasionally also the opposite effect has been observed in that exudative retinal detachment reattached rapidly after resorption of the subretinal fluid.

Incidentally, necrosis of the tumour was associated with massive vitreous haemorrhages, which resorbed slowly or not at all. All eyes with irreversible retinal detachment and

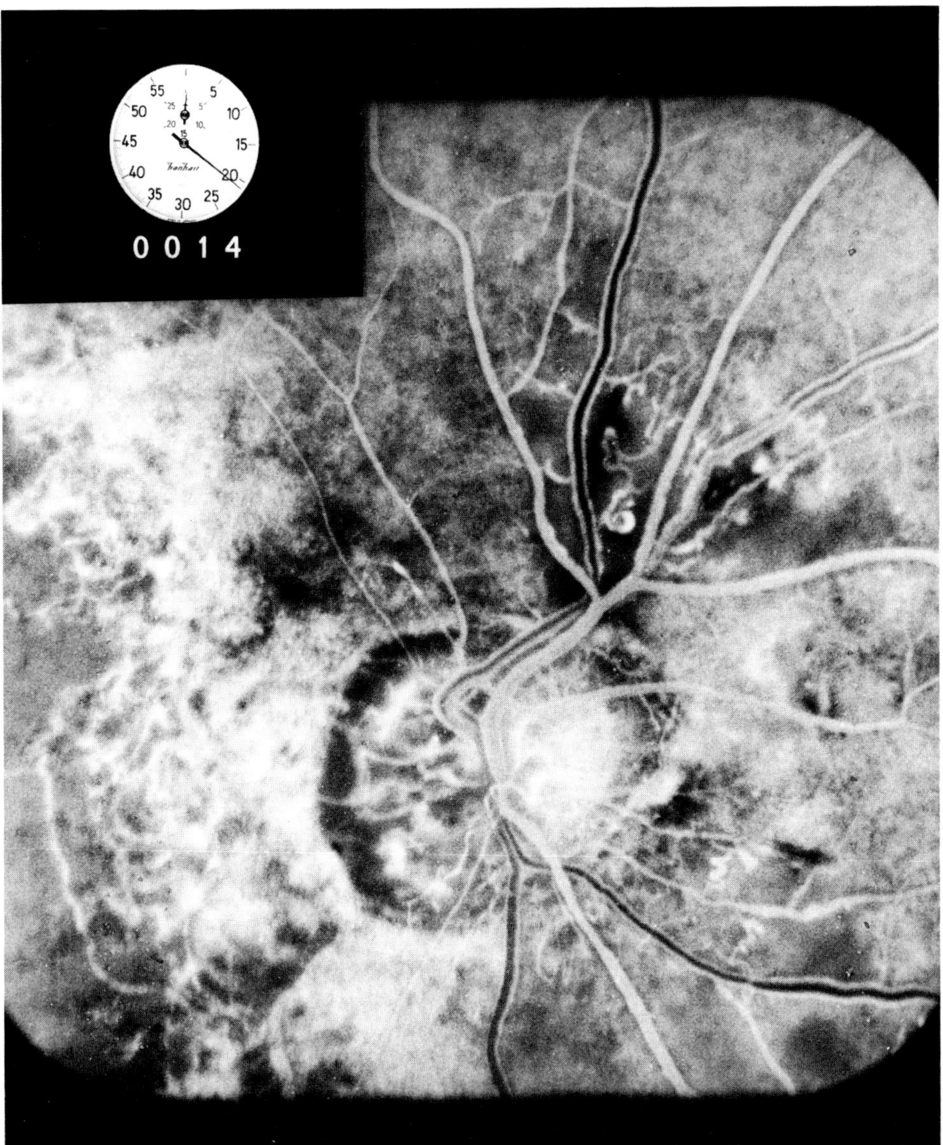

Fig. 9 Fluorescence angiogram of a fundus with irradiation retinopathy.

persisting vitreous haemorrhages were enucleated.

The most important long-term complication is the irradiation retinopathy. Early symptoms are retinal oedema and intraretinal haemorrhages. Later on retinal aneurysms may develop and finally retina and choroid may become totally atrophic with secondary neovascularization. In tumours at the posterior pole the risk of an ischaemic optic atrophy is relatively high. In most of the cases a papilloedema developed in the early post-irradiation period, which regressed after 3-5 weeks and changed into a partial or total optic atrophy (Fig. 9).

The follow-up period is too short for a final evaluation of the irradiation retinopathy. From three up to four years after the irradiation seems to be a critical period in which the condition may again deteriorate further and atrophy of the vessels may increase.

After treatment of ciliary body melanomas we have not observed any damage to the cornea and the iris. One to two years after treatment the first lens opacities due to irradiation developed. Up till now cataract has always been restricted to those parts of the lens that were located in the irradiation field.

Functional results

In our series of 100 patients the average visual acuity prior to the irradiation treatment was 0.56. After the treatment it had decreased to 0.25. There was a large range of individual variations as is shown in the scattergram (Fig. 10). About 25% of the patients had no loss of vision. In some cases with retinal detachment of the macular area visual acuity improved after resorption of the subretinal fluid.

We have performed electroretinography to study the loss of function of the fundus. Amplitude-intensity curves of A and B components of the ERG were determined. In the treatment of the melanomas the irradiation area averaged about 1/4 of the retina. However, the peak values of the A and B

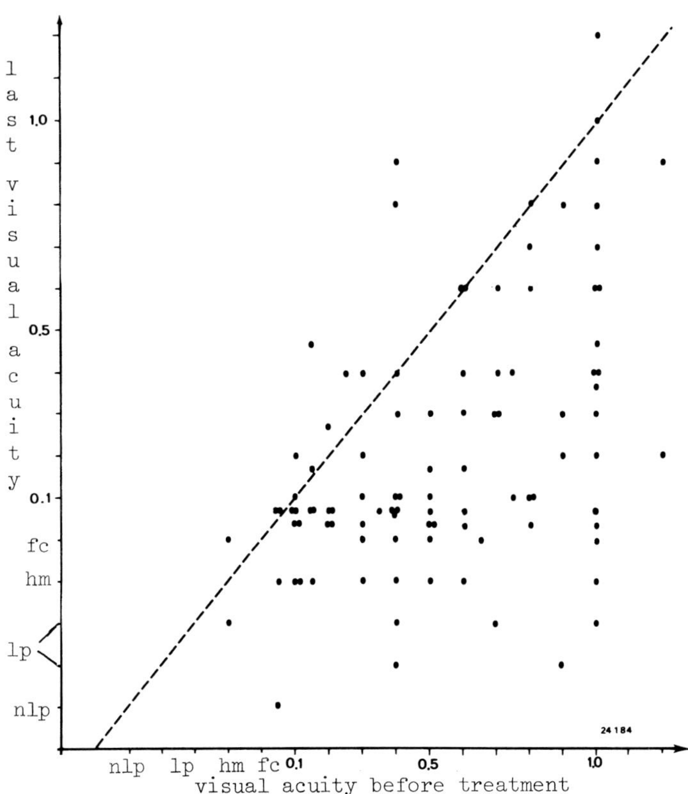

Fig. 10 Visual acuity before and after ruthenium treatment in 100 eyes with malignant melanoma of choroid and ciliary body.

waves were reduced to about 1/2 of the original values. This is indicative of the fact that also non-irradiated parts of the retina are affected by either the irradiation or the toxic action of the necrotic tissue of the tumour. A further decrease of the ERG was observed when a second irradiation treatment was performed. In one case the peak values of the A and B waves decreased to 50% after first and to 22% after the second irradiation treatment. In another patient no ERG responses were obtained after the second treatment. However, this patient still had a visual acuity of 0.1 and no restriction of his peripheral visual field.

Conclusions

For final evaluation of the beta irradiation of malignant melanomas of the choroid we need a longer period of observation. However, from our results so far obtained we may draw some conclusions:

1. The metastatic rate of a malignant melanoma of the choroid after irradiation treatment is not higher, probably even lower, than after enucleation of the eye.
2. The indications for ruthenium irradiation cover a wider field than indicated by Lommatzsch (1977). It is our experience that also tumours with a prominence of up to 7 and even of 10 mm are suitable for ruthenium treatment. This is especially applicable to tumours with a small base and a mushroom-shaped configuration. Successful treatment may also be obtained in ciliary body melanomas.
3. We feel that the scleral surface dosage may be a very suitable irradiation parameter. Our data obtained up till now indicate that the irradiation dosage on the sclera should be at least 700 Gy. At this dosage level not only the tumour but also the nutrient vessels at the base of the tumour are irradiated intensely.

Our future plans will consist of careful planning of the treatment and a detailed recording of the date of beta irradiation in order to increase our knowledge of the fundamental principles and the treatment modalities.

References

Hallerman, D. and Lommatzsch, P.: Langzeitbeobachtungen nach Strahlentherapie des malignen Melanoms der Aderhaut mit dem 106 Ru/106 Rh-Applikator. Ber.Dtsch.Ophthal.Ges. 76: 177-180, 1979.

Kiehl, H., Kirsch, I. and Lommatzsch, P.: Das Überleben nach Behandlung des malignen Melanoms der Aderhaut: Vergleich von konservativer Therapie (106 Ru/106 Rh-Applikator) und Enukleation ohne und mit postoperativer Orbitabestrahlung, 1960 bis 1979. Klin.Mbl.f.Augenheilk. 184: 2-14, 1984.

Lommatzsch, P.: Die therapeutische Anwendung von ionisierenden Strahlen in der Augenheilkunde. VEB G. Thieme, Leipzig, 1977.

Zimmerman, L.E., McLean, I.W. and Foster, W.D.: Does enucleation of an eye containing a malignant melanoma prevent or accelerate the dissemination of tumour cells? Brit.J.Ophthal. 62: 420-425, 1978.

COBALT PLAQUE TREATMENT OF CHOROIDAL MELANOMAS

L. Zografos and Cl. Gailloud

At present opinions as regards radical vs conservative treatment in choroidal melanoma are still controversial. As the death rate due to metastasis is not higher in conservatively treated eyes than in enucleation-treated eyes, it is justified to use one of the various techniques aiming at destruction of these tumours.

In the Ophthalmological Clinic of Lausanne we have been using the ^{60}Cobalt applicators in the conservative treatment of choroidal melanomas since 1969. In the period 1969-1982 we have treated 104 melanoma patients.

The average age of our patients was 55.5 years with a predominance of the 5th and 6th decade. The average age and age distribution is similar to those mentioned in literature. The control period covered at least 5 years for 60 patients treated before 1978 and at least 10 years for 22 patients treated before 1973.

Out of the 60 patients with an observation period of at least 5 years, 5 (8.3%) died of metastasis. For the whole group with an average observation period of 4.6 years the death rate due to metastasis amounted to 6 patients (5.8%). These figures are similar to or even lower than the death rate reported in literature for small melanomas.

Failure of the cobalt plaque treatment necessitating enucleation of the treated eye occurred in 21 patients (20.2% of our series). It was performed because of tumour recurrence in 8 cases, vitreous haemorrhage in 7 cases, glaucoma in 2 cases, functional loss of the eye in 1 case, and for psychological reasons in 3 cases. Out of 10 (9.6%)

Oosterhuis, A. (ed.), Ophthalmic tumors.

ISBN 90-6193-528-8. Printed in the Netherlands.

treated eyes who showed recurrence 8 were enucleated and 2 were treated a second time by means of a cobalt applicator. Of the latter, one had a large melanoma which showed an important recurrence 9 years after irradiation treatment. A second application of cobalt was performed and at present, 2 years later, the patient enjoys a visual acuity of 3/10. The other patient had a melanoma which recurred 7 years after conservative treatment and was treated a second time by cobalt application. One year after the second application the patient enjoys a visual acuity of 3/10.

The average diameter of the melanomas which recurred was 9.2 mm. The majority of the eyes which were enucleated had a melanoma of the spindle A or B cell type.

We have tried to relate the rate of recurrence to the irradiation doses given to the base and the top of the tumour. We found that none of the melanomas treated with an irradiation dose of over 9,000 rad at the top of the tumour showed a recurrence, neither did any of the tumours treated with a irradiation dose of over 35,000 rad at the base of the tumour. We therefore limit our minimum dose of irradiation to 9,000 rad at the top or 35,000 rad at the base of the tumour.

Among the various complications leading to enucleation vitreous haemorrhage comes second in importance. In fact, 12 patients (11.5%) developed a vitreous haemorrhage; in 7 of them the eye was enucleated. In almost all cases of vitreous haemorrhage the retina was destroyed with the tumour herniating into the vitreous cavity. On histological examination of the 7 enucleated eyes with a vitreous haemorrhage we found not occluded vessels in the tumour opening into the vitreous cavity, not covered by retina, which were held responsible for the vitreous haemorrhage in most of the cases. This has induced us to perform photocoagulation prior to the cobalt application to create a fibrous shell over the surface of the tumour in order to avoid bleeding into the vitreous. Of the 54 cases pretreated by photocoagulation only 4 (7.4%) were complicated by a vitreous haemorrhage as against 8 (16%) of the 50 non-coagulated eyes.

In the two cases of enucleation because of a secondary glaucoma histological examination showed many synechiae with closure of the iridocorneal angle.

Our results are summarized in the table. They show that after more than 5 years serious complications may arise. A recurrence of the tumour was observed in 10 patients (16.6%), an enucleation had to be performed in 21 patients (35%).

A period of at least 2 years is necessary to evaluate the rate of destruction of the tumour. The scar developing after radiotherapy can be flat and atrophic, either unpigmented (Fig. 1A) or with partial or irregular pigmentation (Fig. 1B). Progressive decrease in pigmentation can occur if photocoagulation is added to the radiotherapy. After scar formation we very often found the presence of a slight tumorous elevation in the centre of the atrophic scar (Fig. 1C).

The functional results obtained after conservative treatment of melanomas depend on several factors, the most important one being the localization of the tumour. If the tumour is situated in the macular region, it is to be feared that functional results will be very poor after its destruction. Also other side effects of radiotherapy may cause loss of visual acuity after irradiation.

We have studied the tolerance of the optic disc and the macula to ionizing radiation. Seven eyes were treated with a dose of over 20,000 rad on the optic disc and 7 other eyes with a dose of 20,000 rad or more on the macula. No macular complication due to this excessive radiation dose was reported but all 7 eyes having received a dose of over 20,000 rad on the border of the optic disc suffered from severe vascular complications.

The only non-vascular complication due to contact radiotherapy is the development of a secondary cataract. This sometimes actinic cataract was often a side effect to vitreous haemorrhage. It may show as a posterior cortical or a totally white cataract. It was observed more frequently in patients with a long period of observation, as in 10 our of 11 cases the period of observation was more than 5 years.

	Whole series of patients	Patients 5 years after irradiation
Number	104	60
Metastatic death	6 (5.8%)	5 (8.3%)
Recurrence of tumour	10 (9.6%)	10 (16.6%)
Enucleation	21 (21.2%)	21 (35%)

Table. Follow-up results after cobalt plaque treatment.

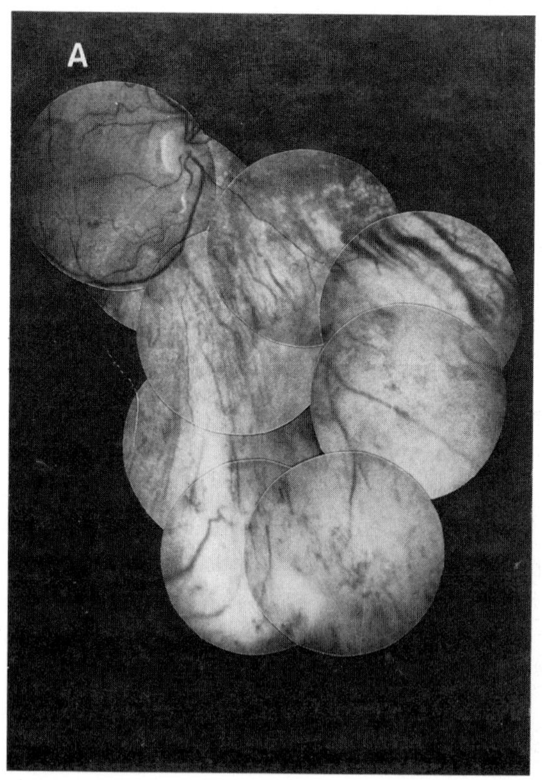

Fig. 1A. Atrophic and unpigmented scar after ^{60}Co treatment of choroidal melanoma.

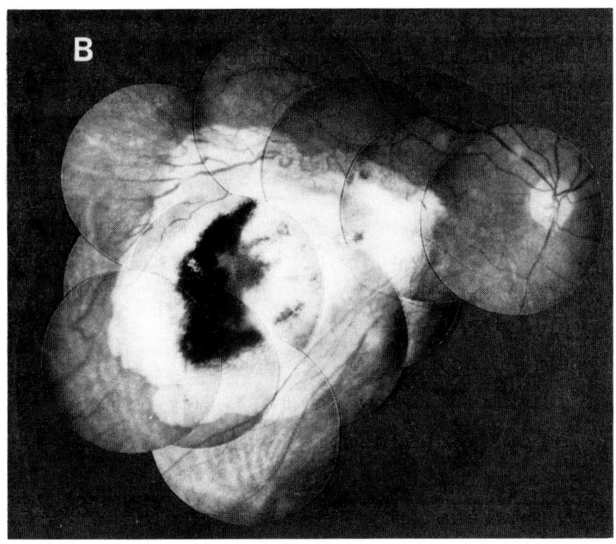

Fig. 1B. Scar with irregular pigmentation after ^{60}Co treatment of choroidal melanoma.

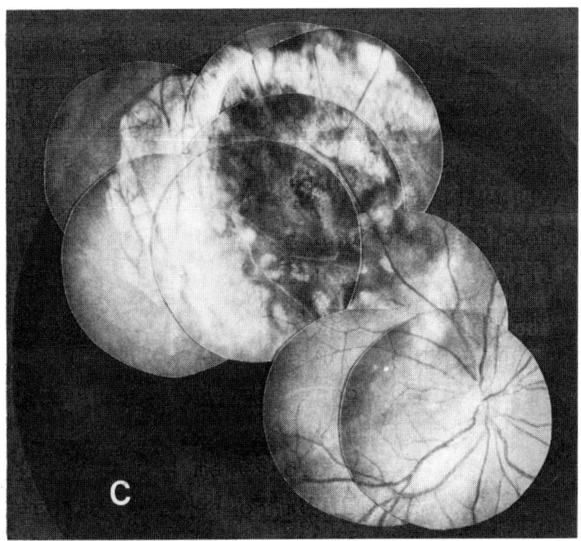

Fig. 1C. Persistent slight elevation of choroidal melanoma in the centre of the atrophic scar after ^{60}Co treatment of the tumour.

The irradiation dose to be used in the treatment of melanomas must be over 9,000 rad at the top of the tumour. The prominence of the tumour is determined by A-ultrasonography. We must be very careful not to exceed an irradiation dose of 20,000 rad on the border of the optic disc adjacent to the tumour. To this purpose precise measurement in disc diameters of the distance between the applicator and the optic disc must be made on photographic slides, to calculate the optimal dose of irradiation. Sometimes we can, by slight decentration of the applicator, avoid administering an irradiation dose which could eventually provoke occlusion of the central retinal artery and vein.

The functional results which we obtained 5 years after treatment in 53 cases are the following. Visual acuity unchanged or higher than the initial visual acuity in 26 cases (49%), decrease of visual acuity in 9 cases (17%), loss of function in 4 cases (7.5%) and enucleation in 14 cases (26.5%).

The various complications which are mainly due to radiotherapy show that the treatment modality is agressive and that it should not be undertaken unless we are certain of the diagnosis. When the diagnosis is not certain it is better to observe the patient and to perform cobalt plaque treatment only when the tumour increases in size.

Tumours likely to respond less favourably to irradiation treatment are those situated very close to the optic nerve and those invading the ciliary body and the root of the iris. For this reason we have recently started to perform surgical excision of these tumours under controlled hypotension as recommended by Professor Foulds of Glasgow. Because of the poor results and the various complications after cobalt plaque treatment in large choroidal melanomas or tumours situated near the posterior pole, we are at present engaged in the development of an accelerated proton beam treatment. This is done in collaboration with the Swiss Centre of Nuclear Research in Villigen.

HAEMATOPORPHYRIN DERIVATIVE PHOTORADIATION OF MALIGNANT MELANOMA IN THE ANTERIOR CHAMBER OF THE RABBIT

J.A. Oosterhuis

This modality of treatment has been studied in cooperation with N.A.P. Franken, J.L. van Delft and D. de Wolff-Rouendaal of the Department of Ophthalmology, Leiden University Medical Centre, T.M.A.R. Dubbelman of the Department of Medical Biochemistry, Medical Faculty of the Leiden University, and W.M. Star and H.P.A. Marijnissen of the Daniel den Hoed Cancer Centre, Rotterdam Therapeutic Institute.

Current therapies for uveal melanoma alternative to enucleation are ionizing radiation, photocoagulation, local resection, and cryotherapy. Photoradiation therapy (PRT) with haematoporphyrin derivative (HpD) may provide a new therapeutic option to the treatment of malignant tumours[1,2]. The dye haematoporphyrin derivative was used as the photosensitizing agent because it preferentially accumulates in tumour tissue[3,4,5,6]. For photoradiation treatment red laser light at 630 nm was used because of its optimal tissue penetration associated with high wavelength[1].

The actual mechanism that causes tumour destruction is not yet clear; tumour cell killing as well as interruption of blood circulation seem to be involved[7,8]. At cellular level deterioration of membrane functions, inhibition of key enzymes, and DNA damage have been observed[9,10]. Singlet oxygen[11] and possibly also superoxide and hydroxyl radicals[12] are the reactive cytotoxic molecules produced during PRT.

Photodynamic destruction by interaction of light and HpD has been demonstrated for various types of malignant tumours in animal models[13,14,15,16].

Oosterhuis, A. (ed.), Ophthalmic tumors.

ISBN 90-6193-528-8. Printed in the Netherlands.

Clinical application of HpD-PRT in humans has been reported for tumours of the bladder, bronchus, lung, eyes, and cutaneous and subcutaneous malignant lesions[17-26]

We have studied the photodynamic action of HpD on melanomas implanted into the anterior chamber of rabbit eyes.

A single piece of tissue of an amelanotic hamster melanoma (Greene's melanoma), measuring about 1 mm^3, was implanted transcorneally onto the iris. After 8 days the tumour had obtained a diameter of about 4-6 mm and was then used for HpD-PRT experiments.

A single intravenous injection of HpD (10 mg/kg body weight) was given. Twenty-four hours later photoradiation therapy was carried out with monochromatic light at 630 $\pm$ 0.5 nm, which was generated by a rhodamine B dye laser, pumped by an argon laser. In all experiments the light irradiance was 60 mW/cm^2, the total light dose was 100 J/cm^2. A diaphragm was used as a mask because determination of porphyrin in tissues had shown that the porphyrin uptake of the iris is 2 to 3 times higher than of the tumour, the uptake of the cornea, lens and vitreous being much lower than of the tumour. In all tissues the porphyrin concentration as well as the porphyrin tumour/iris ratio were found to be highest 24 hours after HpD injection.

Biomicroscopic examination 24 hours after PRT revealed a pale and slightly shrunken tumour in which no vessels were visible any more (fig. 1ab). This aspect remained unchanged throughout the experimental period up to 11 days. The observation period could not be extended because of the development of satellite tumours in the inferior part of the anterior chamber by seeding of tumour cells. The cornea in front of the tumour developed some haziness, which only partly cleared in the subsequent days.

Fluorescein angiography prior to PRT showed a high vascularity of the tumour surface (fig. 2a). Twenty-four hours after PRT fluorescein angiography did not show any sign of circulation in the tumour; non-fluorescent, stagnant

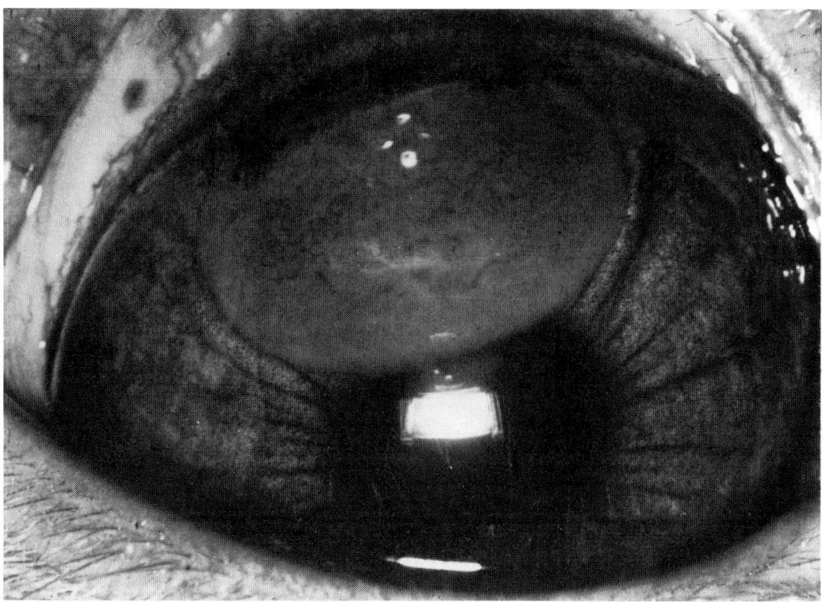

Fig. 1a Anterior chamber of rabbit eye containing a richly vascularised amelanotic Greene hamster melanoma.

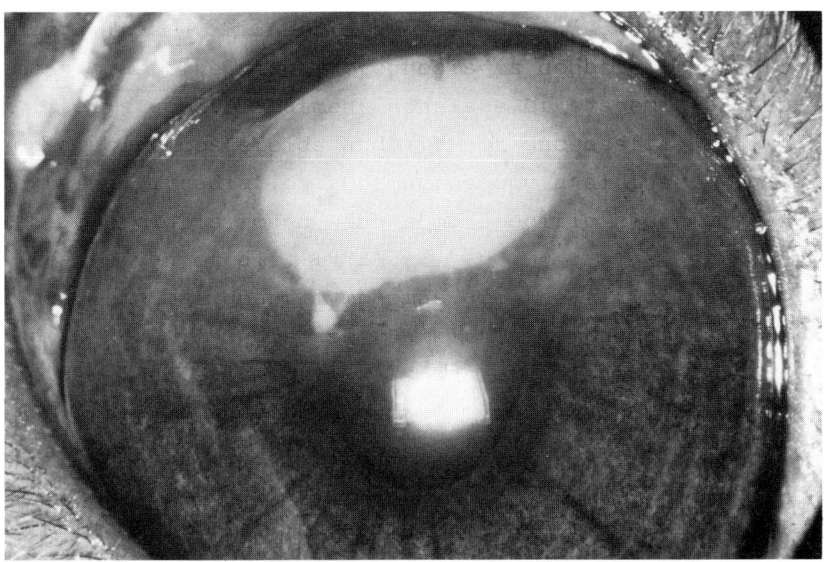

Fig. 1b Same eye one day after haematoporphyrin photoradiation treatment (HpD-PRT). The tumour is pale, slightly shrunken, and tumour vessels are not visible any more.

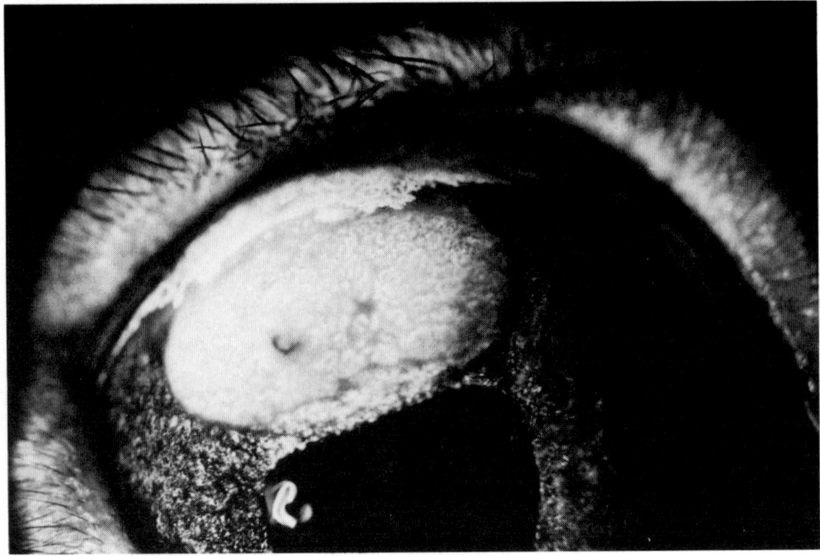

Fig. 2a Fluorescein angiogram of a Greene hamster melanoma implanted onto the iris of a rabbit, showing an intense vascularity of the tumour surface. Note also the dense capillary network of the iris.

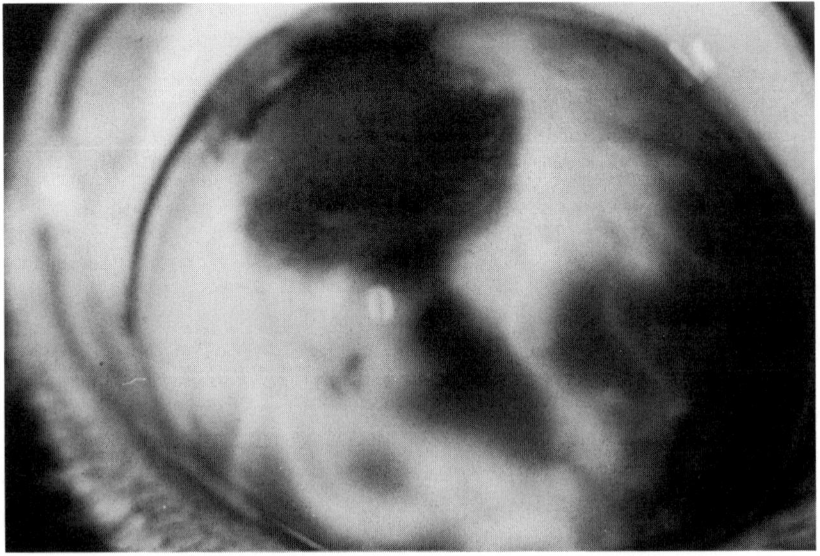

Fig. 2b Fluorescein angiogram one day after HpD-PRT of a Greene hamster melanoma implanted onto the iris of a rabbit, showing non-perfusion of melanoma blood vessels which are visible as black lines. Diffuse fluorescence around the tumour originates from irradiation-damaged iris vessels.

blood showed as black lines (fig. 2b). A diffuse fluorescence around the tumour originated from irradiation-damaged iris vessels.

Histopathologic examination 8 days after implantation onto the iris of the piece of melanoma measuring approximately 1 mm^3 showed that the amelanotic, highly vascularised·tumour had filled a large part of the anterior chamber and had invaded most of the iris tissue in the upper half of the eye; in most eyes the iris pigment epithelium between tumour and lens showed gaps. In only one out of 13 eyes did the HpD-PRT-treated tumour show total necrosis; all others showed only subtotal necrosis.

As early as 24 hours after PRT most of the blood vessels in the necrotic tumour were severely damaged. Vessel walls were disorganised, sometimes with loss of endothelial cells, or had even completely disappeared. Clusters of viable tumour cells were found behind a large haemorrhage or behind iris pigment epithelium, at the tumour periphery, and in some cases also around large blood vessels in the tumour.

The cornea was vascularised and infiltrated by inflammatory cells when tumour touched the cornea or when tumour cells were present in the corneal implantation scar. The aqueous humour contained polynuclear leucocytes and free floating tumour cells. The lens epithelium was damaged and a superficial cataract had developed in the area behind the necrotic tumour except in eyes in which the iris pigment epithelium was not disorganised by the tumour.

In control experiments, consisting of injection of HpD without subsequent irradiation or laser irradiation without previous administration of HpD, no effect on the tumour was observed by either biomicroscopic, fluorescein-angiographic or histopathologic examination.

The photoradiation effect can not be attributed to a rise in temperature as the intratumoral temperature before light exposure was 33.5°C and the rise in temperature during light exposure was only 3°C. In HpD-PRT of the anterior segment of

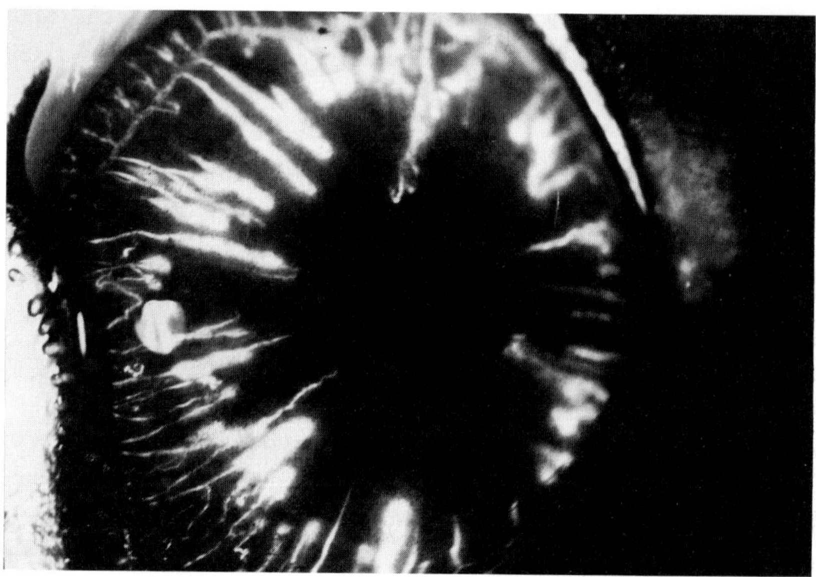

Fig. 3 Fluorescein angiogram 6 months after HpD-PRT of a normal rabbit eye. The capillary bed of the iris is totally occluded; compare with fig. 2a. Only part of the large iris vessels show perfusion and leakage of dye through the damaged vessel wall.

non-tumour-containing eyes the cornea became slightly hazy but recovered within 5 days. Owing to loss of pigment the colour of the iris stroma changed from brown to blue in the course of 15 days and then remained unchanged. The pupil became dilated and did not respond to light any more but recovered to some extent in the course of three months.

Iris fluorescein angiography one hour after PRT showed non-perfusion of the whole capillary bed of the iris and most of the large iris vessels; the vessels that were still perfused leaked profusely. After 6 months some of the larger vessels had reopened but leakage was still present (fig. 3).

Histopathological examination showed extensive atrophy of the iris stroma, thinned iris pigment epithelium, and endothelial cell damage in the few blood vessels that were still present in the deep iris layer.

The parameters, light dose of 100 J/cm^2 delivered and a rather high HpD dose of 10 mg/kg body weight, were chosen to obtain sufficiently evident effects for evaluation of the mechanism of tumour destruction. Penetration of light was sufficient to cause necrosis as far as the base of the tumour; however, clusters of tumour cells that were shielded by iris pigment or by haemorrhage escaped PRT. The survival of cells around blood vessels can not be attributed to insufficient irradiation. Unequal HPD distribution may be caused by the rapid growth rate of the Greene melanoma[15]. Our histopathological finding that tumour necrosis was subtotal in 12 out of 13 eyes is consistent with the high rates of incomplete response to HPD-PRT in clinical oncology[19,20,23,27,28].

HpD-PRT-induced damage to the blood vessels leading to circulatory disorder up to non-perfusion of blood vessels is in agreement with the circulation stop by HPD-PRT of rat tumours in a "sandwich observation chamber"[7] and the impairment of blood flow observed in bladder tumours[8]. HpD-PRT-induced necrosis can partially be explained by a circulation stop. The other mechanism that contributes to tumour response is a direct cytotoxic effect[9,10].

Some factors make intraocular tumours suitable for HpD-PRT: they are small, light can reach them through clear ocular media or sclera, and the laser beam can be targeted to the tumour area. Care has to be taken not to damage the cornea, since we observed transient corneal oedema. Lens proteins can be polymerized by HpD and light[29], which may add to age-related opacification[30]. Lens-epithelial damage and local cataract occurred after HpD-PRT of melanomas, but only if the iris pigment epithelium was disorganised by the tumour. Extreme care must be taken not to irradiate the iris or to damage the retina[31]. The iris accumulates high amounts of HpD, even more than the melanoma; by PRT the iris vascularisation was to a great extent destroyed and the iris became atrophic. HpD-PRT has also been used to destroy newly formed vessels on the iris[32].

Extrapolation of the results to human choroidal melanoma involves uncertainties because the high growth rate of the Greene melanoma with a doubling time of 2 to 3 days[15] differs from the much lower growth rate of the human choroidal melanoma. Other differences are the location and the lack of pigmentation of the experimental melanomas. In a few other studies of Greene's amelanotic melanoma in rabbit eyes tumour necrosis was more pronounced or less so, depending on the HpD and/or light dose, but in most cases it was subtotal[14,15,33].

Two reports have been published on application of HpD-PRT in patients with uveal melanoma[23,24]. Even at high transpupillary light dosis Tse et al.[23] only obtained surface necrosis of the pigmented choroidal melanoma. Bruce[24] obtained a 50% shrinkage in 6 out of 11 rather flat melanomas. However, even in patients with complete clinical tumour resgression, e.g. after xenon arc photocoagulation, recurrences may be observed 10 years after treatment[34].

HpD-PRT is able to induce extensive and immediate tumour necrosis, but in view of the fact that necrosis tends to be subtotal combinations with other ways of treatment have to be explored in order to find a method for total tumour destruction.

References

1. Dougherty, T.J., Kaufman, J.E., Goldfarb, A., Weishaupt, K.R., Boyle, D. and Mittleman, A.: Photoradiation therapy for the treatment of malignant tumors. Cancer Res. 38: 2628-2635, 1978.
2. Dougherty, T.J., Lawrence, G., Kaufman, J.H., Boyle, D., Weishaupt, K.R. and Goldfarb, A.: Photoradiation in the treatment of recurrent breast carcinoma. J.Nat.Cancer Inst. 62: 231-237, 1979.
3. Lipson, R.L., Baldes, E.J. and Olsen, A.M.: The use of a derivative of hematoporphyrin in tumor detection. J.Nat. Cancer Inst. 26: 1-11, 1961.
4. Lipson, R.L., Baldes, E.J. and Gray, M.J.: Hematoporphyrin derivative for detection and management of cancer. Cancer 20: 2255-2257, 1967.
5. Cortese, D.A., Kinsey, J.H., Woolner, L.B., Payne, W.S., Sanderson, D.R. and Fontana, R.S.: Clinical application of a new endoscopic technique for detection of in situ bronchial carcinoma. Mayo Clin.Proc. 54: 635-642, 1979.
6. Gregorie, H.B., Horger, E.O., Ward, J.L., Green, J.F., Richards, T., Robertson Jr., H.C. and Stevenson, T.B.: Hematoporphyrin-derivative fluorescence in malignant neoplasms. Ann.Surg. 167: 820-828, 1968.
7. Star, W.M., Marijnissen, J.P.A., van den Berg-Blok, A.E. and Reinhold, H.S.: Destructive effect of photoradiation on the microcirculation of a rat mammary tumor growing in "sandwich" observation chambers. Clayton Foundation Symp. on Porphyrin Localization and Treatment of Tumors, Santa Barbara, California, 24-28 April, 1983. Alan R. Liss Inc., New York, in press.
8. Selman, S.H., Kreimer-Birnbaum, M.K., Klaunig, J.E., Goldblatt, P.J., Keck, R.W. and Britton, S.L.: Blood flow in transplantable bladder tumors treated with hematoporphyrin derivative and light. Cancer Res. 44: 1924-1927, 1984.
9. Dubbelman, T.M.A.R., van Steveninck, A.L. and van Steveninck, J.: Hematoporphyrin-induced photo-oxidation and photodynamic cross-linking of nucleic acids and their constituents. Biochimica et Biophysica Acta 719: 47-52, 1982.
10. Dubbelman, T.M.A.R. and van Steveninck, J.: Photodynamic effects of hematoporphyrin-derivative on transmembrane transport systems of murine L929 fibroblasts. Biochimica et Biophysica Acta 771: 201-207, 1984.
11. Weishaupt, K.R., Gomer, C.J. and Dougherty, T.J.: Identification of singlet oxygen as the cytotoxic agent in photo-inactivation of a murine tumor. Cancer Res. 36: 2326-2329, 1976.
12. Buettner, G.R. and Oberley, L.W.: The apparent production of superoxide and hydroxyl radicals by hematoporphyrin and light as seen by spin-trapping. FEBS Letters 121: 161-164, 1980.

13. Dougherty, T.J., Grindey, G.B., Fiel, R., Weishaupt, K.R. and Boyle, D.G.: Photoradiation therapy. II. Cure of animal tumors with hematoporphyrin and light. J.Nat. Cancer Inst. 55: 115-121, 1975.
14. Gomer, C.J., Doiron, D.R., White, L., Jester, J.V., Dunn, S., Szirth, B.C., Razum, N.J. and Murphree, A.L.: Hematoporphyrin derivative photoradiation induced damage to normal and tumor tissue of the pigmented rabbit eye. Curr.Eye Res. 3: 229-237, 1984.
15. Sery, T.W. and Dougherty, T.J.: Photoradiation of rabbit ocular malignant melanoma sensitized with hematoporphyrin derivative. Curr.Eye Res. 3: 519-528, 1984.
16. Hayata, Y., Kato, H., Konaka, C., Hayashi, N., Tahara, M., Saito, T. and Ono, J.: Fiberoptic bronchoscopic photoradiation in experimentally induced canine lung cancer. Cancer 51: 50-56, 1983.
17. Benson Jr., R.C., Kinsey, J.H., Cortese, D.A., Farrow, G.M. and Utz, D.C.: Treatment of transitional cell carcinoma of the bladder with hematoporphyrin derivative phototherapy. J.Urol. 130: 1090-1095, 1983.
18. Hisazumi, H., Miyoshi, N., Naito, K. and Misaki, T.: Whole bladder wall photoradiation therapy for carcinoma in situ of the bladder: A preliminary report. J.Urol. 131: 884-887, 1984.
19. Cortese, D.A. and Kinsey, J.H.: Hematoporphyrin derivative phototherapy in the treatment of bronchogenic carcinoma. Chest 86: 8-13, 1984.
20. Hayata, Y., Kato, H., Konaka, C., Amemiya, R., Ono, J., Ogawa, I., Kinoshita, K., Sakai, H. and Takahashi, H.: Photoradiation therapy with hematoporphyrin derivative in early and stage 1 lung cancer. Chest 86: 169-177, 1984.
21. Hayata, Y., Kato, H., Konaka, C., Ono, J. and Takizawa, N.: Hematoporphyrin derivative and laser photoradiation in the treatment of lung cancer. Chest 81: 269-277, 1982.
22. Vincent, R.G., Dougherty, T.J., Rao, U., Boyle, D.G. and Potter, W.R.: Photoradiation therapy in advanced carcinoma of the trachea and bronchus. Chest 85: 29-33, 1984.
23. Tse, D.T., Dutton, J.J., Weingeist, T.A., Hermsen, V.M. and Kersten, R.C.: Hematoporphyrin photoradiation therapy for intraocular and orbital malignant melanoma. Arch. Ophthal. 102: 833-838, 1984.
24. Bruce Jr., R.A.: Photoradiation for choroidal malignant melanoma. In: Porphyrins in Tumor Phototherapy. Eds. Andreoni, A. and Cubeddu, R. Planum Press, New York, 1983, pp 455-461.
25. Zorat, P.L., Corti, L., Tomio, L., Maluta, S., Rigon, A., Mandoliti, G., Jori, G., Reddi, E. and Calzavara, F.: Photoradiation therapy of cancer using hematoporphyrin. Med.Biol.Environnement 11: 511- 516, 1983.
26. Dougherty, T.J.: Photoradiation therapy for cutaneous and subcutaneous malignancies. J.Invest.Dermatol. 77: 122-124, 1981.

27. Dahlman, A., Wile, A.G., Burns, R.G., Mason, G.R., Johnson, F.M. and Berns, M.W.: Laser photoradiation therapy of cancer. Cancer Res. 43: 430-434, 1983.
28. Forbes, I.J., Cowled, P.A., Leong, A.S.Y., Ward, A.D., Black, R.B., Blake, A.J. and Jacka, F.J.: Phototherapy of human tumours using haematoporphyrin derivative. Med.J.Autralia 2: 489-493, 1980.
29. Roberts, J.E.: The photodynamic effect of chlorpromazine, promazine, and hematoporphyrin on lens protein. Invest. Ophthal. Vis.Sci. 25: 746-750, 1984.
30. Best, J.A. van, Tjin A Tsoi, E.W.S.J., Boot, J.P. and Oosterhuis, J.A.: In vivo assessment of lens transmission for blue-green light by autofluorescence measurement. Ophthal.Res., in press.
31. Gomer, C.J., Doiron, D.R., Jester, J.V., Szirth, B.C. and Murphree, A.L.: Hematoporphyrin derivative photoradiation therapy for the treatment of intraocular tumors: Examination of acute normal ocular tissue toxicity. Cancer.Res. 43: 721-727, 1983.
32. Packer, A.J., Tse, D.T., Gu, X.-Q. and Hayreh, S.S.: Hematoporphyrin photoradiation therapy for iris neovascularization. A preliminary report. Arch.Ophthal. 102: 1193-1197, 1984.
33. Liu, L.H.S. and Ni, C.: Hematoporphyrin phototherapy for experimental intraocular malignant melanoma. Arch. Ophthal. 101: 901-903, 1983.
34. François, J.: Treatment of malignant choroidal melanoma by xenon photocoagulation. In: Intraocular Tumors, eds. P. Lommatzsch and F.C. Blodi. Fortschritte der Onkologie, Band 9. Akademie-Verlag, Berlin, 1983, pp 277-285.

DIFFERENTIAL DIAGNOSIS OF NON-PIGMENTED INTRAOCULAR TUMOURS

P.T.V.M. de Jong, G.S. Baarsma and B.C.P. Polak

In this chapter the non-pigmented tumours of iris and ciliary body and the retinoblastomas will be mentioned only briefly as they are discussed in detail elsewhere in this volume. We will discuss the clinical appearance, differential diagnosis, natural course, therapy, and histology of the non-pigmented tumours of the anterior and the posterior segment of the eye.

Cornea and anterior chamber

To our knowledge intraocular tumours originating in the cornea have never been reported. Cysts in the anterior chamber adherent to the cornea generally are of epithelial origin. A cystic diktyoma in the anterior chamber has been reported (Gifford, 1966).

Iris

Non-pigmented tumours in the anterior chamber arising from the iris or the chamber angle have been described as leiomyoma, neurofibroma (Lisch nodules), naevo-xanthoendothelioma or juvenile xanthogranuloma, choristoma (ectopic lacrimal gland tissue) (Gass, 1974), rhabdomyosarcoma, diktyoma, angioma (Gass, 1974), amelanotic iris naevus, metastatic tumour, retinoblastoma, leukaemic infiltrate, and benign lymphoid hyperplasia.

Granulomatous inflammations such as sarcoid, syphilis, tuberculosis, lepra, due to foreign bodies, abscesses, and primary cysts have to be considered in the differential diagnosis.

Oosterhuis, A. (ed.), Ophthalmic tumors.

ISBN 90-6193-528-8. Printed in the Netherlands.

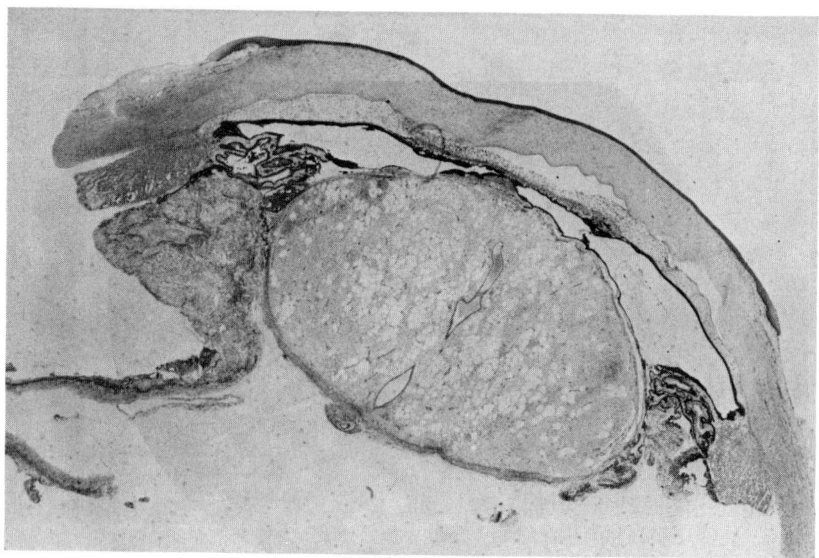

Fig. 1 Pseudophakia lipomatosa. Massive replacement of lens by adipose tissue, covered by wrinkled lens capsule within connective tissue. Thirteen year old boy. Haematoxylin and eosin; 15x. (Courtesy Prof. Manschot).

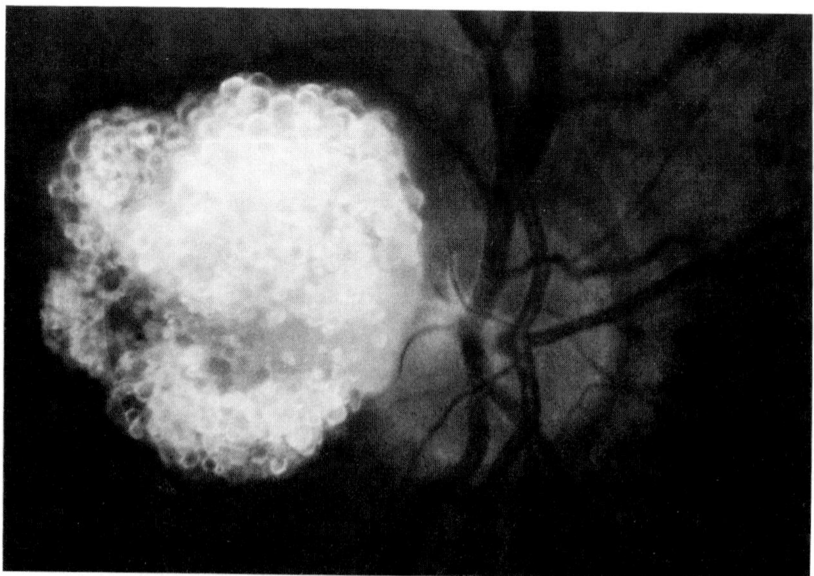

Fig. 2 Astrocytic hamartoma with mulberry appearance in a patient with tuberous sclerosis (fig. 3).

The iris tumours are described in detail by Foulds elsewhere in this volume.

Lens

Primary tumours of the lens are not known.

Ciliary body

Tumours of the non-pigmented epithelium of the ciliary body are usually classified as congenital and acquired tumours (Shields, 1983).

The *congenital* tumours are glioneuroma, non-teratoid medullo-epithelioma or diktyoma, and teratoid medullo-epithelioma or teratoneuroma; the diktyomas and terato-neuromas may be benign or malignant.

The *acquired* tumours are the pseudo-adenomatous hyper-plasia with reactive hyperplasia or senile hyperplasia (Fuchs' adenoma), the adenoma that may be solid, papillary, or pleomorphic, and the adenocarcinoma or malignant epi-ehlioma that has the same subdivision.

The tumours of the ciliary body are described in detail by Foulds elsewhere in this volume.

Vitreous body

Duke-Elder (1969) states that there are no primary tumours in the vitreous. One wonders, however, whether in some cases of persistent hyperplastic primary vitreous (PHPV) one is not justified to talk of primary vitreous tumours when mesenchymal tissue is found that has differentiated into fat tissue, rhabdomyoblasts, cartilage, or brain tissue (fig. 1). It is possible that these tissues are derived from a medullo-epithelioma, which normally grows in the iris or ciliary body at the average age of five years but may also start in the optic disc or retina (Broughton and Zimmerman, 1978). In any case one should keep in mind that PHPV may be concomitant with a medullo-epithelioma that is either benign or malignant. The combination of PHPV with a retinoblastoma has been described in one patient (Morgan and McLean, 1981).

Retina

The non-pigmented retinal tumours are divided into tumours of the neuroretina, those of vascular origin, and pigment-epithelial neoplasms.

Neuroretinal tumours are retinoblastomas, astrocytomas or benign hamartomas, massive gliosis, glioneuromas, and mixed glial tumours. Retinoblastomas and astrocytomas are the most common ones, while the spontaneously involuted or arrested so called retinomas or retinocytomas will be seen less frequently.

In the differential diagnosis of retinoblastoma one should consider metastasis, medullo-epithelioma, pigment-epithelial hamartoma, incontinentia pigmenti; furthermore, Coats' disease, congenital cataract, toxocara, toxoplamosis, coloboma of the choroid, optic disc dysplasia, PHPV, retinopathy of prematurity, dominant exudative vitreo-retinopathy, X-linked congenital retinoschisis with or without vitreous haemorrhage, Norrie's disease, myelinated nerve fibres, metastatic endophthalmitis, herpes or cyto-megalovirus retinitis, bleached vitreous haemorrhage, old perforation, and uveitis must be considered. For a more elaborate discussion on retinoblastoma see the chapter by Tan and Schipper elsewhere in this volume.

The hamartomas, astrocytomas or astrocytic hamartomas are solitary tumours or may appear in association with the autosomal dominantly inherited tuberous sclerosis (Bourne-ville-Pringle) (Fig. 2) or neurofibromatosis (Reckling-hausen). One may see white-yellowish tumours in the retina or on the optic disc, sometimes with a mulberry or spawn appearance due to calcification.

The diagnosis can be difficult if the tumour looks like an amelanotic dome-shaped mass with dilated blood vessels on top of it or if it is small and looks like an ill-defined, transparent thickening of the nerve fibre layer. Astrocytomas mostly originate in the second to third decade. Diagnosis is usually made by ophthalmoscopy or by biomicroscpy. Especially for the small transparent tumours fluorescein angiography is useful, showing hypofluorescence in the arterial phase with a lacework of fine vessels in the venous phase and early leakage.

In the differential diagnosis in young patients retinoblastomas should be considered in the first place. The chalky bodies of retinoblastomas, however, are duller, those of astrocytomas more glistening. Retinoblastomas often have more prominent feeder vessels and show more seeding of tumour cells. The presence of general symptoms of tuberous sclerosis, especially sebaceous adenoma of the facial skin (fig. 3), or neurofibromatosis may help. In older patients one should consider drusen of the optic disc (both drusen and astrocytomas may be accompanied by haemorrhages), aspecific granulomas, myelinated nerve fibres, and amelanotic melanomas. Visual prognosis generally is good and treatment is not necessary except in very rare cases when the tumour shows rapid growth or when an exudative retinal detachment develops. In that case, therapy is the same as for capillary angiomas, which are discussed later.

Histologically one finds an eosinophylic mass in the neuroretina with well-defined fibrous astrocytes with oval or round nuclei and slight eosinophylic cytoplasm.

Massive gliosis is the final stage of many disorders resulting in glaucoma or atrophy of the eye. Clinically the diagnosis is seldom made. The disease is usually unilateral and the fundus often can not be examined, e.g. after trauma, inflammation, congenital anomaly, or secondary glaucoma. In those rare cases where the fundus could be visualised the diagnosis retinoblastoma or

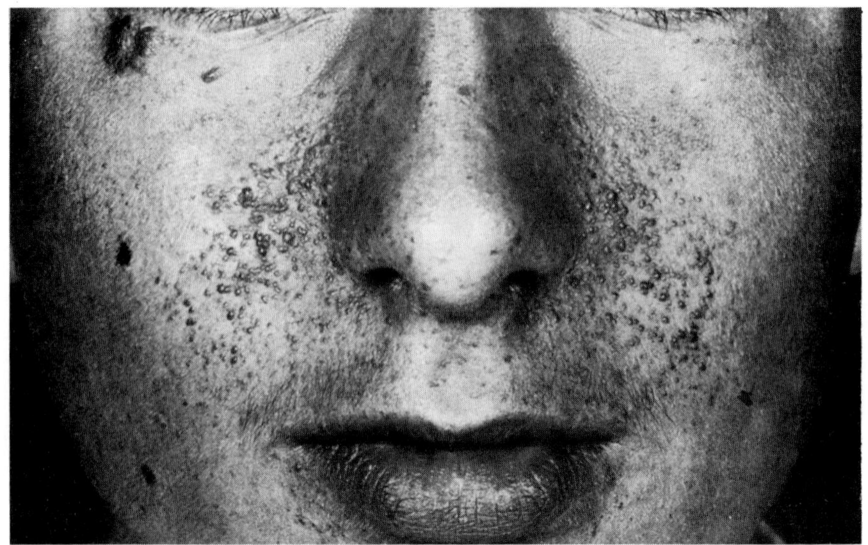

Fig. 3 Adenoma sebaceum of the facial skin in tuberous sclerosis (Bourneville-Pringle).
(Courtesy Prof. Suurmond).

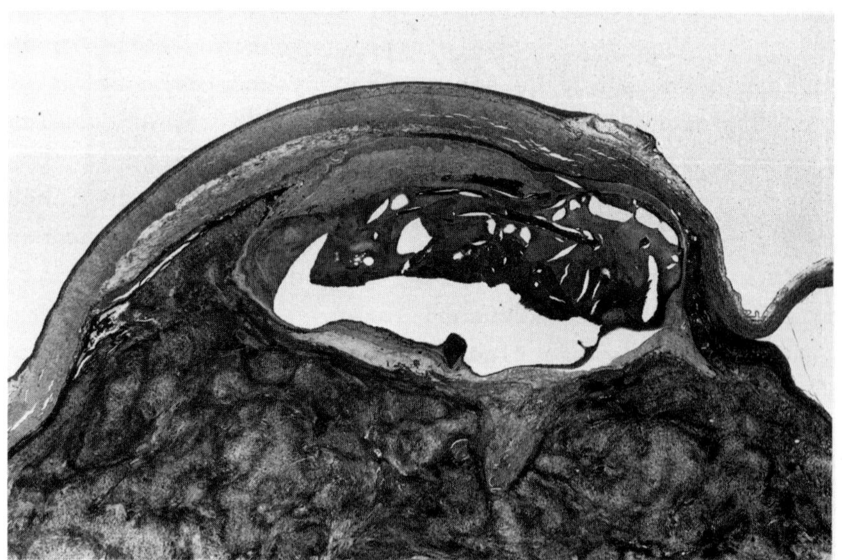

Fig. 4 Massive gliosis (low grade intraocular glioma). Lens dislocated by benign mass of glial cells which fills the eye. Twenty-six year old man; birth weight 1.250 grams. Haematoxylin and eosin; 15x.
(Courtesy Prof. Manschot).

amelanotic melanoma was made. There are no specific diagnostic criteria. Ultrasound examination shows an aspecific intraocular mass with high reflectivity resembling these two tumours; CT scanning does not give additional information. There is no therapy available; pain or suspicion of another tumour may necessitate enucleation.

Histologically the retina is locally thickened and has partly or totally been substituted by glial tissue with abnormal blood vessels (fig. 4). The tumour is benign, non-invasive, and consists of well-differentiated glial cells.

Glioneuroma is a very rare choristomatous, benign tumour mostly discovered in the chamber angle shortly after birth. It arises from the medullary epithelium at the anterior border of the primitive optic cup. Sometimes it is present in the retina. Most eyes are enucleated on suspicion of a retinoblastoma.

Mixed glial tumours are tumours that are not really glial in origin but have a considerable glial component. An example is the capillary haemangioma, which will be discussed below.

Vascular tumours can be divided into two types, viz. the capillary haemangioma (von Hippel) and the cavernous haemangioma. The so-called racemose haemangioma such as the Wyburn-Mason syndrome is an arteriovenous malformation and not really a tumour.

Capillary (haem)angioma (fig. 5abc) starts as a very small, red tumour, hardly bigger than a microaneurysm (fig. 5a). When the tumour grows, arteriovenous fistulas are formed and gradually big, round, pink to red tumours appear with large vessels. If no treatment is applied, a serous retinal detachment develops and mostly at this stage the patient with a capillary angioma becomes aware that something is amiss. Capillary angiomas of the retina may grow from the inner retinal layers into the vitreous

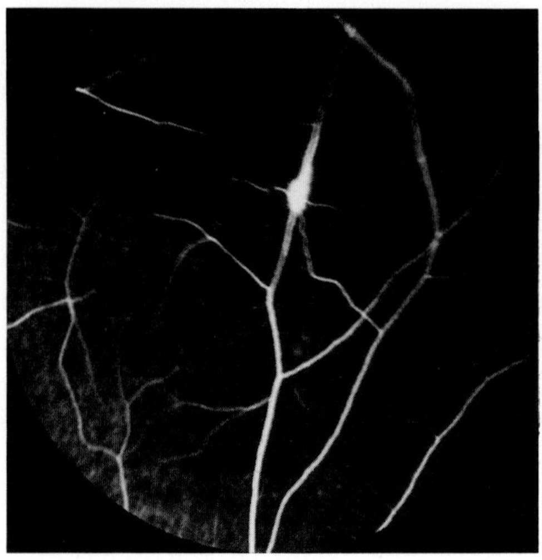

Fig. 5 a. Fluorescein angiogram of smallest capillary haemangioma we have ever seen. On ophthalmoscopy it was hardly visible. Male patient aged 30 years.

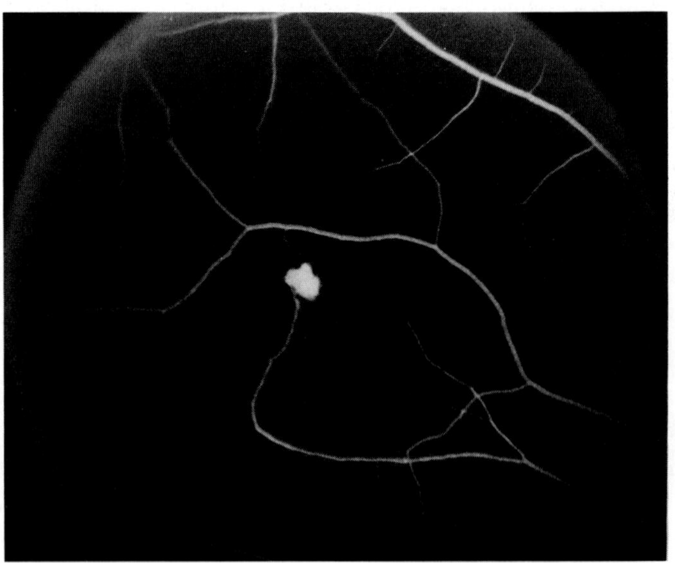

b. Same patient. Slightly bigger haemangioma in the other eye.

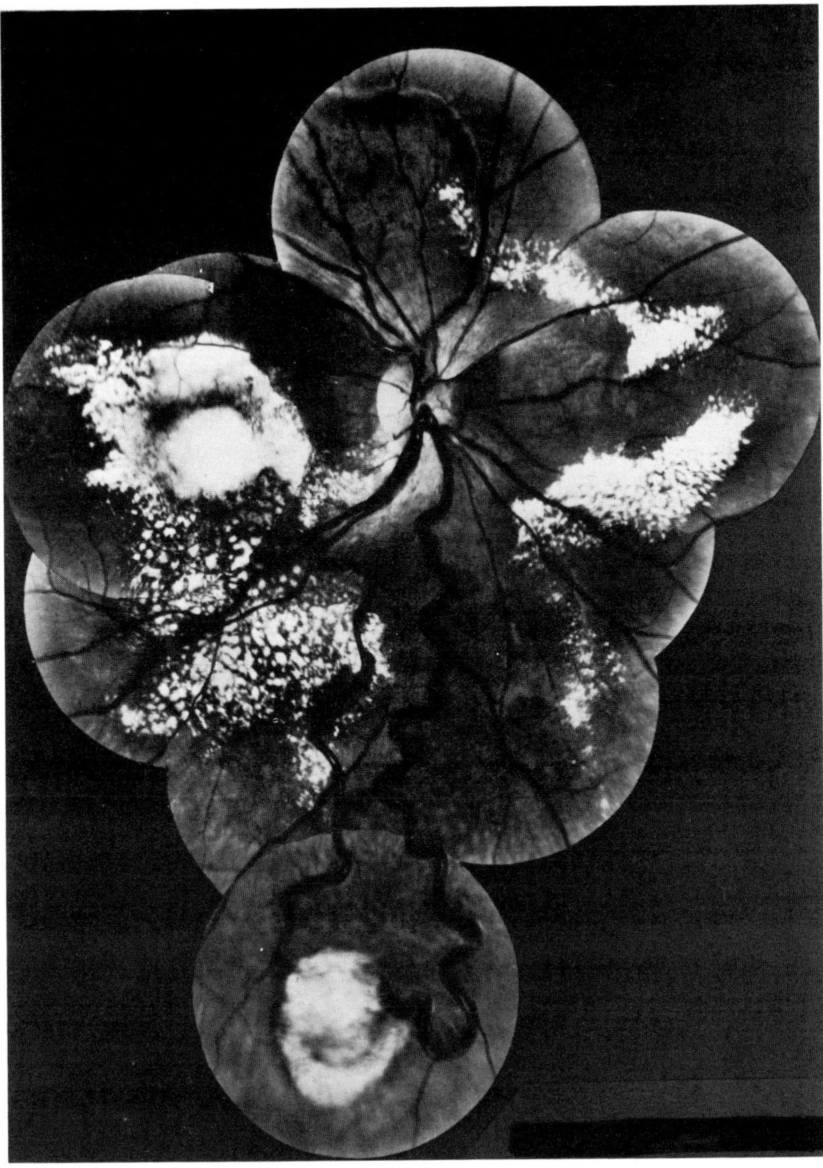

c. Fullgrown capillary haemangioma at 6 o'clock position with secondary peripapillary exudation. Large exudate in the macular area. (Courtesy Dr Riaskoff).

cavity in an endophytical way or they may grow exophytically from the outer retinal layers into the choroid or the optic disc. Recently, a young patient with a bilateral exophytic parapapillary growth has been described (Yimoyines et al., 1982). The haemangioma may be located on and adjacent to the optic disc (fig. 6abcd). One of our patients had an optic atrophy due to an angioma in the intracranial part of the optic nerve. Capillary angioma is transmitted as an autosomal dominant trait. If cysts are present in the cerebellum, spinal cord, kidneys, pancreas, or other organs, it is called von Hippel-Lindau's disease.

Early diagnosis in patients from afflicted families is made primarily with fundoscopy and biomicroscopy for the very small tumours (fig. 5ab). In the differential diagnosis one should consider the arteriovenous malformation of the racemose angioma (fig. 7); this remains stationary and does not show round tumours, hard exudates, retinal detachments, nor does it show leakage on the late angiogram. At a later stage one should exclude Coats' disease (fig. 8), macroaneurysmata, cavernous haemangioma, proliferative retinopathy due to diabetes, hypertension or sickle cell anaemia, and peripheral disciform reactions. Most entities in the differential diagnosis of retinoblastoma are also included in the differential diagnosis of capillary angiomas and the other non-pigmented intraocular tumours. The end stages are massive gliosis, secondary glaucoma, and phthisis bulbi. We have seen two patients with a completely calcified sclera resulting in a stone hard atrophic eye.

Therapeutical results for tumours smaller than 2.5 disc diameters are equally favourable after photocoagulation, cryotherapy, or diathermy. For larger tumours repeated freeze-thaw cryotherapy is advocated, while partial thickness scleral diathermy with a buckling procedure is advised when secondary detachments have developed.

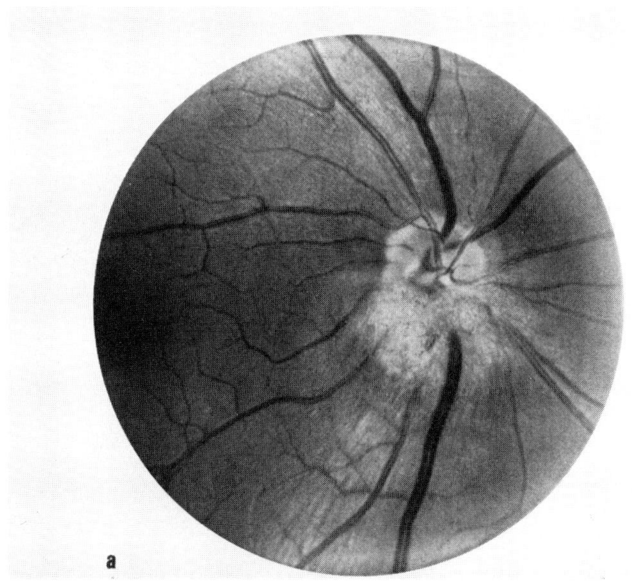

Fig. 6 a. Capillary haemangioma on and adjacent to the inferior half of the optic disc.

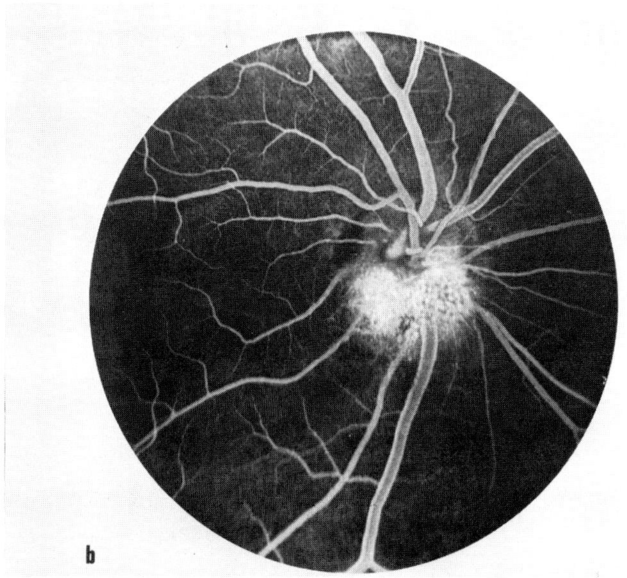

b. Fluorescein angiogram of same fundus, showing dense network of capillaries.

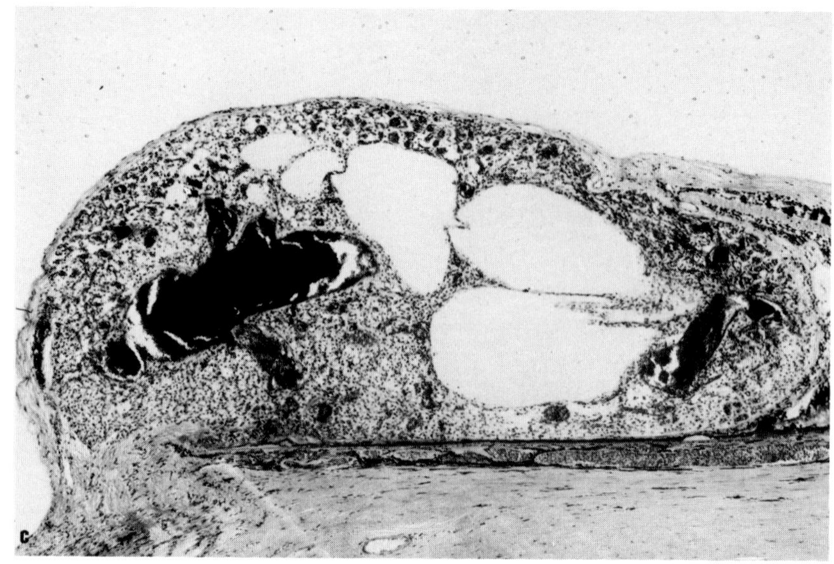

c. Histologic specimen of a juxtapapillary retinal angiomatosis in 76-year old man; haematoxylin and eosin; 60x.
(Courtesy Prof. Manschot).

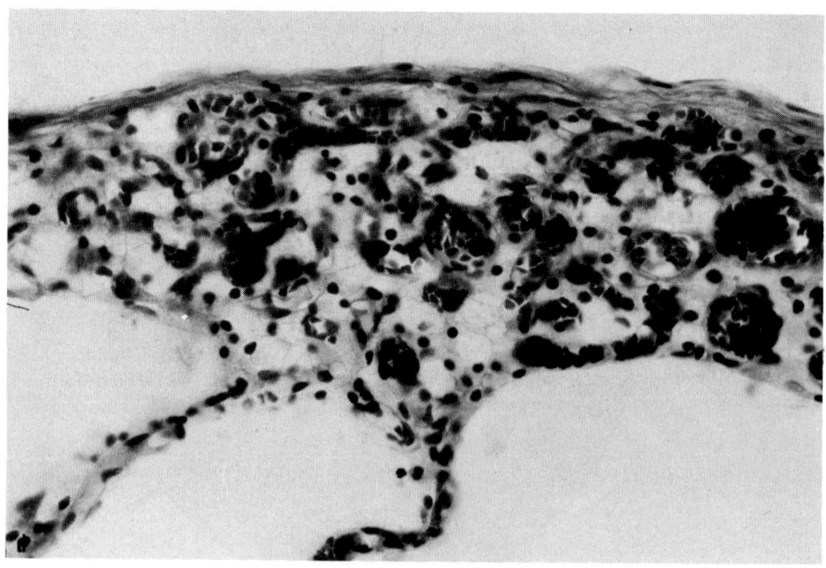

d. Detail of fig. 6c, showing capillary and cavernous spaces; 380x.
(Courtesy Prof. Manschot).

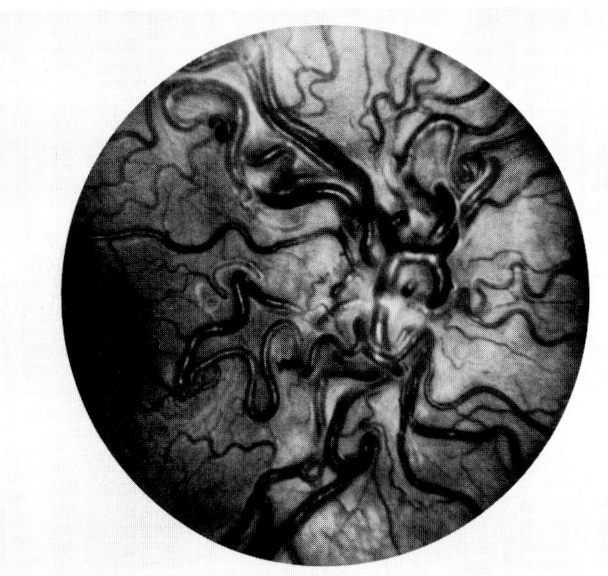

Fig. 7 Fundus aspect of a retinal racemose angioma (Wyburn-Mason syndrome).

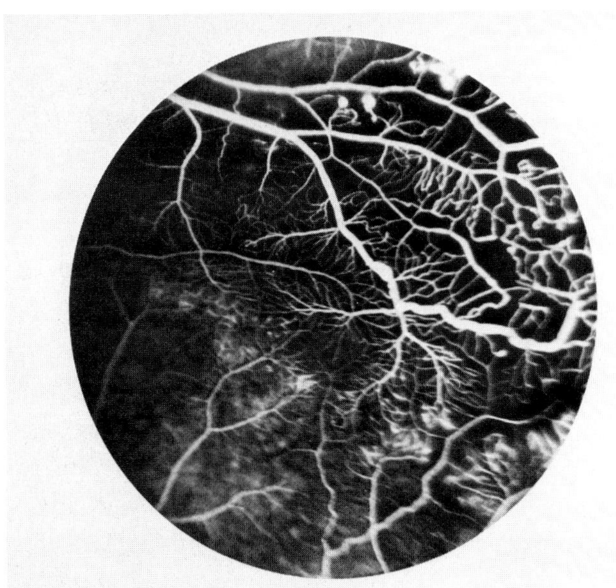

Fig. 8 Typical fluorescence pattern in Coats' disease, showing a coarse capillary pattern and irregular dilatation of the large vessels.

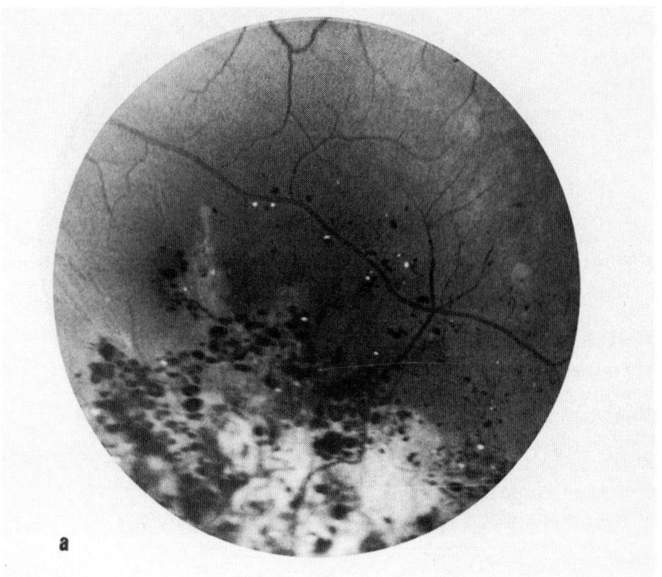

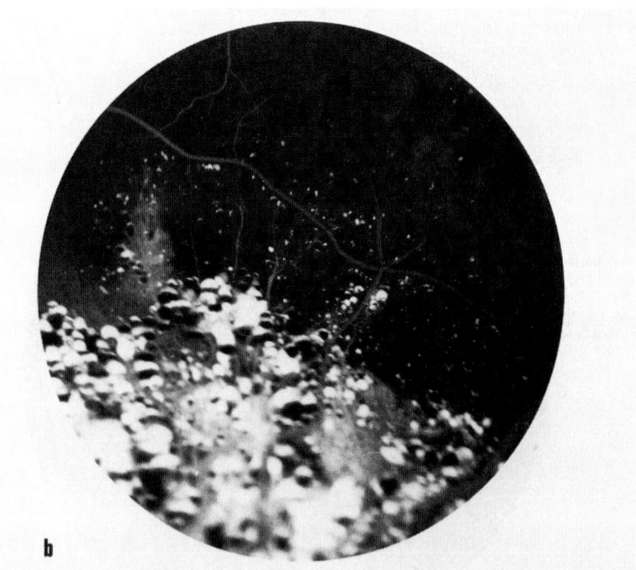

Fig. 9 a. Cavernous haemangioma of the retina with white glial tissue.
b. Late phase fluorescein angiogram of same fundus, showing the fluorescein-blood interfaces in the caverns. (Courtesy Dr Bos).

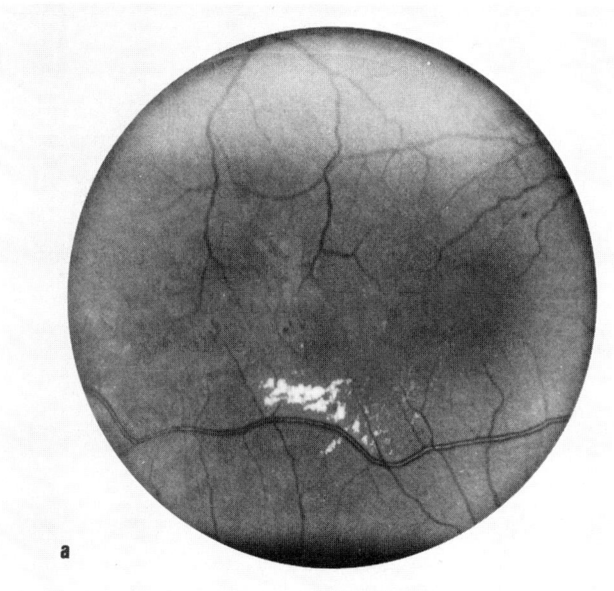

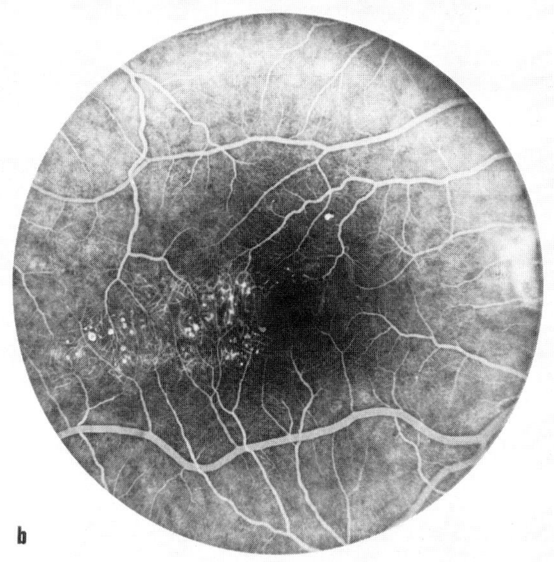

Fig. 10 a. Leber's miliary retinal aneurysms.
b. Fluorescence angiogram of same fundus, showing hyperfluorescent retinal capillaries and microaneurysms temporal to the central avascular zone.

Histology shows normal capillaries with proliferating endothelial cells and pericytes combined with many interstitial glial cells and big vacuoles.

The cavernous (haem)angioma of the retina is most often a coincidental finding in patients with cutaneous haemangiomas. Ophthalmoscopically it resembles clusters of microaneurysms, sometimes covered with glial tissue. It is a non-progressive tumour with an unknown heredity but sometimes familial occurrence. The fluorescein-blood interface in the aneurysms in the late phase fluorogram is the most typical diagnostic tool (fig. 9ab). Differential diagnosis covers Coats' disease (fig. 8), teleangiectasis or Leber's miliary aneurysms (fig. 10ab), macroaneurysms, and the more common retinal diseases with microaneurysms such as diabetes, hypertension, etc. Photocoagulation is hardly ever indicated unless vitreous haemorrhages have developed.

Pigment-epithelial hyperplasia may be jet black but may also be hypopigmented, sometimes with a white rim. It is a non-elevated lesion, often seen on routine ophthalmoscopy, probably congenital, and it does not require treatment.

Pigment-epithelial hamartomas, congenital retino-pigment-epithelial malformations or juxtapapillary hamartomas, are unpigmented or greenish blue or slate coloured, often parapapillary lesions with a non-pigmented apex on the vitreous side and a pigmented base (fig. 11abc). They all show tortuosity of the retinal vessels, sometimes not in accordance with the visible amount of glial membranes on their surface. Usually the lesion will be found unilaterally in healthy, hypermetropic children or teenagers; it is not hereditary, not progressive, and is considered to be a congenital anomaly of the pigment epithelium and the overlying neuroretina. Birth trauma, e.g. a subretinal haemorrhage with resulting periretinal

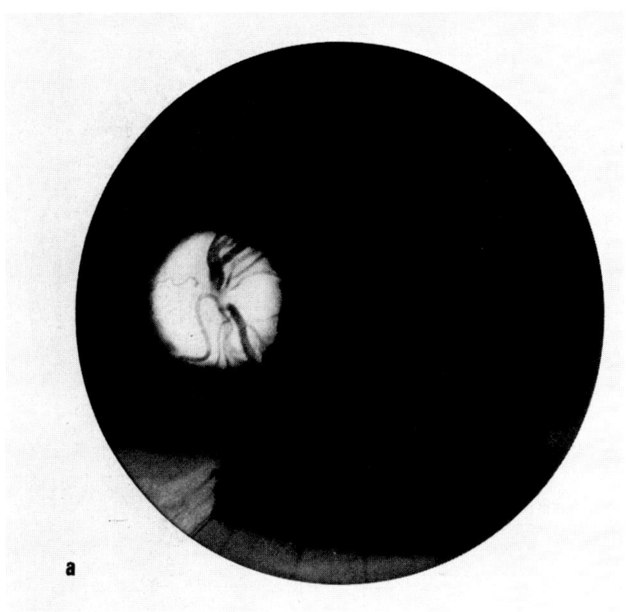

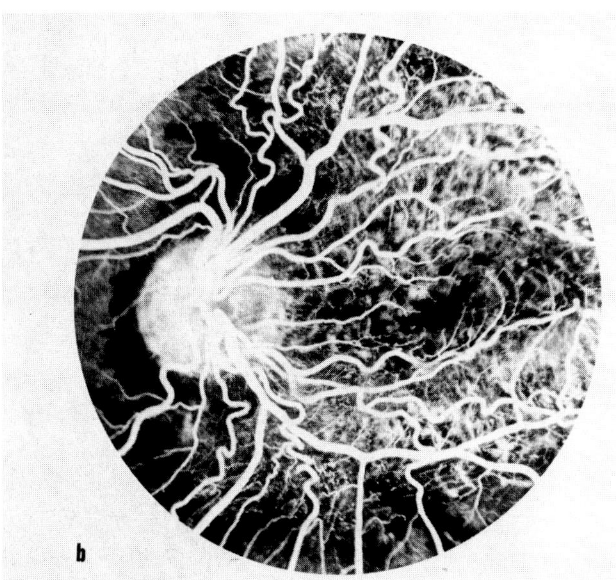

Fig. 11 a. Juxtapapillary pigment-epithelial hamartoma.
b. Typical early fluorescence pattern of same fundus.

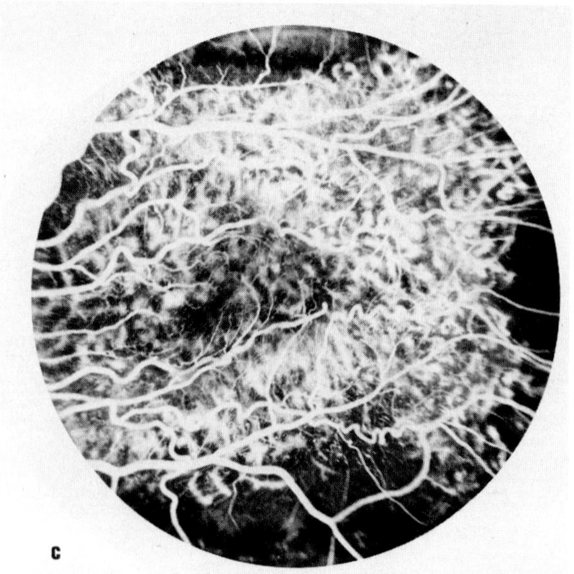

c. Late phase fluorescence pattern of same fundus.

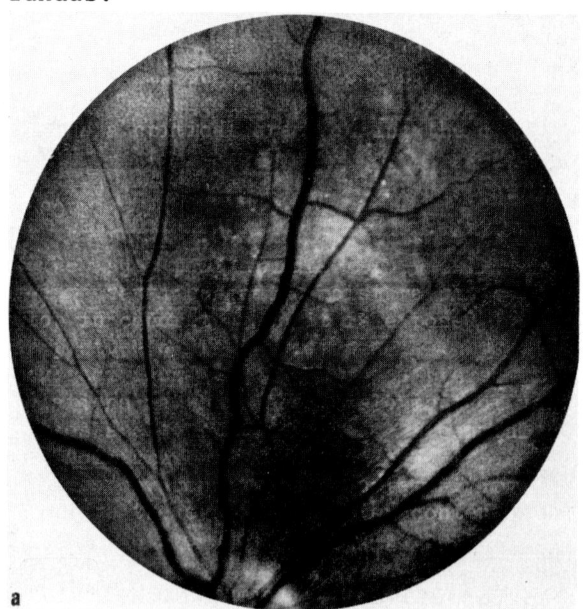

Fig. 12 a. Haemangioma of the choroid.

fibrosis and reactive pigment-epithelial hyperplasia may also be an explanation for this tumour. The differential diagnosis covers preretinal fibrosis with reactive pigment-epithelial hyperplasia, granulomatous tumours, disciform lesions, melanoma, and toxocariasis. The prognosis for the eye is favourable, for the visual acuity, however, it is poor. Treatment is not indicated. The fluorescein angiogram shows a typical picture.

Histologically the top of the lesion is made up by thickened and malformed retina with intraretinal gliosis; the base is formed by hyperpigmented and hypertrophic pigment epithelium. There is no unanimity regarding the histological subdivision of the lesions with respect to the presence or absence of pigment-epithelial cells and strands in the neuroretina (Laqua and Wessing, 1979).

Choroid

Non-pigmented choroidal tumours are the haemangiomas, amelanotic naevi and melanomas, metastases, choristomas, neurilemmomas or schwannomas, reticuloses, and lymphomas.

Choroidal haemangiomas are benign vascular hamartomas; hamartomas are local tumours formed by differentiated cells normally encountered in the same tissue (fig. 12abc). In the choroid there are localised and diffuse haemangiomas, the latter often concomitant with encephalofacial haemangiomas (Sturge-Weber). As a rule, the diffuse haemangiomas are discovered around the age of eight years, the localised ones in the fourth decade (Witschel and Font, 1976). An eye with a diffuse tumour has a much redder fundus reflex than the fellow eye and this makes diagnosis easy. Usually the tumours are discovered on routine control of children with a Sturge-Weber syndrome or by a drop of visual acuity due to a serous detachment or cystoid macular oedema. Localised tumours also present themselves with metamorphopsia or a serous detachment. In those cases differentiation from

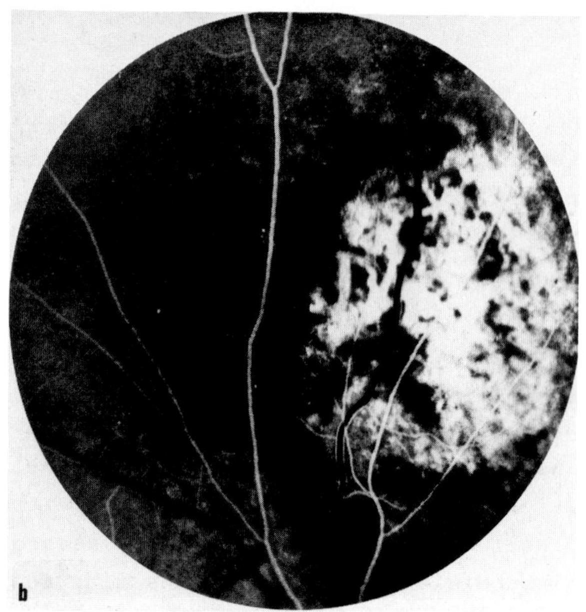

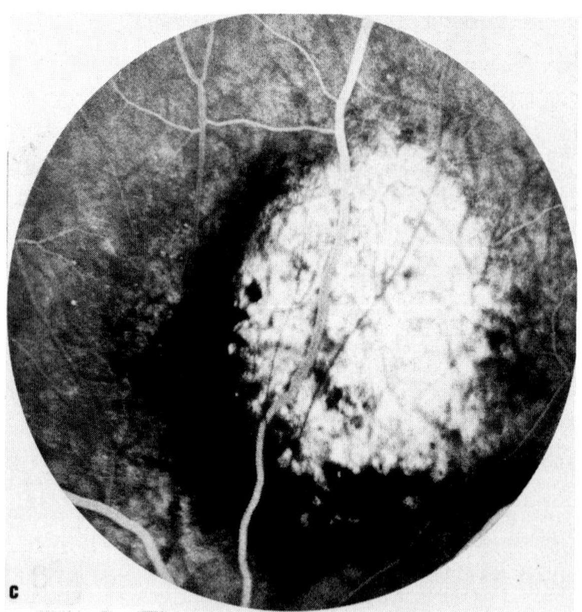

b. Early phase fluorescence angiogram of same haemangioma, showing filling of its vascular structure.
c. Late phase fluorescence angiogram of same haemangioma, showing diffuse intense staining of the tumour; note absence of pigmentation.

melanomas, metastases, choristomas, posterior scleritis, sympathetic uveitis, retinal detachment, Harada's disease, choroidal effusions, central serous chorioretinopathy, and pigment-epithelial detachment may be difficult. This also holds true for granulomatous inflammations, reticuloses, colobomata, and retinoschisis, and sometimes a posterior staphyloma may mimic a tumour on ophthalmoscopy. Haemangiomas are often solitary, pink, poorly demarcated, rather flat, and they may bleach on pressure on the eye (blanching phenomenon). Amelanotic melanomas and metastases, on the other hand, are more yellow, better demarcated, and more elevated. Choroidal metastases of distant tumours are often multifocal or bilateral. Central serous chorioretinopathy or pigment-epithelial detachments have a typical fluorescein angiographic pattern. Ultrasonography can help to differentiate between haemangioma (high reflectivity), melanoma (choroidal excavation), and choristoma (high reflectivity with shadowing), and P32 is useful to differentiate between the first and the second.

Treatment with photocoagulation is only indicated in case of an exudative detachment. The aim should be not to eradicate the tumour but to create a chorioretinal scar on the tumour large enough to keep the retina attached and to serve as a barrier against penetration of the subretinal fluid. At this moment argon laser treatment seems to be the best modality. In case of a big retinal detachment one should try to exchange the subretinal fluid with intravitreal Ringer's solution or air and to perform photo- or cyrocoagulation (Sanborn et al., 1982).

On histological examination the solitary haemangiomas are most often of the cavernous type, whereas the diffuse ones usually have a mixed cavernous-capillary appearance. Pure capillary choroidal haemangiomas are very rare.

For the diagnosis of unpigmented naevi and melanomas see the chapter on pigmented intraocular tumours in this volume.

Metastatic tumours of the choroid are usually not diagnosed until the patient has visual complaints. In 80% of the females breast carcinoma is the primary tumour; in the males lung carcinoma accounts for 30%, unknown tumours for 28% and skin carcinoma for 17%. The metastases are often multifocal and bilateral, and usually grow faster than haemangiomas or melanomas. The differential diagnosis has been discussed under the heading of choroidal haemangiomas. In 75% a serous detachment develops. When no primary tumour is known or found, one can perform external irradiation with 3000 Rad to assess the diagnosis ex juvantibus if the tumour regresses afterwards. P32 examination can only differentiate metastases from benign tumours, not from malignant ones. In very difficult cases one may consider needle biopsy.

Therapy is indicated when visual symptoms arise, and will consist of external irradiation. Enucleation is only indicated in case of severe pain due to secondary glaucoma or if one can not differentiate between metastasis and a malignant primary tumour. Diagnostic enucleation to find the nature of the primary tumour is not advocated as the location of the primary tumour is rarely identified histologically.

Choristomas are tumours of ectopic tissues. In the eye there are five types of choristomas, viz. limbal dermoid, glioneuroma of the anterior chamber angle, iris choristoma with lacrimal gland tissue, PHPV with ectopic tissue, and choroidal choristoma with osseous tissue. The latter is a benign tumour, often encountered unilaterally in young women. Its colour is orange-yellow with brown pigment clumps due to pigment-epithelial proliferation; its borders are sharply demarcated and slow progression over the years has been documented. Differential diagnosis covers organised subretinal haemorrhages, amelanotic naevi or melanomas, metastases, and choroidal haemangiomas. Choroidal choristoma has been described after trauma, posterior scleritis (Trimble and Schatz, 1983) and an unknown fatal disease with eosinophylic granuloma (Kline et al., 1982). Diagnosis is easy because of the reflectivity and density of the osseous tissue on ultrasonography and CT scan. Therapy is not advocated unless subretinal neovascular membranes or serous detachments make photocoagulation necessary. Histology shows well differentiated osseous tissue in the choroid.

Neurilemmomas or *schwannomas* are not easily differentiated from amelanotic melanomas or solitary dome-shaped astrocytomas on examination. The only way of differentiation would be a needle biopsy, which has its drawbacks (Shields et al., 1981).

Non-pigmented choroidal *reticuloses* may be benign or malignant. The benign reactive lymphoid hyperplasia is usually encountered unilaterally around the age of 55 due to complaints of visual loss. On ophthalmoscopy an amelanotic choroidal tumour with serous detachment is often found. From time to time a salmon-pink mass is found in the conjunctiva and the diagnosis can be made from a biopsy. Further signs are elevated intraocular pressure, retinal detachments, and iridocyclitis. For the differential diagnosis see choroidal haemangiomas. The visual prognosis is doubtful, the prognosis for life is good. Treatment consists of systemic or subtenonial corticosteroids and, if not successful, a low dose of external irradiation. On macroscopy a diffuse thickening of the choroid is found with some specific histological features (Ryan et al., 1972).

Among the malignant *lymphomas* are the reticulum cell sarcoma, Hodgkin's disease, Burkitt's lymphoma, and mycosis fungoides. Reticulum cell sarcomas often show keratitic precipitates, a varying amount of vitreous cells, or subretinal white tumours. Diagnosis is often made by a vitreous biopsy. The differential diagnosis covers panuveitis, disseminated choroiditis, leukaemia, amelanotic naevi or melanomas, haemangiomas, and benign lymphoid reactive hyperplasia. Treatment consists of external irradiation with 1500 to 3000 Rad. Leukaemias become manifest by vascular sheathing, nerve fibre infarcts, venous engorgement, haemorrhages, and Roth's spots. Also yellowish retinal or choroidal infiltrates may be seen. Often the diagnosis is already known from systemic signs. In case of doubt the differentiation between mycotic endophthalmitis, viral retinitis, and leukaemia can be made by vitreous biopsy.

Optic disc

Most non-pigmented tumours have already been discussed. Capillary and cavernous haemangiomas of the optic disc show the same characteristics as the retinal ones. The arterio-venous malformations or racemose haemangiomas always extend from the disc; they have been mentioned with the retinal vascular tumours. The differential diagnosis with astro-cytoma covers retinoblastoma and drusen of the optic disc. All three may reveal deep parapapillary haemorrhages. Myelinated nerve fibres may resemble beginning astrocytomas or retinoblastomas. The combined pigment-epithelial hamarto-ma has also been discussed. A juvenile xanthogranuloma of the optic disc, retina and choroid has been described (Wertz et al., 1982). Parapapillary amelanotic melanoma may resemble an optic disc tumour. Metastases, reticulum cell sarcoma, and leukaemias may arise in the optic disc. From the optic nerve astrocytomas and meningiomas may grow into the optic disc. The differential diagnosis in these cases consists of morning glory disc, coloboma, and granulomatous inflammation.

Sclera

No primary scleral tumours are known.

Acknowledgements

We would like to thank Messrs. D. de Bruijn, B.C.P. Smit, and C. van Oostende for photographic help, and Mrs. C.H.M. Muijlwijk-Planting for bibliographical and secretarial assistance.

References

Broughton, W.L., and Zimmerman, L.E.: A clinicopathologic study of 56 cases of intraocular medulloepitheliomas. Amer.J.Ophthal. 85: 407-418, 1978.

Duke-Elder, S.: System of Ophthalmology, vol. XI. Kimpton, London, 1969, p. 334.

Gass, J.D.M.: Differential Diagnosis of Intraocular Tumors. A Stereoscopic Presentation. Mosby, St. Louis, 1974, pp. 358-359.

Gifford, H.: A cystic diktyoma. Survey Ophthal. 11: 557-561, 1966.

Kline, L.B., Skalka, H.W., Davidson, J.D. and Wilmes, F.J.: Bilateral choroidal osteomas associated with fatal systemic illness. Amer.J.Ophthal. 93: 192-197, 1982.

Laqua, H. and Wessing, A.G.: Congenital retino-pigment epithelial malformation, previously described as hamartoma. Amer.J.Ophthal. 87: 34-42, 1979.

Morgan, K.S. and McLean, I.W.: Retinoblastoma and persistent hyperplastic vitreous occurring in the same patient. Ophthalmology 88: 1087-1091, 1981.

Ryan, S.J., Zimmerman, L.E. and King, F.M.: Reactive lymphoid hyperplasia: an unusual form of intraocular pseudotumor. Trans.Amer.Acad.Ophthal.Otolaryngol. 76: 652-671, 1972.

Sanborn, G.E., Augsburger, J.J. and Shields, J.A.: Treatment of circumscribed choroidal hemangiomas. Ophthalmology 89: 1374-1380, 1982.

Shields, J.A.: Diagnosis and Management of Intraocular Tumors. Mosby, St. Louis, 1983.

Shields, J.A., Sanborn, G.E., Kurz, G.H. and Augsburger, J.J.: Benign peripheral nerve tumor of the choroid. A clinico-pathologic correlation and review of the literature. Ophthalmology 88: 1322-1329, 1981.

Trimble, S.N. and Schatz, H.: Choroidal osteoma after intraocular inflammation. Amer.J.Ophthal. 96: 759-764, 1983.

Wertz, F.D., Zimmerman, L.E., McKeown, C.A., Croxatto, J.O., Whitmore, P.V. and LaPiana F.G.: Juvenile xanthogranuloma of the optic nerve, disc, retina, and choroid. Ophthalmology 89: 1331-1335, 1982.

Witschel, H. and Font, R.L.: Haemangioma of the choroid. A clinicopathologic study of 71 cases and a review of the literature. Survey Ophthal. 20: 415-431, 1976.

Yimoyines, D.J., Topilow, H.W., Abedin, S. and McMeel, J.W.: Bilateral peripapillary exophytic retinal hemangioblastomas. Ophthalmology 89: 1388-1392, 1982.

DIFFERENTIAL DIAGNOSIS OF PIGMENTED INTRAOCULAR TUMOURS

P.T.V.M. de Jong, J.A. Oosterhuis and P.J. Ringens

In this chapter we give an "overview" of pigmented intraocular tumours of the anterior and posterior segment of the eye.

Anterior chamber and iris

Pigmented tumours in the anterior chamber originate in most cases from the iris or the ciliary body. They are discussed by Foulds elswhere in this volume. They may be naevi, melanomas, melanocytomas, iris cysts, flocculi, metastases from cutaneous melanomas, iris adenomas, epithelial cysts, and foreign bodies. Iris melanocytoma, heterochromia, siderosis and iris naevus syndrome may simulate diffuse melanoma.

Ciliary body

Pigmented ciliary body tumours are also discussed by Foulds in this volume. Here we only mention naevi, malignant melanomas, sometimes ringshaped, melanocytomas, adenomas, adenocarcinomas, and solid or cystic hyperplasia (Goder, (1983).

Vitreous

Pigmented tumours in the vitreous are of uveal origin and will be described under that heading.

Retina

Lesions due to congenital hypertrophy of the retinal pigment epithelium are usually found on routine ophthalmoscopy, as they do not cause complaints. They are sharply

Oosterhuis, A. (ed.), Ophthalmic tumors.

ISBN 90-6193-528-8. Printed in the Netherlands.

demarcated, completely flat, jet black to mottled gray, often with more or less round focal areas of depigmentation; they may be surrounded by a small, light halo of hypopigmentation (fig. 1). Congenital hypertrophy is benign and treatment is not indicated. Sometimes the lesions occur in patches; they are then called congenital grouped pigmentations or, because of their configuration, "bear tracks" (fig. 2).

Reactive hyperplasia is a phenomenon familiar to most ophthalmologists who perform photocoagulation or cryo treatment. It may occur in any kind of inflammation or trauma. The "high water marks" in longstanding retinal detachment are an example of reactive hyperplasia.

The hamartoma of the retina and retinal pigment epithelium has a varying amount of pigmentation; it is discussed in the chapter on non-pigmented intraocular tumours in this volume.

Pigment-epithelial adenomas and carcinomas are very rare. They are jet black, sharply demarcated and slightly elevated, sometimes they show vitreous seeding of tumour cells, and they mostly occur in coloured people.

Choroid

Naevi, benign melanocytic tumours, of the choroid are present in six per cent of the population. Ninety per cent of them are located behind the equator. Most of them have a diffuse, slate gray appearance of an evenly distributed pigmentation and are not or hardly elevated. Slight metabolic disturbance due to the presence of melanocytic cells induces the development of drusen overlying Bruch's membrane in more than half of the naevi (fig. 3). The degree of pigmentation may vary considerably; most naevi show a hyperpigmentation but sometimes a partly hypopigmented naevus is seen, in which localized drusen outside the area of hyperpigmentation is the only indication of the hypopigmented naevus area (fig. 4ab). Incidentally one may even observe a

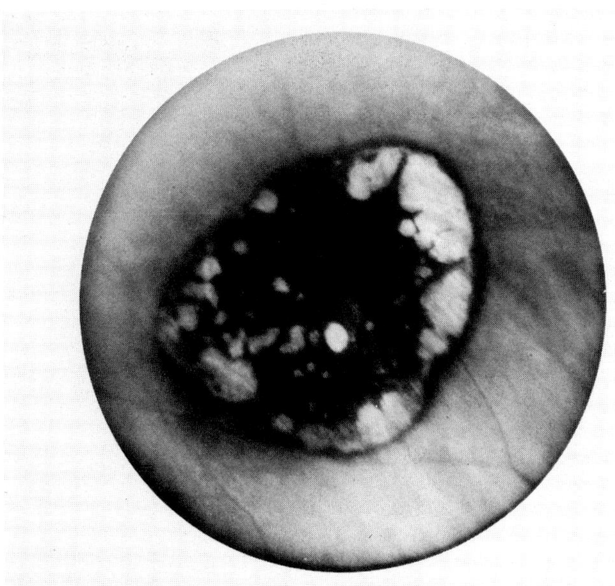

Fig. 1 Fundus aspect of a congenital hypertrophy of the retinal pigment epithelium.

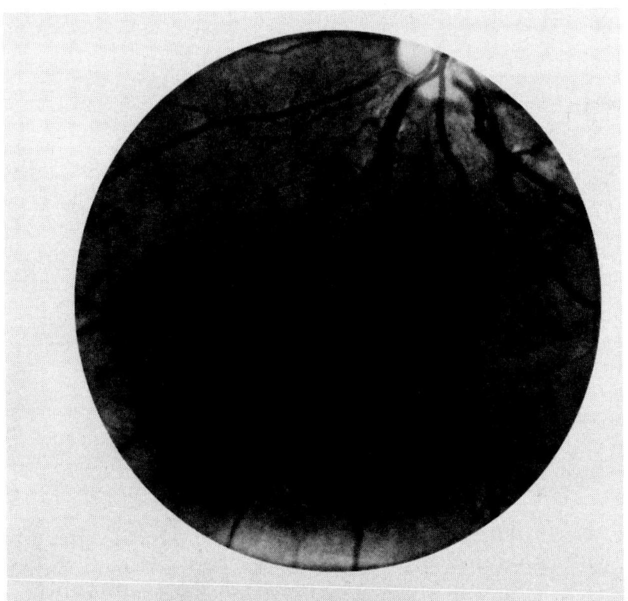

Fig. 2 Grouped pigmentations, "bear tracks", of the retinal pigment epithelium.

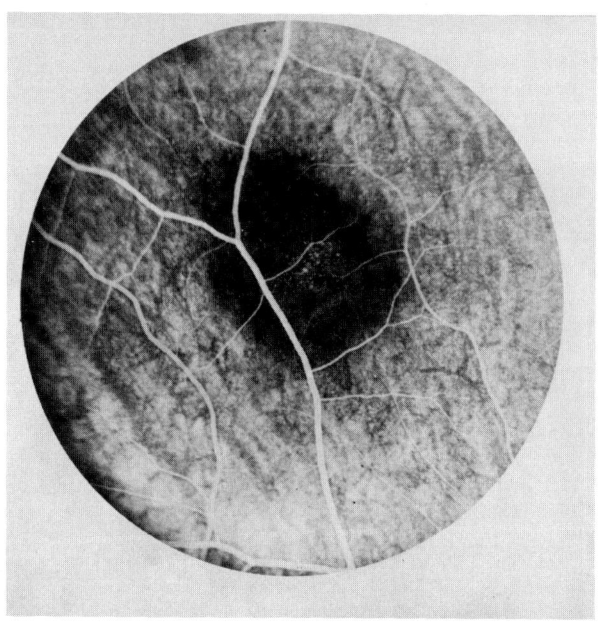

Fig. 3 Fluorescence angiogram of choroidal naevus with drusen of Bruch's membrane; naevus pigment blocks choroidal fluorescence.

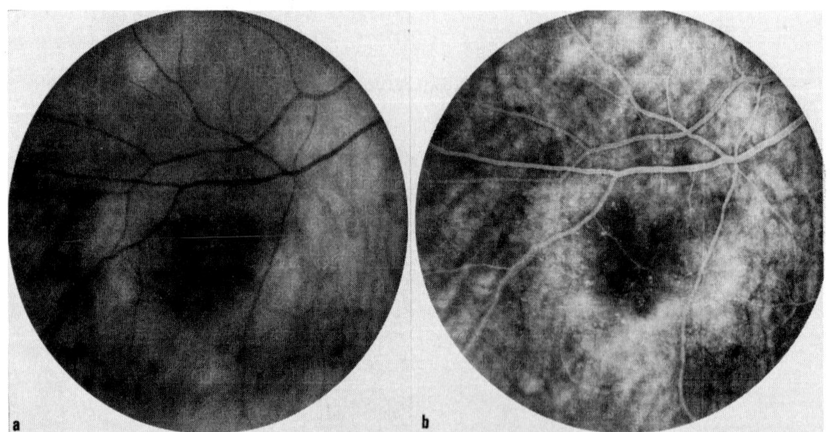

Fig. 4 a. Choroidal naevus with hyperpigmented centre surrounded by hypopigmented zone.
b. Fluorescence angiogram of same naevus, showing hypofluorescent centre and hyperfluorescent periphery; in both areas drusen of Bruch's membrane are present.

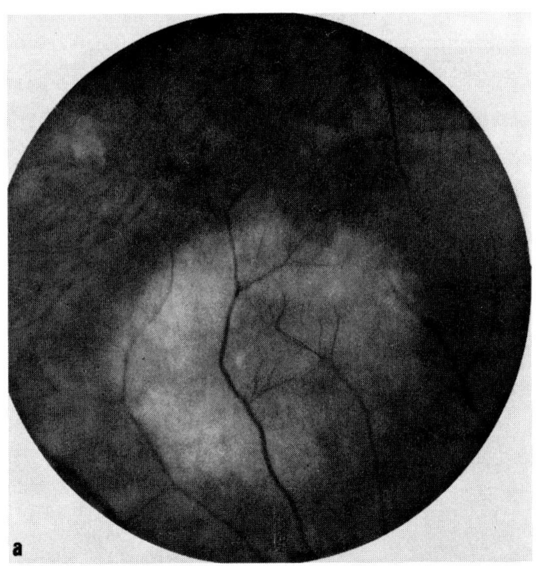

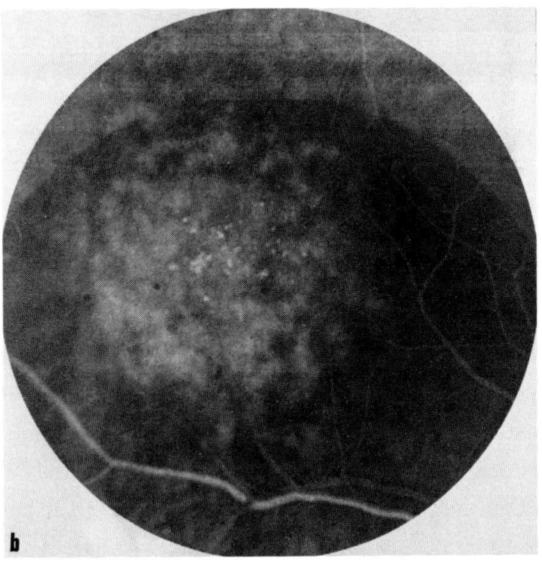

Fig. 5 a. Diffusely hypopigmented choroidal naevus.
b. Fluorescence angiogram of same fundus, showing hyperfluorescence in the naevus area; drusen of Bruch's membrane are present.

totally hypopigmented naevus (fig. 5ab) (Oosterhuis and von Winning, 1979). Focal leakage through the damaged pigment epithelium may lead to subretinal pooling of fluid and retinal oedema (fig. 6). In these cases the ophthalmoscopic aspect may be indistinguishable from that of a malignant melanoma of the choroid. The way to differentiate between naevi and small melanomas is described by Oosterhuis and de Wolff-Rouendaal elsewhere in this volume. In the differential diagnosis of small pigmented tumours also subretinal haemorrhages, reactive hyperplasia and congenital hypertrophy of the retinal pigment epithelium are to be considered. In the vicinity of the optic disc a melanocytoma may be present, which however, as a rule, is jet black and not slate gray (fig. 7ab).

Malignant melanoma of the choroid may or may not be pigmented but usually it is unilateral; in literature only a few bilateral cases have been mentioned (Oosterhuis et al., 1982). It is rather rare in coloured people. Rather small and flat tumours located at the posterior pole are found owing to early visual complaints. Peripherally located tumours may become large before being noticed by the patient. Malignant melanoma can grow in a diffuse or a nodular way, and in a mushroom shape when it ruptures through Bruch's membrane. In the latter case the tumour is usually surrounded by an exudative detachment. We have seen patients, however, with a rhegmatogenous detachment who also had a malignant melanoma. On top of the melanoma orange pigment or lipofuscine is often seen and around the base clumps of pigment, "taches noirâtres", are a common finding.

The diagnosis can usually be firmly established by the presence of visual complaints, ophthalmoscopic and biomicroscopic examination, ultrasonography, fluorescein angiography and visual field examination. With these diagnostic modalities the incidence of misdiagnosis, which formerly has been up to 20%, could be reduced to as low as 1.7% (Davidorf et al., 1983). Only exceptionally, mainly in very small tumours, is a P32-uptake test required for confirmation

Percentual distribution of conditions simulating melanoma of the choroid (Shields et al., 1980)

		per cent
choroidal naevus	suspicious	26.5
	non-suspicious	1.75
exudative haemorrhagic chorioretinopathy (disciform degeneration)	central	12.5
	peripheral	11
congenital pigment-epithelial hypertrophy		9.5
choroidal haemangioma		8
retinal pigment-epithelial reactive hyperplasia		6
melanocytoma of optic nerve		3
choroidal detachment		3
haemorrhagic pigment-epithelial or sensory retinal detachment		2.75
vitreous haemorrhage		2.75
rhegmatogenous retinal detachment		2.5
posterior scleritis		1.5
metastatic carcinoma		1.25
miscellaneous		11
		100

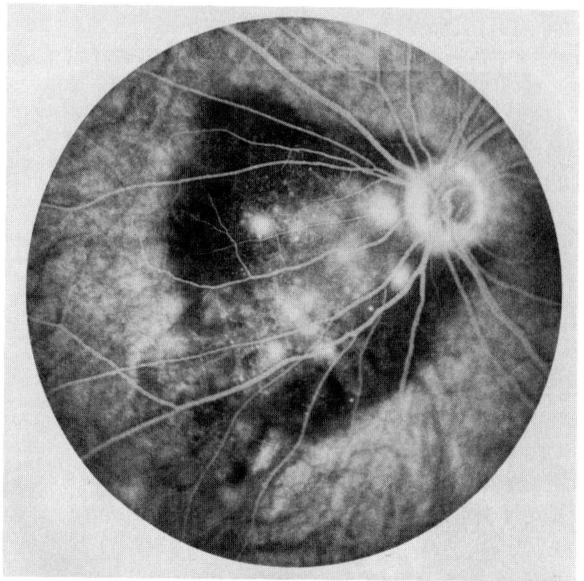

Fig. 6 Fluorescence angiogram of a choroidal naevus, showing multifocal leakage of dye through the pigment epithelium.

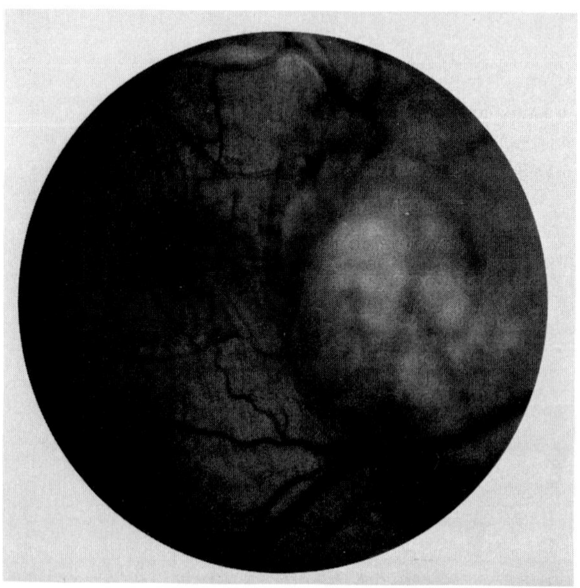

Fig. 8 Choroidal melanoma covering the optic disc, simulating an optic disc tumour.

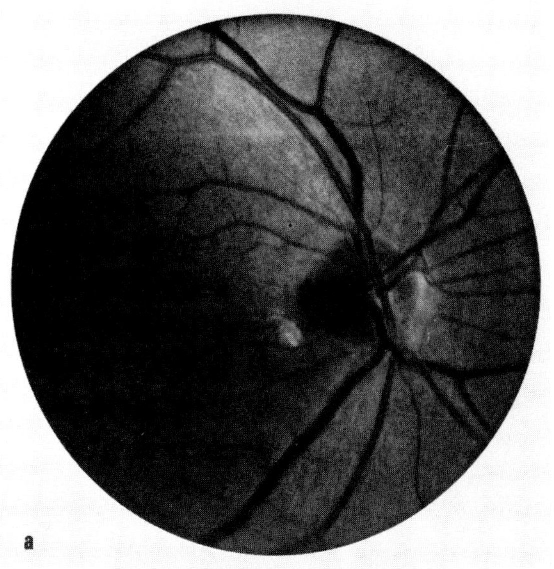

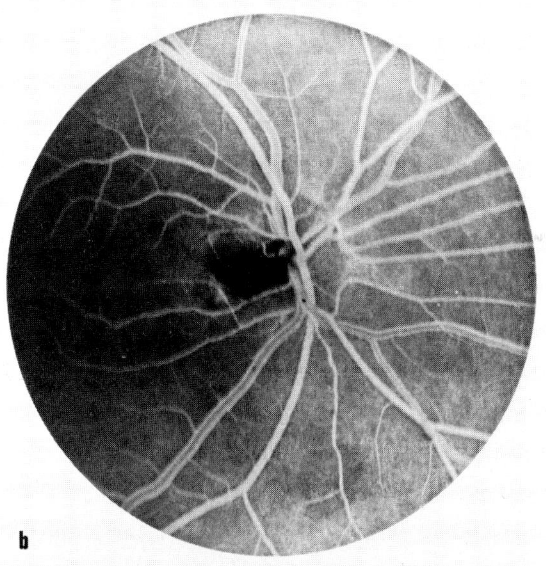

Fig. 7 a. Melanocytoma of the optic disc.
b. Fluorescence angiogram of the same fundus.

of the diagnosis. When the ocular media are not clear, ultrasonography is the primary diagnostic tool. The most frequently misdiagnosed lesions clinically supposed to be a choroidal melanoma according to Shields et al. (1980) are given in the table. In general, in case of doubt as to the diagnosis of a choroidal melanoma it is advisable to obtain the opinion of ophthalmologists who are familiar with and have gained experience in tumour diagnosis, also in view of their different therapeutic modalities.

Optic disc

The only primary pigmented tumour of the optic disc is the melanocytoma. It is a benign tumour with a gray to black aspect, eccentrically located on the optic nerve head, with hair-like extensions; in half of the cases there is an adjacent choroidal naevus (fig. 7ab). It is rare in Caucasians, its incidence being highest in coloured people, while the Mediterranean population has an intermediate position. Concomitant signs may be a Marcus Gunn pupillary defect, arcuate visual field defects, and sometimes visual loss due to nerve fibre compression. Over the years there may be very slow growth. Therapy is not indicated.

Pigmented secondary tumours of the optic disc may be either overgrowth from an adjacent choroidal melanoma (fig. 8), or metastasis from a cutaneous melanoma, which is extremely rare.

References

Davidorf, F.H., Letson, A.D., Weiss, E.T. and Levine, E.: Inicdence of misdiagnosed and unsuspected choroidal melanomas. Arch.Ophthal. 101: 410-412, 1983.

Goder, G.J.: Tumors of the ciliary body. In: Intraocular Tumors, eds. Lommatzsch, P.K. and Blodi, F.C. Springer Verlag, Berlin, 1983, pp 129-137.

Oosterhuis, J.A. and von Winning, C.H.O.M.: Naevus of the choroid. Ophthalmologica 178: 156-165, 1979.

Oosterhuis, J.A., Went, L.N. and Lynch, H.T.: Primary choroidal and cutaneous melanomas, bilateral choroidal melanomas, and familial occurrence of melanomas. Brit.J. Ophthal. 66: 230-233, 1982.

Shields, J.A., Augsburger, J.J., Brown, G.C. and Stephens, R.F.: The differential diagnosis of posterior uveal melanoma. Ophthalmology 87: 518-522, 1980.

RETINOBLASTOMA

K.E.W.P. Tan and J. Schipper

Introduction

Retinoblastoma is a rare malignant tumour of the retina occurring in about 1 : 15,000 children. It is generally thought that the tumour originates in the retinoblasts, the embryonic retinal cells.

The disease occurs in two forms:

1. a solitary sporadic form which, like most other tumours, appears without apparent reason;
2. a basically multifocal form related to a genetic mutation, which is dominantly hereditary; this category, comprising about one third of all cases, is of special importance: there are few situations more tragic than that of a child doomed to blindness because of malignant tumours in both eyes.

The enormous technical advances achieved during the last fifty years have made it possible to cure many eyes afflicted with retinoblastoma. There is now an almost 100% chance of a complete cure if the treatment is carried out in the early stages at one of the retinoblastoma centres. The story is a classic example of how excellent results can be obtained when dedicated eye specialists, radiotherapists, paediatricians, radiophysicists and oncologists work in close co-operation in a treatment centre (Fig. 1).

The fact that the predisposition for retinoblastoma is hereditary is of great interest from the oncogenetic point of view. In addition, manifestations of chromosomal abnormalities occur in some cases of retinoblastoma.

Oosterhuis, A. (ed.), Ophthalmic tumors.

ISBN 90-6193-528-8. Printed in the Netherlands.

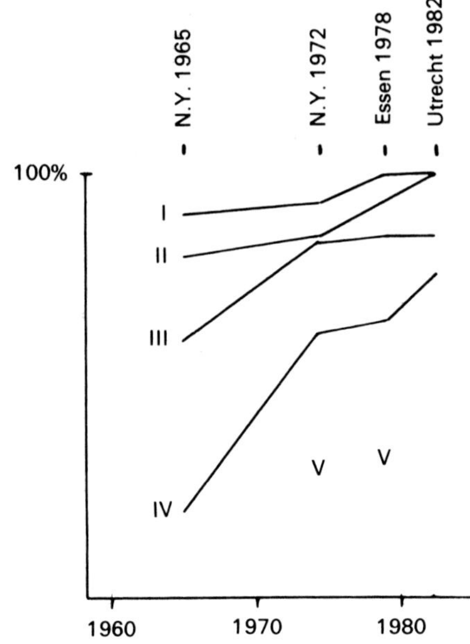

Fig. 1 Improvement of the cure rates of the various retinoblastoma stages according to the Reese classification over the period 1960 to 1980.

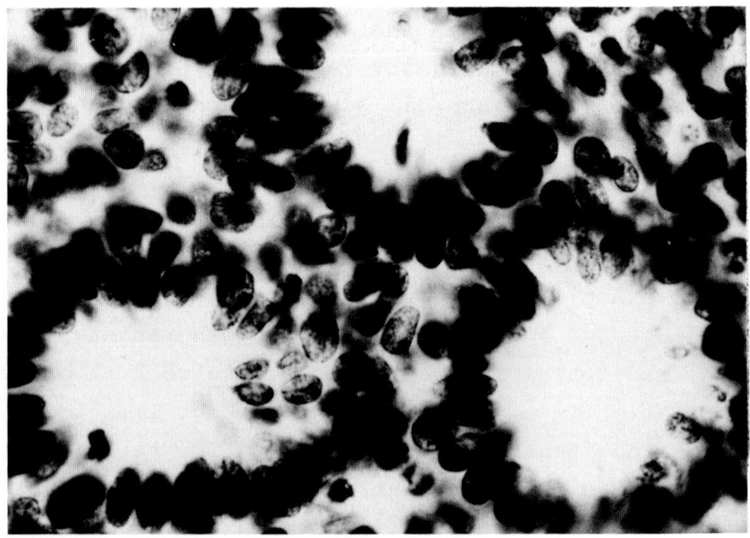

Fig. 2 Flexner-Wintersteiner rosettes.

From the pathological-anatomical angle the tumour consists of small round cells with scanty protoplasm and little stroma. The differentiation often changes from place to place in the tumour. A very typical pattern occurs in the form of the so-called Flexner-Wintersteiner rosettes where the tumour apparently tries to form optic cups (Fig. 2). In rare cases a photoreceptor differentiation is present.

In many tumours viable areas are present beside extensive necrotic regions and calcium deposits are often found here. Tumour growth occurs mainly in the area around the blood vessels and in one outer layer of the tumour where the oxygenation via the vitreous humour appears to be sufficient to keep active cells alive (Fig. 3).

On a more macroscopic scale one finds various types of growth:

1. an endophytic growth if the tumour originates from the internal layer of the retina (Fig. 4a);
2. an exophytic growth if the tumour originates from the external layers of the retina; this type of tumour lifts the retina from the underlying sclera (Fig. 4b);
3. a rare, diffused type of growth; this clinical diagnosis is frequently overlooked (Fig. 4c).

In advanced stages the original growth is usually not identifiable; the picture then shows an eye totally destroyed and largely filled with tumorous tissue (Fig. 4d).

Extraocular extension occurs relatively late. There are three possibilities:

1. growth through the optic nerve to the brain (about two thirds of all cases of extraocular extension);
2. growth through the sclera;
3. haematogeneous metastasis.

These conditions are seldom seen in the Netherlands or in other countries with well-developed health services. If the tumour has reached the brain or if haematogenic metastasis has occurred, the disease is incurable.

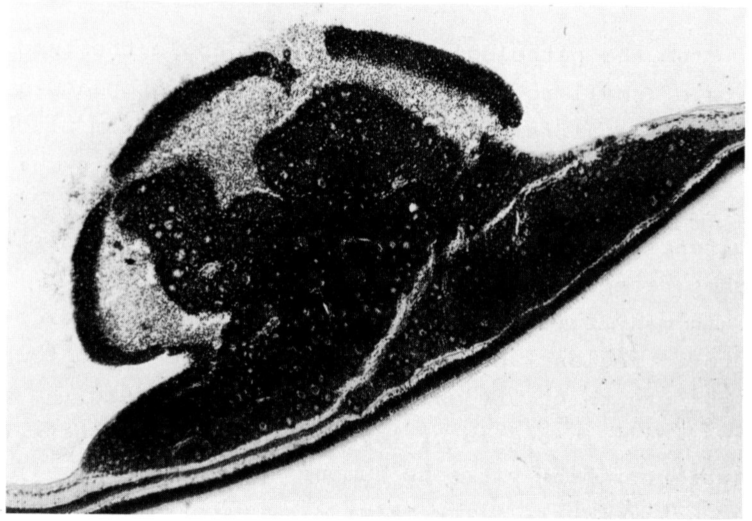

Fig. 3 Section of a small retinoblastoma. It is possible to distinguish adjacent areas of viable and necrotic cells.

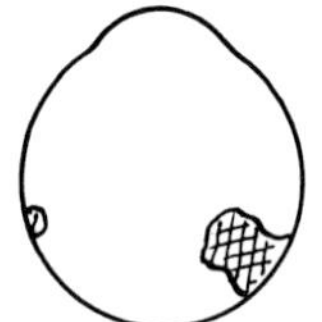

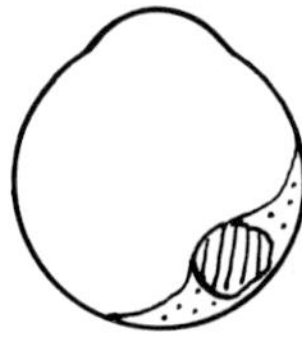

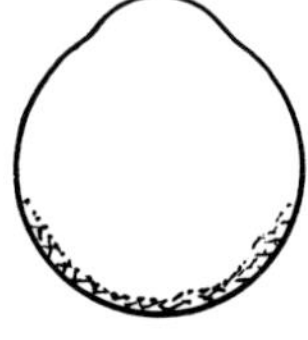

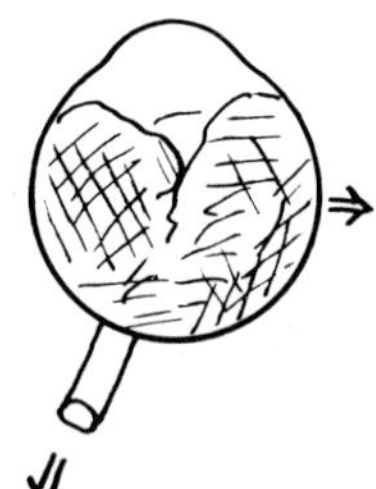

Fig. 4a Endophytic growth.

Fig. 4b Exophytic growth.

Fig. 4c Diffuse growth.

Fig. 4d The growth type is no longer distinguishable.

While the mortality rate in the United States for instance is about 9%, it is practically 100% in under-developed countries.

Clinic

The growth of the tumour practically always commences in the first year of the child's life. The symptomatology is changeable and depends on the localization and spread of the tumour. Roughly one may say that in the developed countries 60% of the cases have a leucocoria, that is to say, a large white tumour which is visible through the pupil (Fig. 5), 30% have strabismus if the tumour grows in the macular region or if the macula is covered, 10% have a varied symptomatology. In underdeveloped countries the disease often manifests itself by a cauliflower-like tumour which grows out of the eye.

From the differential-diagnostic angle a number of other abnormalities are recognized in the symptomatology of leucocoria such as persisting primary vitreous and retrolental fibroplasia. Correct diagnosis is sometimes extremely difficult, especially as biopsy is not possible. Careful examination under general anaesthesia by an ophthalmologist acquainted with retinoblastoma seems to be the most reliable way to assess the diagnosis.

The problem is different when the symptom is a strabismus. Roughly 1 in 2,000 children with strabismus will have a retinoblastoma and about 1 in every 1,000 will have an intraocular abnormality. It is important in all children with strabismus to exclude any disease in the macular region by funduscopy. This can often be done without anaesthetic if the pupil is well dilated.

If the family history contains proof of hereditary retinoblastoma, then regular and detailed examination is essenial from about the first or second week after birth.

Therapy

Nowadays there are various possibilities to destroy the tumour and save the eye:

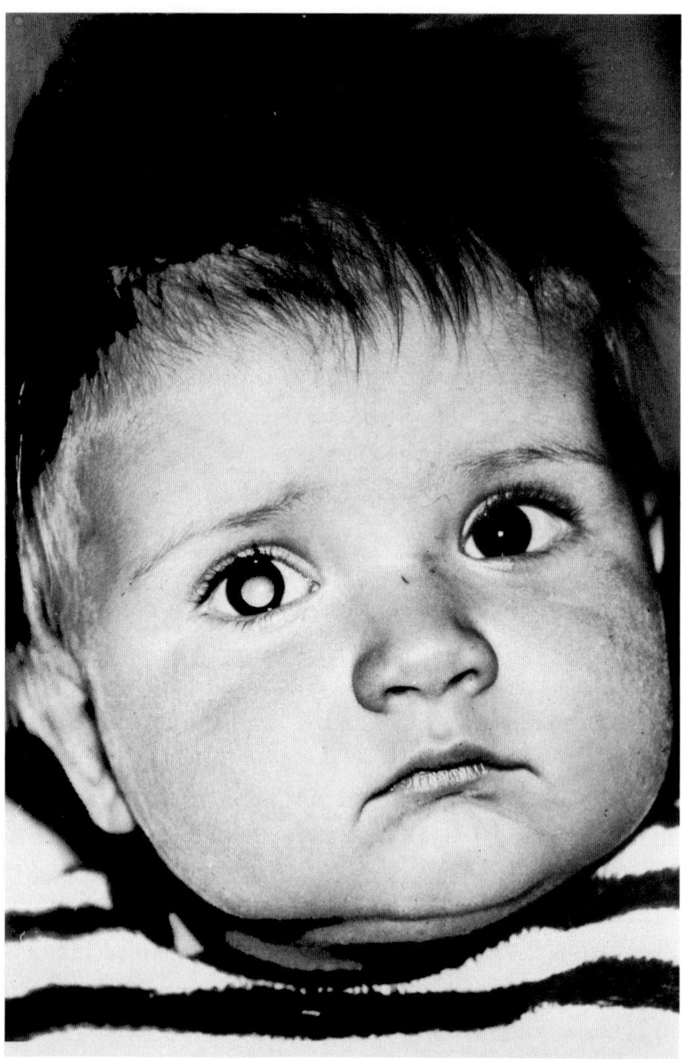

Fig. 5 Leucocoria. The large white tumour is visible through the pupil.

1. radiotherapy
2. photocoagulation
3. cryotherapy
4. chemotherapy

In most cases it is necessary to use a combination of these therapies. Needless to say that this requires specialized knowledge and it is generally accepted that the treatment should be carried out in centres. These centres of retinoblastoma treatment are often places where, in the past, pioneers in the field of retinoblastoma treatment used to work and where now, depending of course on the stage of development of the tumour, good and even extremely good results are achieved.

Radiotherapy

Radiotherapy usually is the first method of treatment that comes to mind. The tumour, or the greater part of the tumour, generally is extremely sensitive to radiation and 45 Gy (4,500 rad) can be considered correct as a therapeutic dose. Radiotherapy is also of value in small tumours that are still in the "statu nascendi". As the smallest visible tumour consists of about 1,000,000 tumour cells, the presence of still invisible small tumours in cases of multifocal retinoblastoma certainly is not just imagination.

Radiotherapy can, in principle, be administered in two ways:

1. by external beam irradiation
2. by radioactive applicators.

Preference is generally given to the first possibility because of easy control and uniformity of the dosage. Radioactive applicators are particularly indicated in recurrences where the area has already been irradiated.

Problems in radiotherapy are:

1. the very high sensitivity of the eye lens to radiation: as little as 8 Gy (800 rad) may cause a cataract;
2. the sensitivity to radiation of the anterior eye

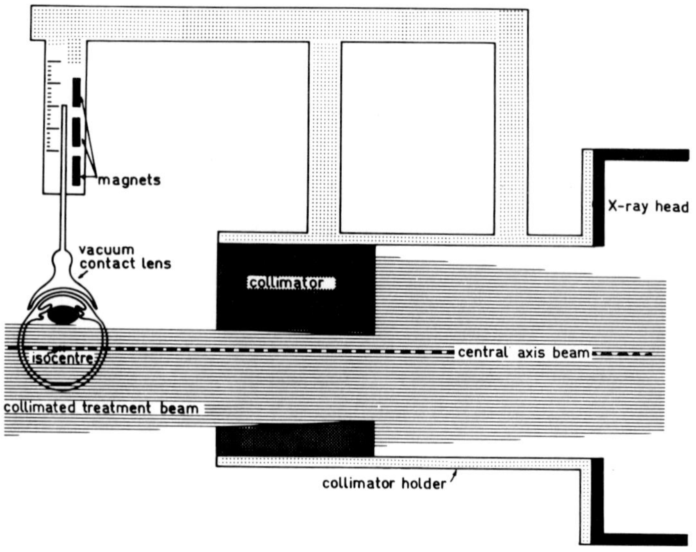

Fig. 6 Diagram showing the irradiation technique used.

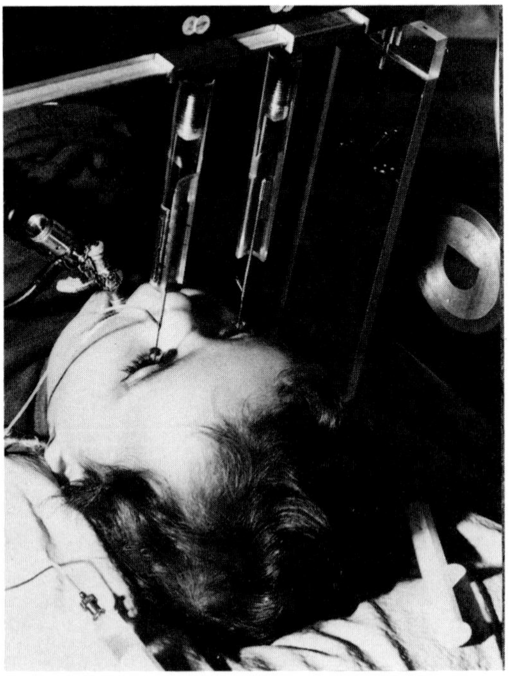

Fig. 7 The irradiation technique used on a patient with a bilateral retinoblastoma.

segment; about 20 Gy (2,000 rad) may already result in radiokeratitis and glaucoma;

3. the radiation damage to the retina and the optic nerve, which can be expected above 50 Gy (5,000 rad);
4. the development of secondary tumours (for example, sarcomata) in the irradiated area.

Needless to say that it is possible to minimize damage by the use of methods which ensure that the retina receives the correct dose of radiation while the surrounding areas are adequately shielded. The method developed by Schipper in Utrecht goes a long way towards achieving this (Figs 6,7). By using a linear accelerator it is possible to obtain a sharply demarcated field of irradiation. Because a contact lens is used to fixate the eye, the position of the eye in relation to the tumour mass can be adjusted with an accuracy of about 0.3 mm. Thus the surrounding tissues and especially the lens of the eye receive only the dosage that is unavoidable if the whole of the retina is to be within the field of radiation.

It can be expected that radiotherapy has the greatest effect on a well-oxygenated tumour, i.e. a tumour which has a satisfactory blood circulation. For this reason radiotherapy has to be administered preferably prior to photo- or cryo-coagulation. In the latter two modalities of treatment - which will be discussed later - large areas of the vascular bed are destroyed; also in a tumour treated for the first time, poorly oxygenated and partially necrotic areas will be present, which is one of the reasons why a good fractionation is so important. By reason of the dying off of the quickly growing, well oxygenated cells around the blood vessels, the poorly nourished cells will obtain more oxygen; they can then be destroyed by a subsequent fraction.

Regression of the tumour sometimes appears to be insufficient; fortunately, in these cases there is a possibility of additional treatment: photocoagulation or cryotherapy. The importance of this is shown by the percentage of cases in which additional therapy was judged to be necessary: New York 53%, Essen 80%, Utrecht 60%.

Since it is not possible to carry out biopsy, the judgement of the viability of the tumour(s) is highly subjective; this is apparently the reason for the differences in percentage of additional treatment.

Photocoagulation

Xenon arc photocoagulation is only possible if the ocular media are sufficiently clear and the tumour does not lie too far in the periphery of the retina. A problem is the whiteness of the tumour, which reflects almost all the light directed upon it. This means that tremendous light power is necessary. If there is a high degree of absorption at just one site, then, due to the excessive heat which develops, a vapour bubble can develop, causing the tumour to explode with the disastrous consequence of spreading of tumour cells throughout the vitreous.

The procedure of photocoagulation usually is as follows: At the first treatment a cordon of coagulations is placed around the tumour. Owing to partial vascular obliteration a haemorrhagic necrosis develops. This bleeding is made use of during further treatments in order to obtain a more intensive absorption of the light. Four to six sessions are often needed to destroy the tumour. Because biopsy is not possible, evaluation of the result is difficult. If the tumour is not completely destroyed, it will grow again after a few months.

In Essen, the cradle of photocoagulation, this method is used regularly to destroy small tumours without previous radiotherapy. The only problem is that tumours in "statu nascendi" are not affected and that occasionally new tumours are detected a few weeks later, sometimes in difficult positions.

Cryotherapy

It is possible to treat small tumours in the periphery of the retina with cold. Experience gained with this method has shown, however, that it is not entirely favourable. A problem is the difficulty to evaluate whether the tumour has

	Reese classification	"cure rate"	
I	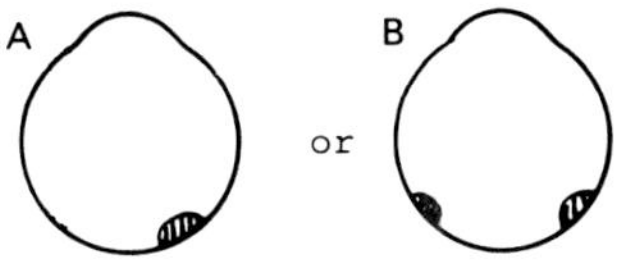 A or B	12/12	100%
II	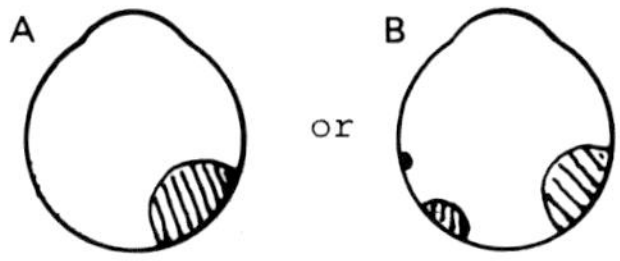 A or B	9/9	100%
III	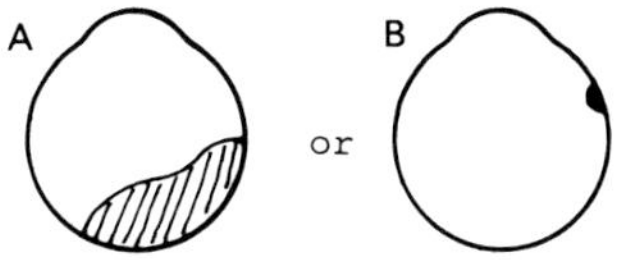 A or B	10/12	83%
IV	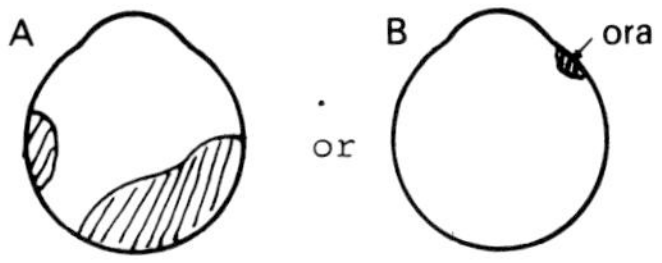 A or B (ora)	11/14	79%
V	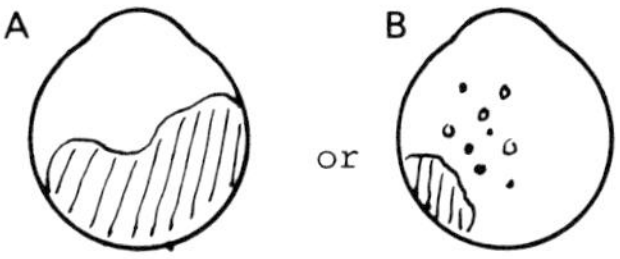 A or B	0/5	0%

Fig. 8 Results of radiotherapy, if necessary supplemented by photocoagulation or cryotherapy, over the period 1970-1980 with a minimum follow-up of one year, grouped according to the Reese classification.

been completely destroyed or not. Various times in the past tumours have reappeared after months or even years, apparently developing from tumours which were earlier thought to have been destroyed.

It is obvious that the success of the treatment largely depends on the stage at which the disease is diagnosed and the therapy begun. The "cure rates" at given stages of the disease are shown in figure 8.

Chemotherapy

Chemotherapy is extremely effective in the treatment of various types of tumours which occur during childhood and the role of chemotherapy in the treatment of retinoblastoma is evident.

In 1953 tri-ethylene-melamine (TEM) was introduced by the New York group as an adjuvant to radiotherapy in the treatment of retinoblastoma. This example was followed by many others. On evaluation in 1969, after two children had died as a result of chemotherapy, no significant difference was found in the results of treatment with or without chemotherapy, neither have other studies shown any influence on the final result. A dramatic effect of a combination of chemotherapeutic drugs on a far advanced tumour has frequently been seen but it was never permanent. One of the problems might be that penetration of the drugs into the eye is limited due to the so-called blood-retina barrier but this can not be the only explanation, since in case of a haematogeneous metastasis of retinoblastoma the mortality rate, in spite of chemotherapy, is still practically 100%.

Clinical experimental work in the field of chemotherapy of retinoblastoma is seldom possible in the Netherlands or other western countries; in the early stages of retinoblastoma the results of radiotherapy, if necessary in combination with photocoagulation or cryotherapy, are so successful that experimental changes in the treatment are considered to be ethically unjustified. The far advanced cases fortunately are so rare that it is hardly possible to form an opinion.

The underdeveloped countries with many advanced cases but without well-equipped radiotherapeutic centres could possibly stimulate further investigation.

Double tumours

It has become clear in recent years that carriers of hereditary retinoblastoma have an increased risk of developing second tumours in later life. At present the extent of the risk is not precisely known but the percentage is not insignificant. In principle, there are three categories:

1. tumours in the irradiated area;
2. tumours of the epiphysis;
3. tumours elsewhere in the body.

The first category is often the result of very high doses of radiation at an earlier date. This is due to the fact that with earlier orthovoltage X-ray beams, contrary to modern megavolt X-ray beam technique, the absorption in the bone is about twice that in the soft tissues. It is hoped that with modern radiotherapy this problem will, to a great extent, belong to the past, but no definite judgement can be passed at present because the incubation period is often 10 years or longer.

In rare instances a retinoblastoma-like tumour occurs alongside a hereditary retinoblastoma in the epiphysis of the brain. In cases of pinealomas, which are sometimes called trilateral retinoblastomas, the gene appears to "remind itself" of the phylogenetic optical origin of the epiphysis.

The third category is the most intriguing and also the most puzzling one. About 60% of the tumours elsewhere in the body are osteogenic sarcomas of the lower extremities. It is not clear whether this is a less common expression of the retinoblastoma gene or the manifestation of a generally increased susceptibility to other malignant tumours.

Genetic counselling

As has been pointed out in the Introduction, two forms of retinoblastomas occur: a solitary sporadic retinoblastoma without known cause, and a basically multifocal retinoblastoma related to a dominant genetic mutation.

It is often difficult to give genetic advice because in practice it is frequently impossible to determine to which group a patient with a solitary tumour belongs. It is possible that for fortuitous reasons only one tumour has developed in multifocal type retinoblastoma but it is also possible that a number of tumours developed in one eye only and that these merged into one solitary tumour at a later stage.

If the condition is bilateral or if there is another sufferer among close relatives, then genetic counselling is simple: the descendants have a 50% chance of becoming once again carriers of the hereditary disease, in about 49% retinoblastoma will appear and in 1% the gene will not express itself.

It is considered essential that children born to carrier parents are examined in the first or second week of life, although this does not guarantee that the disease can be successfully treated because some children are born with fully developed retinoblastoma in both eyes. At present there is no possibility of prenatal diagnosis.

Chromosome investigation

With the development of the banding technique in chromosome research the way seemed clear to visualize the genetic mutations. In general, however, this was not the case. Only in a small percentage a deletion of the long arm of chromosome 13 was visible. It was assumed for various reasons that the retinoblastoma gene does indeed lie in the long arm of chromosome 13 but that it is not yet possible to detect the abnormality because of its minute size (fig. 9).

At the moment efforts are being made to establish the presence of a sub-microscopic deletion by means of DNA probes, which are in principle related to one locus.

Finally, the importance of retinoblastoma in the search for a cancer cure. Knudson has based his "two-hit" theory on the statistical division of the number of tumours in multifocal retinoblastoma. In general, two mutations would be necessary for the development of a tumour. In multifocal retinoblastoma the first mutation would be genetically present and thus the tumour would develop at any place where a second mutation occurs. It would appear, however, that the problem is in fact far more complex. Predisposition to retinoblastoma and to other tumours might be a key to the cancer riddle, which is a compelling reason for focussing attention upon this rare tumour.

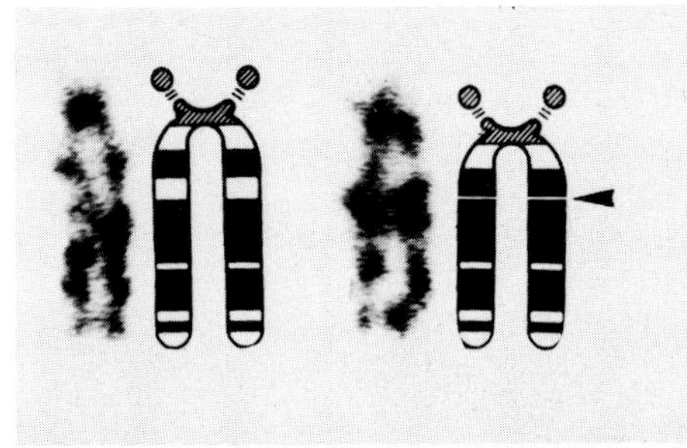

Fig. 9 Small 13q14 deletion (by courtesy of Dr. C.H.C.M. Buys, Groningen University).

MANAGEMENT OF CONJUNCTIVAL TUMOURS

D. de Wolff-Rouendaal

Introduction

Most conjunctival tumours in routine ophthalmological practice are innocuous, benign swellings which can easily be diagnosed and excised if necessary, but a few tumours may give rise to diagnostic and therapeutic problems. As malignant tumours on the bulbar conjunctiva as a rule can be locally excised as long as they are small and have not infiltrated into the fornices, the eyelids or the caruncula, it is important that an early diagnosis is correctly made.

Clinical examination and diagnosis

Careful history taking may reveal that a conjunctival tumour grew after a trauma or surgery on the outer eye, e.g. a strabismus operation, so the tumour may be an exuberance of granulation tissue. Sudden fast growth in a conjunctival swelling may simulate a malignancy. The tumour may be associated with systemic disease such as sarcoidosis or malignant lymphoma, which makes an inquiry into the general health indispensable.

On inspection of the conjunctiva with and without biomicroscopy a differentiation may be made between an epithelial growth with a rough and cracked surface or a subepithelial tumour or cyst covered by smooth and undisturbed conjunctival epithelium; however, some tumours which develop in the subepithelial tissue may give rise to pseudo-epitheliomatous lesions, which may give a wrong impression of the origin of the growth. Leukoplakia, a whitish-glistening appearance in patches of the conjunctiva, may be associated with malignant epithelial conjunctival tumours but also with

Oosterhuis, A. (ed.), Ophthalmic tumors.

ISBN 90-6193-528-8. Printed in the Netherlands.

benign conjunctival lesions which may produce keratinization in the conjunctival epithelium. Enhanced vascularization gives the impression of malignancy but also haemangiomas and inflammatory nodules often are accompanied by local increase in vascularization.

The tumour may be pigmented; clinically, the density of the pigmentation is generally not indicative of the degree of malignancy of the conjunctival tumour. Pigmented tumours contrast readily with the white sclera but in case non-pigmented tumours are surrounded by a heavily vascularized area it is difficult to estimate the margins of the lesions.

Many solid benign and malignant tumours of the bulbar conjunctiva show a flat infiltration into the surrounding healthy conjunctiva; scleral infiltration is rare. In the tarsal conjunctiva, the fornices and the caruncula, however, the malignant tumours may invade the deeper layers much more easily. This makes it difficult to estimate their extension, which creates special therapeutic problems.

Examination of the eye and orbit is necessary to differentiate a primary conjunctival tumour from an extrascleral extension of an intraocular tumour or a forward extension of an intraorbital process. A pigmented tumour may be an extraocular extension of a melanoma of the ciliary body. A haemangioma of the conjunctiva may have a large extension into the orbit and may be difficult to excise.

Photography is indispensable for documentation prior to treatment or for assessment of growth of the tumour.

Malignant conjunctival tumours

Clinical findings in a conjunctival tumour may point to malignancy, but establishing the diagnosis itself is not rewarding as it remains hazardous in the majority of the tumours. If a malignant conjunctival tumour is suspected, exfoliative cytology may be of great help to differentiate between superficial benign, malignant and premalignant lesions and therefore to decide on the treatment to be performed. The cytology procedure is easily tolerated by the patient and can be repeated if necessary. A dry cottonwool swab is rubbed over the surface of the tumour (Fig. 1) and the detached cells are spread out on a glass slide, stained according to Papanicolaou or Giemsa, and studied under the light microscope. Local anaesthesia may deform the tumour cells and is not allowed in this test. The value of exfoliative cytology is demonstrated in the following two case histories.

Case history 1

A 48 year old male patient presented with a pigmented tumour in the nasal part of the conjunctiva of his left eye. It had been observed by his ophthalmologist for 16 years without any change or growth, so the clinical diagnosis was benign conjunctival naevus. Recently, the tumour had started to grow rapidly and to be surrounded by many dilated vessels.

Exfoliative cytology prior to excision revealed atypical pigmented cells very suspicious of malignant melanoma. Histology of the excised tumour showed malignant melanoma without residual naevus tissue (Figs. 2a,b).

Case history 2

A 60 year old female patient had a highly vascularized tumour with glistening surface in the temporal bulbar conjunctiva of her left eye. The clinical diagnosis was Bowen's disease of the conjunctiva.

Exfoliative cytology showed many inflammatory cells but a certain amount of atypical epithelial cells were present too. Histology after excision showed no malignancy but granulation tissue. This was not in accordance with the findings on exfoliative cytology; therefore, further histological investigation was carried out and then an intraepithelial carcinoma of the conjunctiva was found.

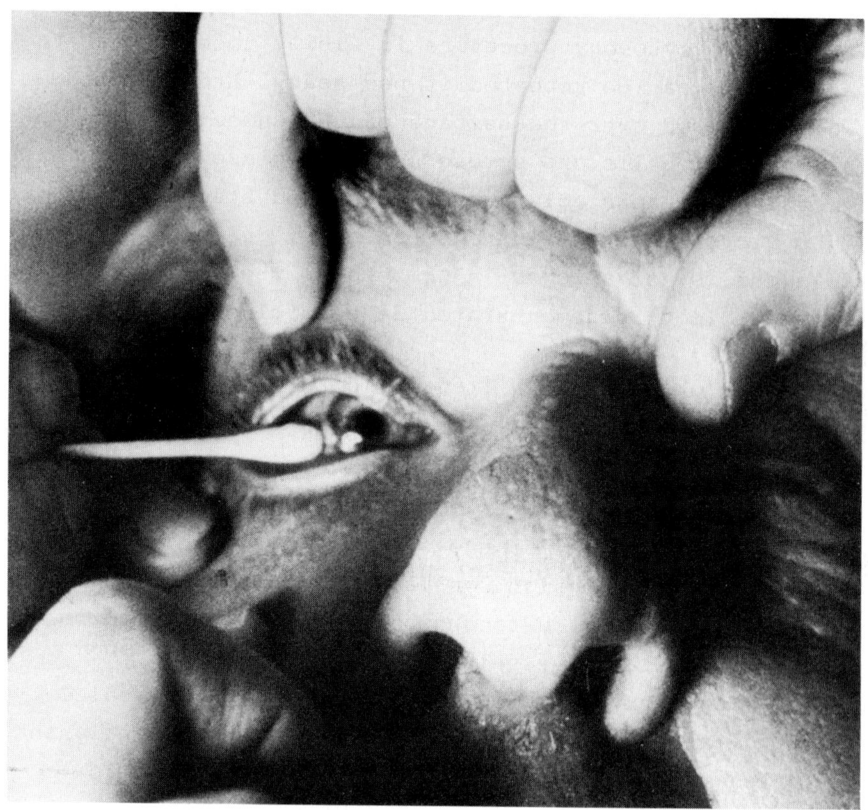

Fig. 1 For exfoliative cytology a dry cottonwool swab is rubbed over the surface of the tumour.

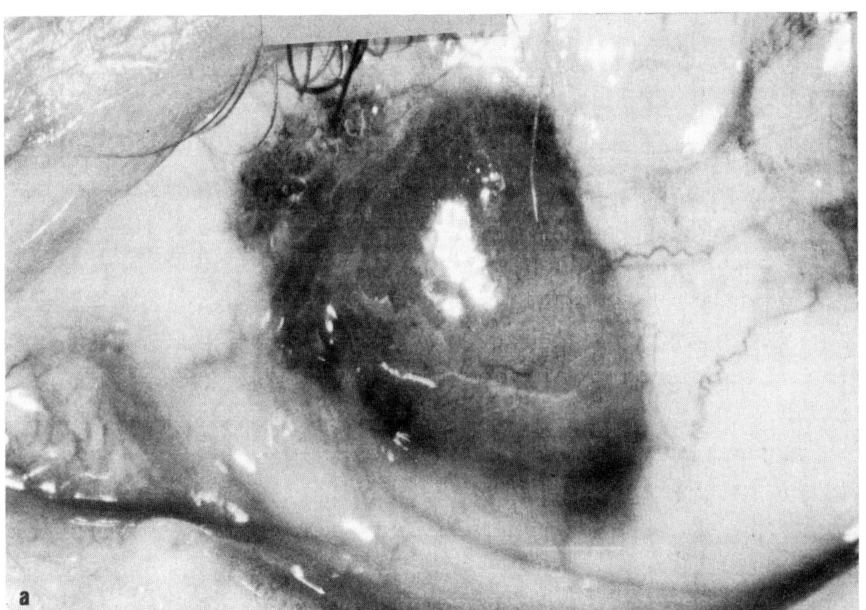

Fig. 2a Pigmented tumour which had been present for 16 years before it started to grow rapidly and to be surrounded by dilated blood vessels.

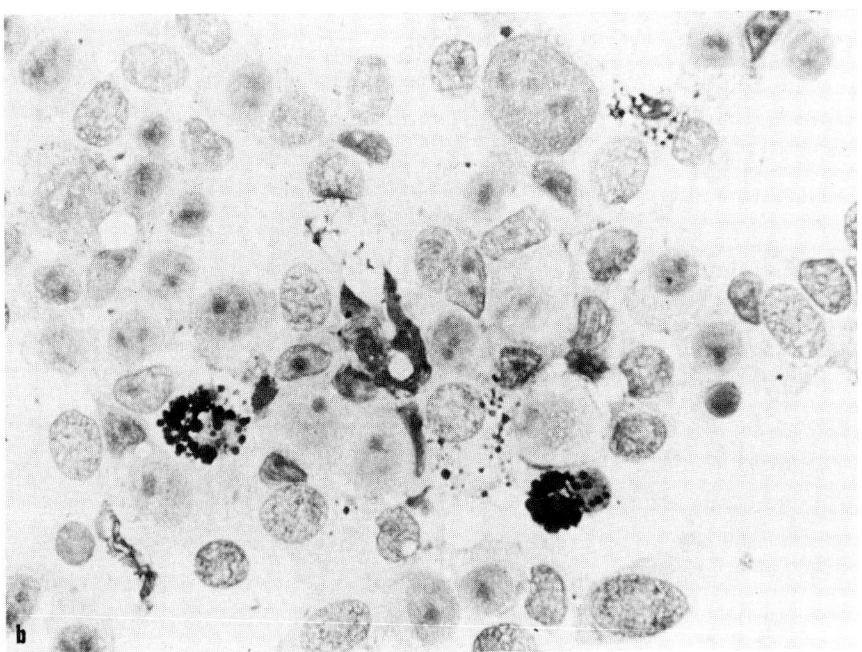

Fig. 2b Cytology: enlarged anisokaryotic and anisochromatic nuclei; dense chromatin structure, enlarged nucleoli; sometimes mitoses are found. Suspicious of malignant melanoma.

If malignant cells are found on exfoliative cytology, examination of the lymph nodes in the preauricular and the submandibular region is required, as they may reveal regional metastasis. Distant metastases may be very difficult to find on general examination, amongst others chest X-rays and liver function tests. They rarely occur in conjunctival carcinoma but are frequent in Meibomian gland carcinoma of the eyelid[11] and in conjunctival malignant melanoma[2,14,16]. In the latter, metastatic disease may develop many years after treatment of the primary tumour. All malignant conjunctival tumours have a high tendency to recidivate after local excision, especially when they arise in carcinoma in situ and acquired melanosis. In the presence of metastasis extensive mutilating surgery should not be performed.

Premalignant conjunctival lesions

Precancerous epithelial conjunctival lesions show clinical and histological similarities to precancerous skin lesions. Clinically, one may observe patches of thickened, sometimes fleshy conjunctiva; sometimes leukoplakic lesions are seen (Fig. 3a). Both may spread superficially in the conjunctiva and give rise to invasive, sometimes ulcerating carcinomas in an unknown percentage. Enhanced vascularization may be a sign of active growth, malignant change or invasion into the subepithelial tissue.

In *intra-epithelial carcinoma* the conjunctival epithelium is thickened and on histology it shows atypical cells from the basal layers up to the surface; mitotic activity is enhanced; parakeratosis and dyskeratosis may be present. The pathological keratinization may show clinically as leukoplakia. As long as polarity of the cells is preserved, the lesion is called dysplasia and shows resemblance to Bowen's disease of the skin. When polarity of the cells within the epithelium is lost, the lesion is identical to carcinoma in situ (Fig. 3b). As long as the malignant cells do not penetrate the basal membrane of the epithelium, the lesion behaves as a benign tumour without tendency to infiltrate

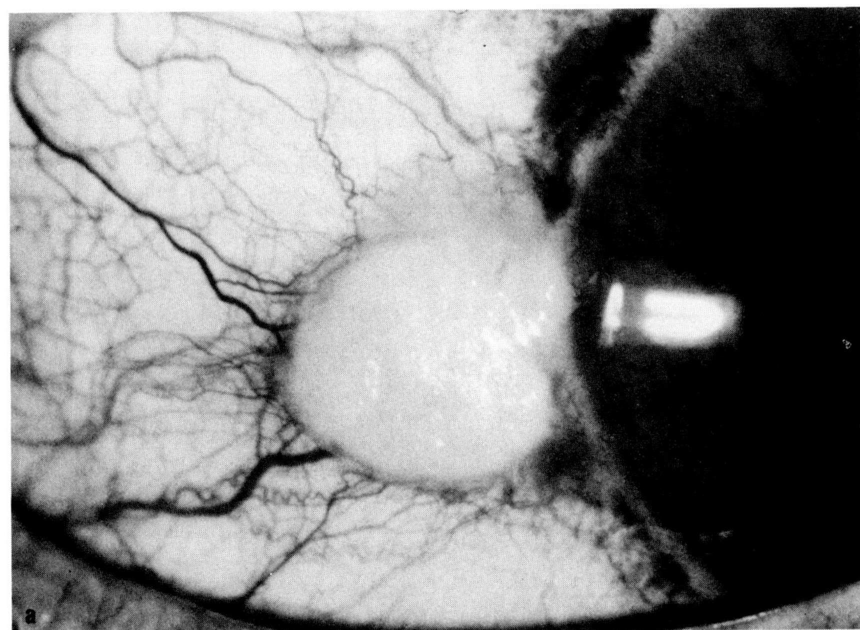

Fig. 3a Whitish glistening flat conjunctival tumour with dilated blood vessels, suspicious of m. Bowen.

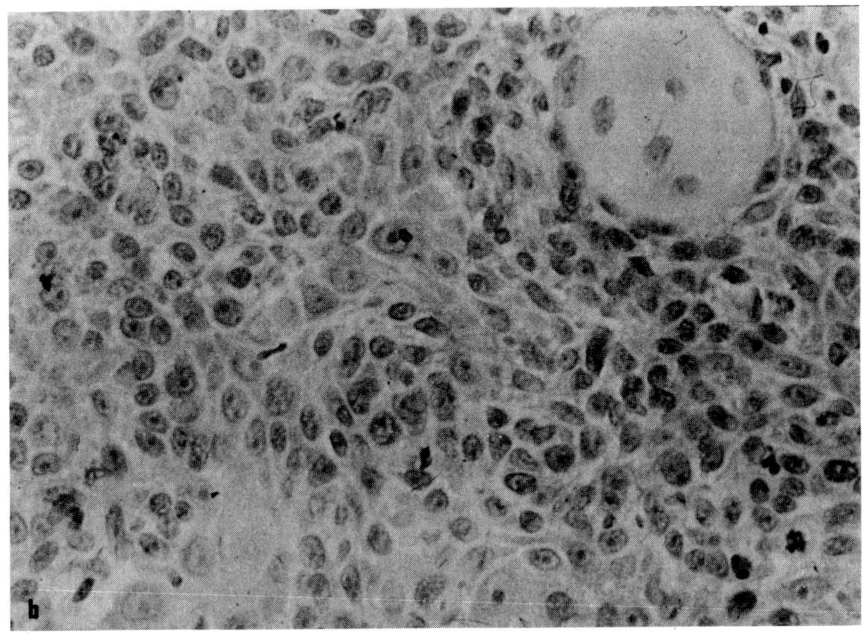

Fig. 3b Histology: carcinoma in situ. Epithelial cells with irregular nuclei, prominent nucleoli, mitoses and individual keratinization (not in photograph: no invasion of subepithelial tissue).

or metastasize. A change into malignancy shows by penetration through the basal membrane and infiltration into deeper structures. When the tumour is localized in the bulbar conjunctiva, invasion into the eye is rare and occurs mostly along the blood vessels. When located in fornix, eyelid or caruncula, the tumour invades deeper tissues more easily than the sclera; all tumour tissue has to be totally excised to prevent further infiltration into the orbit.

Local excision combined with cryosurgery in conjunctival carcinoma is presently being advocated[4]. As the conjunctival carcinoma is radiosensitive, radiotherapy by X-ray or radioactive applicators, with or without previous local excision, may destroy the tumour completely[9]. Lymphogenic or haematogenic metastases are rare and occur only in 5% of the cases[11]. Orbital exenteration may be inevitable when local excision in combination with radiotherapy fails to eliminate the tumour.

In _precancerous or acquired melanosis_ a flat pigmentation of the conjunctiva develops in adult life in one eye only. Pigment is either finely distributed over the whole conjunctiva or part of it, or present in dark patches. The pigmentation may fluctuate in intensity and in localization. According to Reese[12] invasive melanomas arise in 17% of acquired melanosis cases. Increase of pigmentation in itself is not necessarily a sign of malignant change, but enhancement of vascularization or tumour formation in the conjunctiva are alarming signs which stress the need of further investigation by either exfoliative cytology or biopsy.

The histological findings in acquired melanosis may also vary in intensity in the course of time and localization but there is no exact information on this variability.

When flat pigmented patches are combined with enhanced vascularization, histological investigation may reveal intra-epithelial melanoma (Fig. 4a). On histology atypical melanotic cells are seen originating from the basal cell layers, which may proliferate diffusely or in loosely packed nests on the lower border of the conjunctival epithelium,

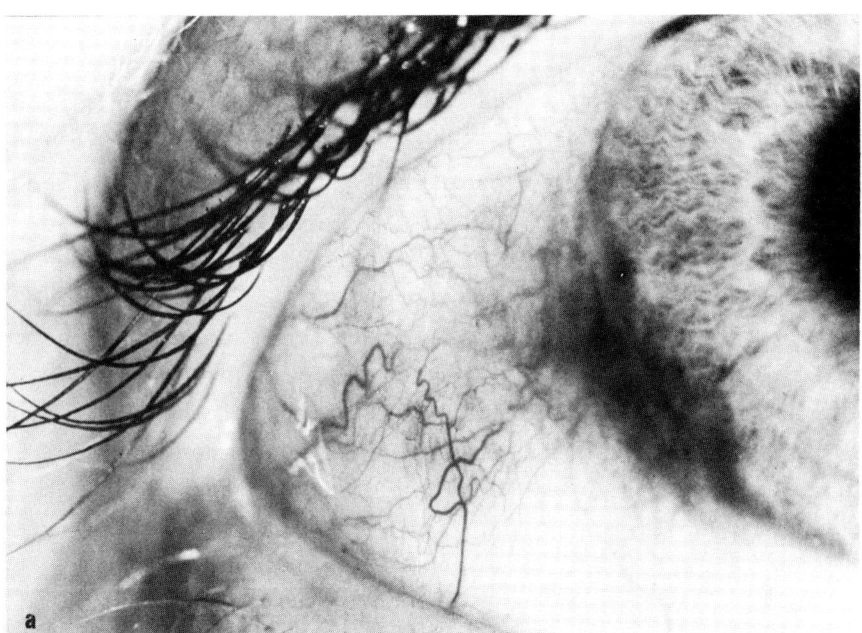

Fig. 4a Flat pigmentation in limbus, cornea and conjunctiva, suspicious of precancerous melanosis.

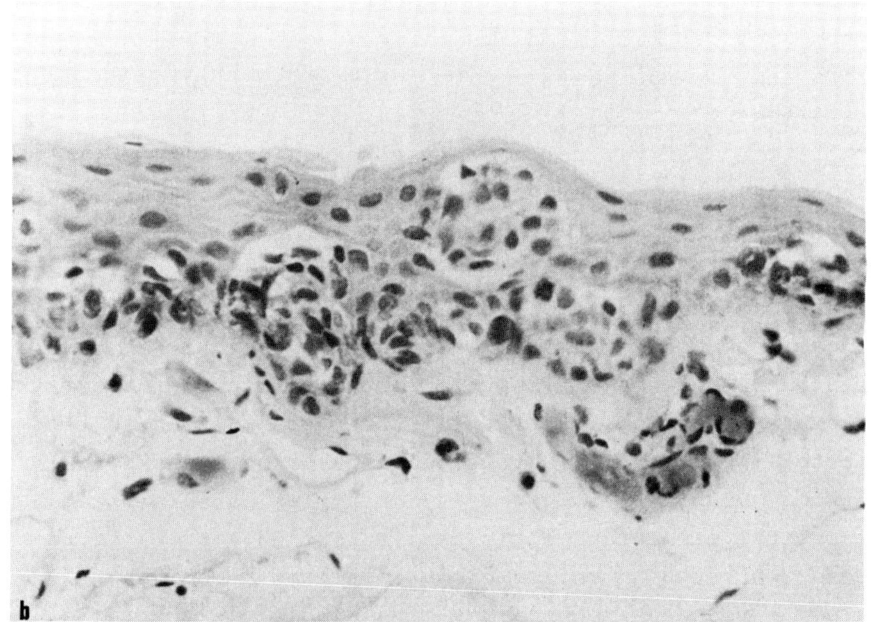

Fig. 4b Histology: intraepithelial melanoma. Nests of partly pigmented atypical cells and mitoses. Migration of nests and individual cells towards the surface. No invasion of subepithelial tissue.

thereby disturbing the architecture (Fig. 4b). As a rule, the conjunctival epithelium is not thickened. Individual cells or groups of cells may migrate to the surface, which does not occur in benign pigmented proliferations of the conjunctiva. Mitoses may be present. As long as the basal membrane is intact, which is difficult to establish, the melanoma cells are not in contact with lymphatic canals or blood vessels and the lesion does not metastasize. A change into malignancy shows by penetration through the basal membrane and infiltration into more deeply located structures.

The melanoma shows little tendency to penetrate the cornea or the sclera and Bowman's membrane seems to be a good barrier. In the bulbar conjunctiva the melanoma tends to grow laterally into the adjacent conjunctiva, limbus and cornea; in the fornices, the tarsal conjunctiva and the caruncula the penetration into the deeper layers is unpredictable and complete excision therefore is far more difficult. The conjunctival melanoma has a high tendency towards lymphogenic spread to preauricular or submandibular lymph nodes and towards haematogenic metastasis, leading to death in 14 to 42%[2,7,14].

In conjunctival melanoma local excision is the therapy of choice but high recurrence rates have been reported: Liesegang & Campbell 72%[7], Brooks Crawford 79%[2], de Wolff & Oosterhuis 69%[14]. In melanomas originating from precancerous melanosis the recurrence rate is 100%[7,15].

Melanomas originating in the bulbar conjunctiva can be treated by local excision; the survival in these cases is excellent. When the primary or recurrent melanoma is located in fornix, tarsal conjunctiva or caruncula, the risk of metastasis is high. In our series of 59 patients an orbital exenteration was carried out in 40% (23 patients) because of such an unfavourable localization or - more rarely - frequent recurrences of a bulbar conjunctival melanoma; metastatic death occurred in 47% (11 patients) (see Table).

Localization	local excision		orbital exenteration		irradiation		total	
	no.	†	no.	†	no.	†	no.	†
Bulbar conjunctiva	24	0% (0)	7	0% (0)	0	0% (0)	31	0% (0)
Fornix) Tarsal conjunctiva) Caruncula) Orbit)	7	14% (1)	17	64% (11)	4	75% (3)	28	54% (15)
Total	31	3% (1)	24	46% (11)	4	75% (3)	59	25% (15)

Table. Localisation, treatment and mortality in conjunctival melanoma.

Lederman[6] and Lommatzsch[8] have advocated irradiation of conjunctival melanomas. In our series, radiotherapy was not a standard procedure. Up till now radiotherapy was the first treatment in 7 patients, but a variety of radiotherapeutic methods has been used. In 5 patients the tumour recurred. In 3 patients radiotherapy was combined with local excision, 2 of which had no recurrences. In 3 patients irradiation of a melanoma that had recurred after local excision was not successful.

Favourable prognostic factors in conjunctival melanomas according to Zimmerman[15] are a small diameter, a thickness of less than 2 mm, localization near the limbus, a circumscript and solitary tumour, and the absence of a regional nodal metastasis. Thus, an early diagnosis when the tumour is still small facilitates treatment and gives a better prognosis than at a later stage.

metastasis. Thus, an early diagnosis when the tumour is still small facilitates treatment and gives a better prognosis than at a later stage.

The reason of the high recurrence rate after local excision of a conjunctival melanoma is poorly understood. Small tumour remnants or seeding of malignant cells during surgery may play a role[12]. To restrict local seeding we currently treat the surface of the tumour prior to excision with 4% formaldehyde solution and subsequently rinse the operating field with 0.5% sodium hypochlorite (Dakin's) solution to kill the free floating tumour cells[3]. The rinsing procedure is repeated after excision of the tumour. The bare sclera is not covered by a conjunctival flap in order to prevent burying of any tumour cells.

Treatment and control of patients with conjunctival malignant melanoma require special experience and should preferably be carried out in specialized centres.

References

1. Brownstein, S., Jakobiec, F.A., Wilkinson, R.D., Lambords, J. and Jackson, B.: Cryotherapy for precancerous melanosis (atypical melanocytic hyperplasia) of the conjunctiva.

Arch.Ophthal. 99: 1224, 1983.
2. Brooks Crawford, J.: Conjunctival melanomas, prognostic factors and analysis of a series. Trans.Amer.Ophthal.Soc. 78: 467-502, 1981.
3. Van Delft, J.L., De Wolff-Rouendaal, D. and Oosterhuis, J.A.: Irrigation with mercury chloride and sodium hypochlorite to prevent local recurrence after excision of conjunctival melanoma. An experimental study. Docum. Ophthal. 56: 61-67, 1983.
4. Frauenfelder, F.T. and Wingfield, D.: Management of intraepithelial conjunctival tumors and squamous cell carcinomas. Amer.J.Ophthal. 95: 359-363, 1983.
5. Jakobiec, F.A., Brownstein, S., Albert, W., Schwarz, F. and Anderson, R.: The role of cryotherapy in the management of conjunctival melanoma. Ophthalmology 89: 502-515, 1982.
6. Lederman, M.: Radiotherapy of cancerous and precancerous melanosis. Trans.Ophthal.Soc.UK 78: 147-169, 1958.
7. Liesegang, T.J. and Campbell, R.J.: Mayoclinic experience with conjunctival melanomas. Arch.Ophthal. 98: 1385-1389, 1980.
8. Lommatzsch, P.K.: Beta-irradiation of conjunctival melanomas. Trans.Ophthal.Soc.UK 97: 378-380, 1977.
9. Lommatzsch, P.K.: Beta-ray treatment of malignant epithelial tumors of the conjunctiva. Amer.J.Ophthal. 81: 198-206, 1976.
10. Lopes Cardozo, P., Oosterhuis, J.A. and De Wolff-Rouendaal, D.: Exfoliative cytology in the diagnosis of conjunctival tumours. Ophthalmologica (Basel) 182: 157-164, 1981.
11. Naumann, G.O.H.: Pathologie des Auges. Springer-Verlag, Berlin-Heidelberg-New York, 1980.
12. Reese, A.B.: Pigmented tumors. In : Tumors of the Eye. Harper & Row Publishers, Hagerstown, 1976, pp. 25-27.
13. Oosterhuis, J.A. and De Wolff-Rouendaal, D.: Local metastasis in conjunctival melanoma. Docum.Ophthal. 56: 55-59, 1983.
14. De Wolff-Rouendaal, D. and Oosterhuis, J.A.: Conjunctival melanomas in the Netherlands: a follow-up study. Docum. Ophthal. 56: 49-54, 1983.
15. De Wolff-Rouendaal, D. and Oosterhuis, J.A.: Conjunctival melanomas in the Netherlands. II. Short communication, in press.
16. Zimmerman, L.E.: Melanocytic tumors of interest to the ophthalmologist. Ophthalmology 87: 497-502, 1980.

THE DIAGNOSIS AND MANAGEMENT OF TUMOURS OF THE IRIS AND CILIARY BODY

Wallace S. Foulds

My subject is the diagnosis and management of tumours affecting the iris or ciliary body, and is based on experience of ninety malignant melanomas of the anterior uvea seen in the twenty year period 1964 to 1983, and on a small number of other tumours affecting the tissues of this area.

Although iris tumours may expand posteriorly into the ciliary body, or ciliary body tumours expand anteriorly into the iris, it is easier to consider the diagnosis and management of tumours arising in these two situations separately.

In general, patients with iris tumours present because of the abnormal appearance of the affected eye, while patients with ciliary body tumours tend to complain of blurred vision, often associated with distortion or displacement of the lens. In both cases, presentation tends to occur earlier than with choroidal tumours and tumours of the anterior segment tend to be smaller at presentation than choroidal tumours, unless the latter have been diagnosed in an asymptomatic eye during routine ophthalmoscopy or unless they directly affect macular vision.

Taking iris tumours first, the differential diagnosis includes benign heterochromia, iris naevus, iris cysts and inflammatory granuloma. By far the commonest tumour is the malignant melanoma (Ashton, 1964), but very occasionally other tumours may occur, such as the leiomyoma which varies greatly in its malignancy. Other benign tumours include melanocytoma and angioma.

In benign heterochromia of the iris the diagnosis can usually be made confidently on clinical grounds. The condition

Oosterhuis, A. (ed.), Ophthalmic tumors.

ISBN 90-6193-528-8. Printed in the Netherlands.

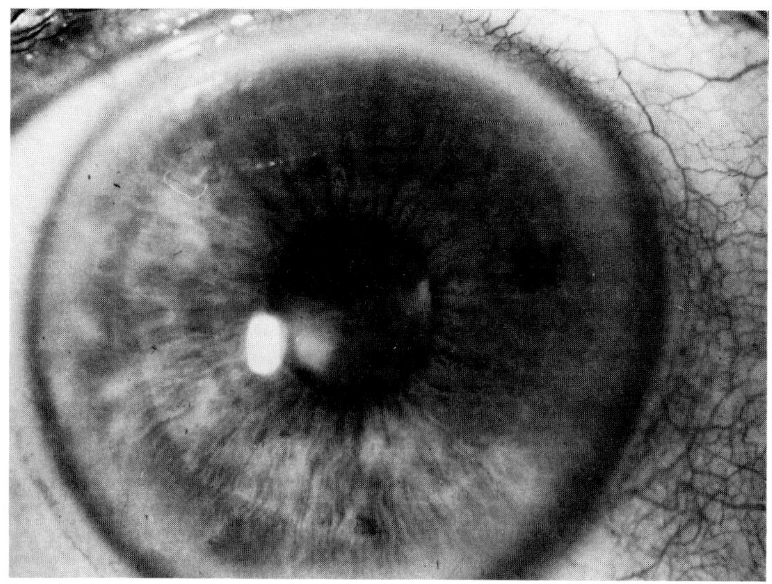

1a

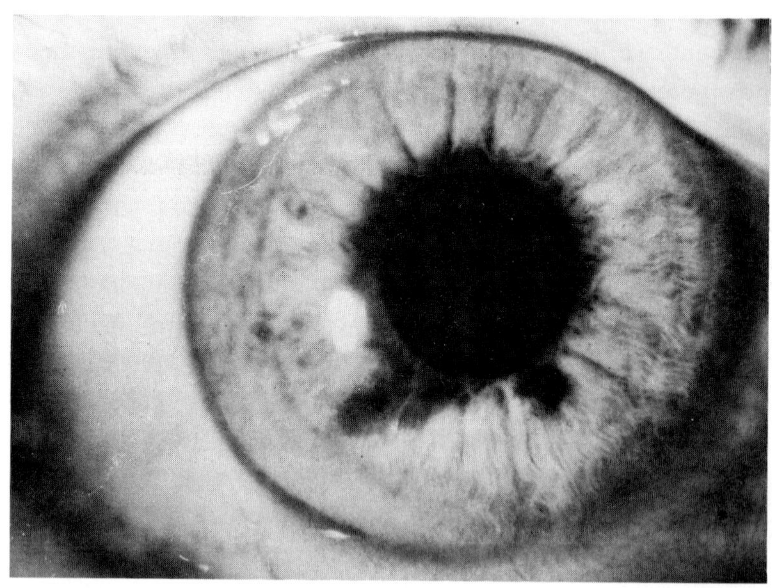

1b

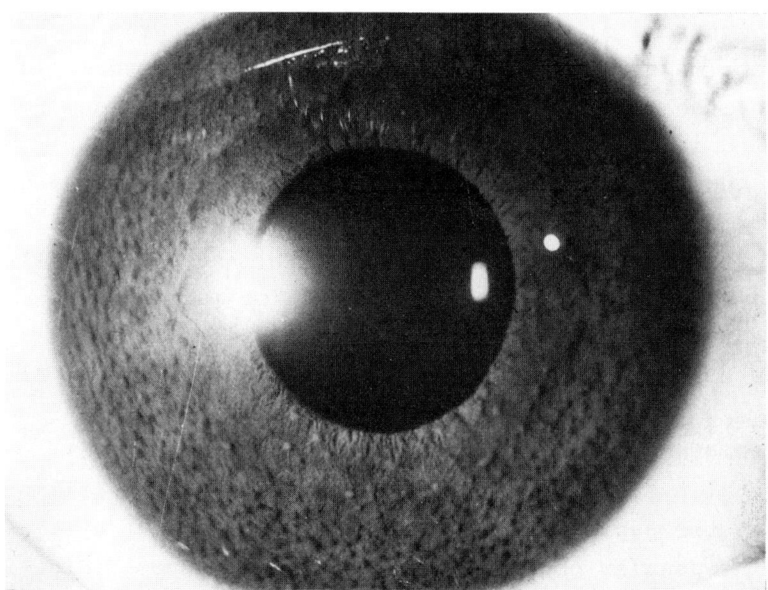
1c

Fig. 1 Benign pigmented lesions of the iris.
a. Benign heterochromia
b. Iris freckle
c. Iris in melanocytosis oculi.

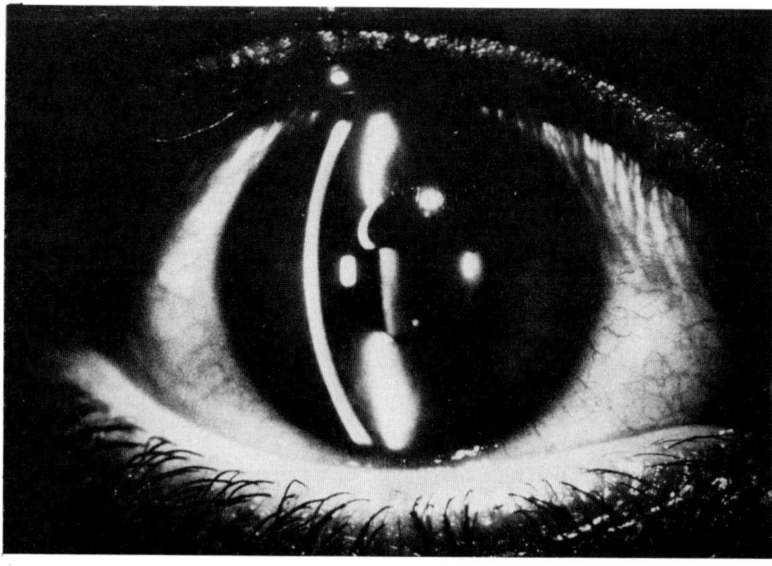

Fig. 2 Congenital cysts of the iris epithelium at the pupil margin.

is non-progressive and not associated with any distortion of the iris stroma or of the pupil. The affected area may represent merely a localised variation in the normal pigmentation of the iris stroma (Fig. 1a) or there may be a more localised increase in pigmentation giving rise to the condition known as iris freckle (Fig. 1b). Widespread benign hyperpigmentation of the iris may be seen in congenital melanocytosis oculi (Font et al., 1967), and occasionally this is complicated by the development of malignancy. Malignant transformation is especially associated with oculodermal melanocytosis (naevus of Ota) (Naumann et al., 1967).

Iris cysts too, pose little diagnostic difficulty. Congenital cysts of the pigment epithelium of the iris may occur at the pupil margin where their translucent cystic nature is usually obvious on slit-lamp microscopy (Fig. 2). Less commonly pigment epithelial cysts may occur on the posterior surface of the iris where they may be mistaken for the anterior extension of a ciliary body tumour. Such cysts have a characteristic smooth contour and may be multilocular. The surface of the cyst has the relatively homogeneous pigmented appearance characteristic of normal iris pigment epithelium and lacks the variable pigmentation and vascularity which characterise ciliary body tumours. Technically it may be difficult to demonstrate transillumination of these cysts and aid in the diagnosis may come from fluorescein angiography for these cysts do not fluoresce on angiography nor do they show late leakage of dye.

Differentiation of cysts of the posterior surface of the iris from a malignant tumour is important. In a recent case the patient had been advised enucleation for this benign congenital defect (Fig. 3). Acquired cysts of the iris may also occur and these include implantation cysts, in relation to which a history of trauma is obviously helpful. Implantation cysts again have a characteristic clinical appearance, distorting the iris stroma and in a phakic eye causing displacement, distortion or opacity of the lens (Fig. 4).

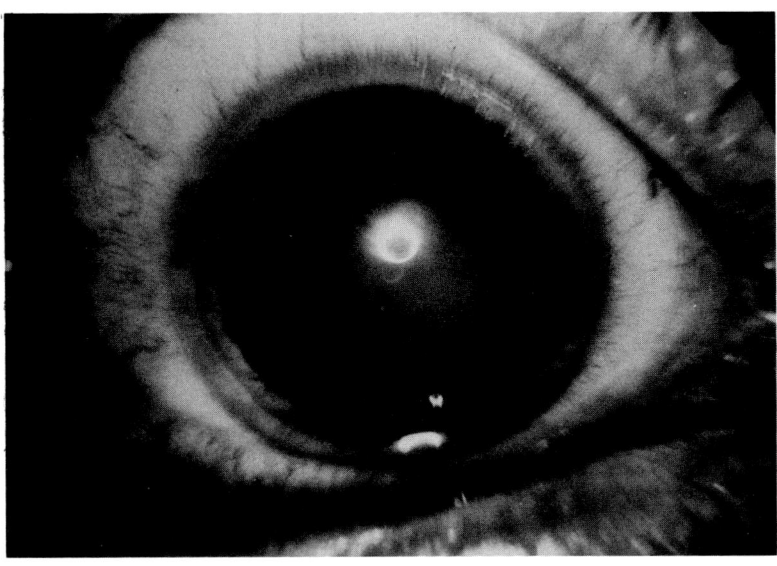

Fig. 3 Congenital cyst of the iris epithelium mistaken for ciliary body melanoma.

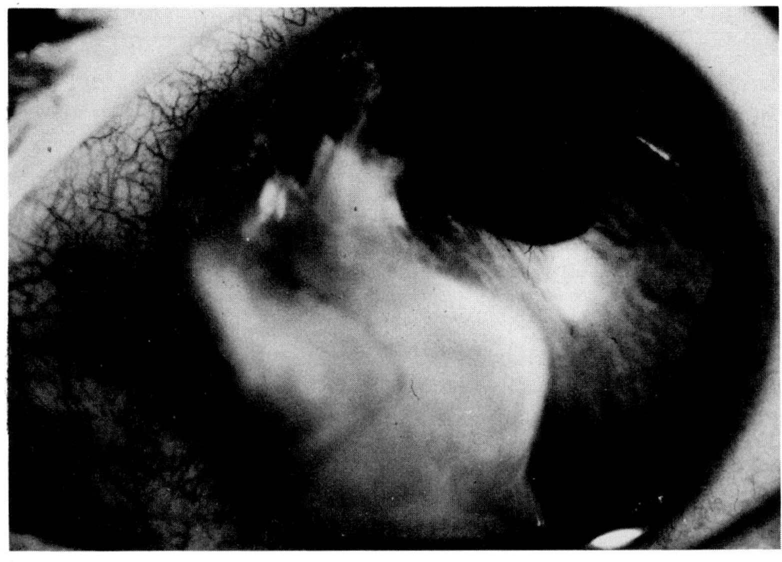

Fig. 4 Implantation cyst of the iris.

Excision of an implantation cyst with or without lensectomy by similar techniques as are used for the excision of iris or ciliary body tumours may be curative.

The main diagnostic problem in the case of iris tumours is between a malignant melanoma on the one hand and a benign naevus on the other. In my experience benign leiomyoma is so rare as hardly to enter into the differential diagnosis.

Of all the clinical signs, the most useful in differentiating a malignant melanoma from an iris naevus is a recorded increase in size of the lesion. It is not unusual however for naevi to become more pigmented at puberty and this may give rise to a misleading history. Malignant melanoma of the iris may be very slow growing and one must be careful that the patient is not lost to follow-up only to present at a subsequent date with an inoperable tumour (Fig. 5).

A study carried out on patients seen during the period 1965 to 1980 compared the clinical features of thirty suspect iris lesions of which nineteen were proven melanomas, and eleven on the basis of clinical experience and subsequent behaviour, were presumed to be benign naevi. In general, naevi tend to be relatively flat and avascular, while malignant melanomas tend to be raised and often show the presence of abnormal vessels. In the study alluded to, all the eleven naevi were avascular, while in nineteen cases of malignant melanoma, eleven (fifty-eight per cent) showed abnormal vessels. The degree of pigmentation of a malignant melanoma is very variable and certainly colour is not a good guide to whether the lesion is malignant or benign. The majority of naevi in the study quoted were pigmented (nine out of eleven - eighty-two per cent), while eleven of the malignant melanomas were pale in colour (fifty-eight per cent) with only eight out of nineteen cases showing obvious pigmentation (forty-two per cent). Figure 6 shows an example of a malignant melanoma which is pale and almost entirely non pigmented, although complicated by a spontaneous hyphaema. Figure 7 shows a deeply pigmented melanoma of the iris. All intermediate grades of pigmentation are seen. Similarly,

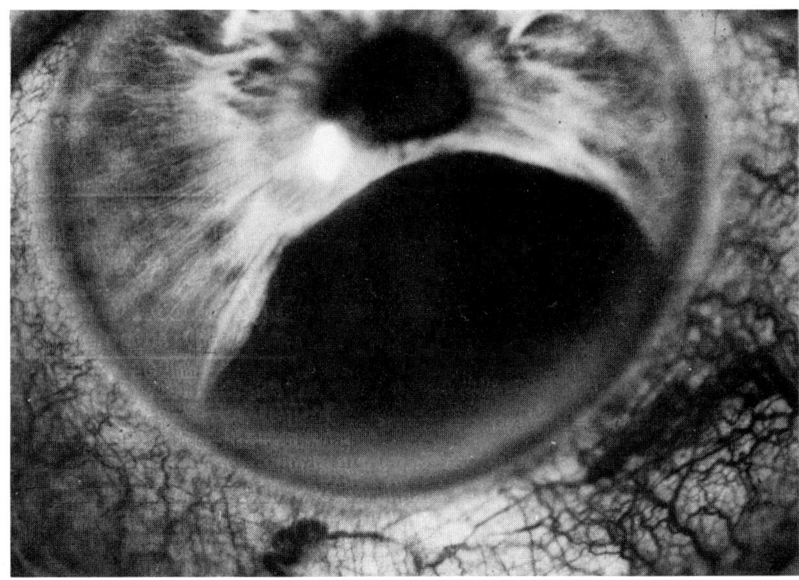

Fig. 5 Inoperable tumour of iris and ciliary body in a patient lost to follow-up for ten years. Secondary glaucoma had supervened in the interval.

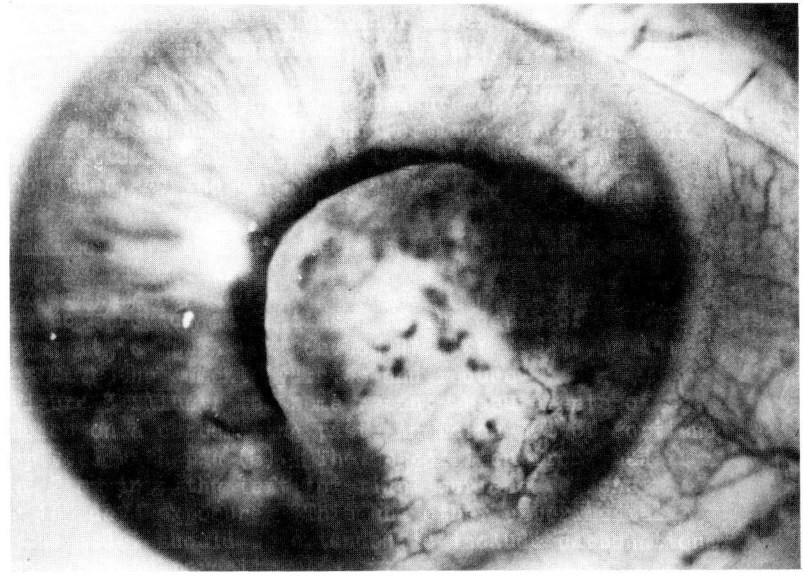

Fig. 6 Pale, non-pigmented malignant melanoma of the iris.

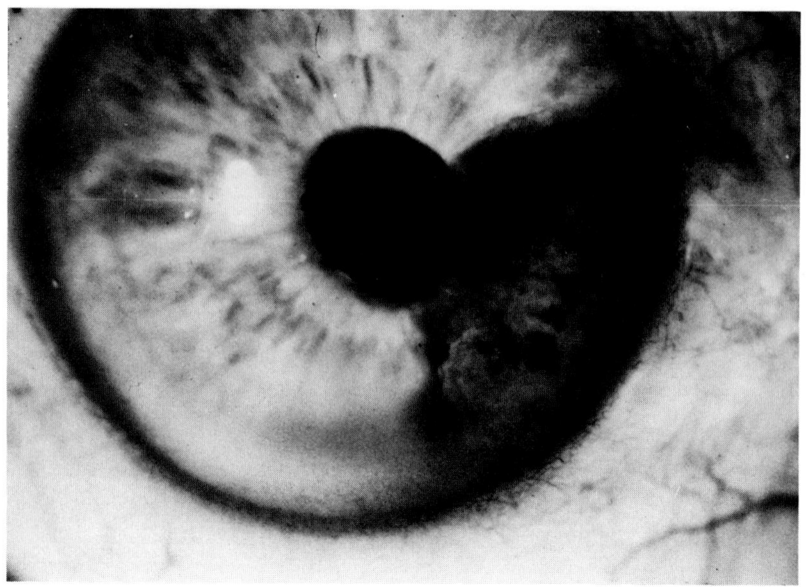

Fig. 7 Deeply pigmented malignant melanoma of the iris.

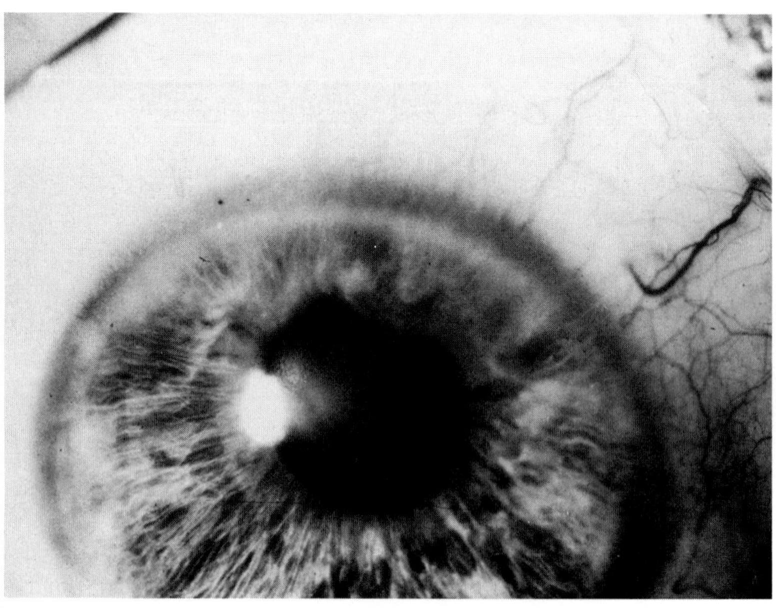

Fig. 8 Pale, non-pigmented naevus of the iris.

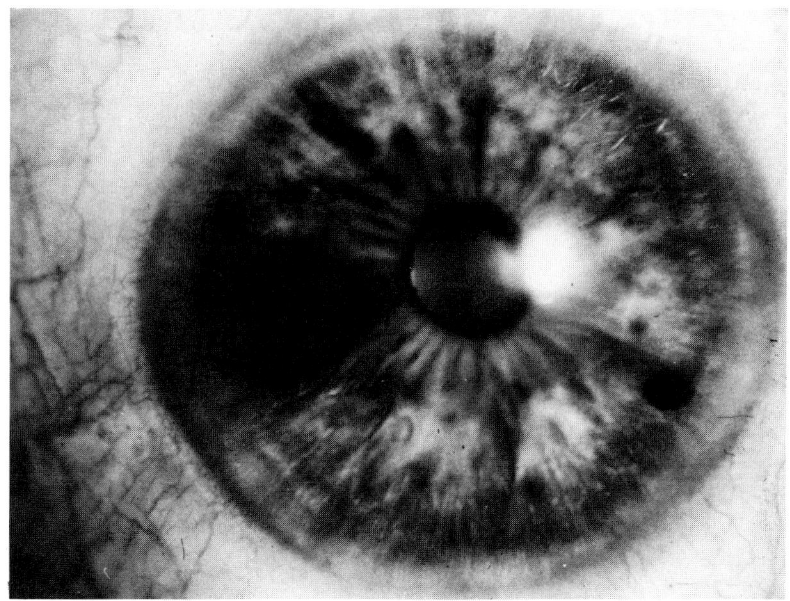

Fig. 9 Deeply pigmented naevus of the iris.

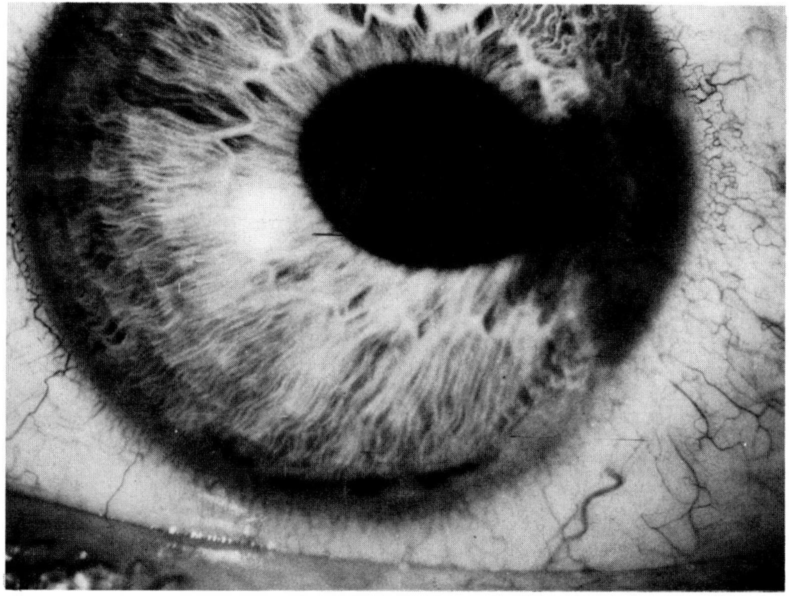

Fig. 10 Ectropion uveae in malignant melanoma of the iris.

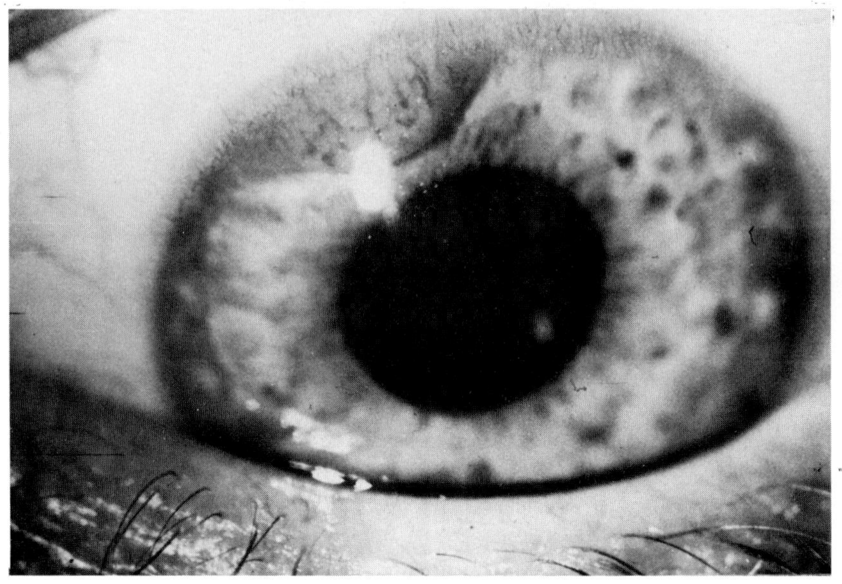

11a

Fig. 11 Fluorescein angiography of lightly pigmented iris tumour.

a. Clinical photograph
b. Vascular pattern of tumour fluoresces early.
c. Late leakage of dye.

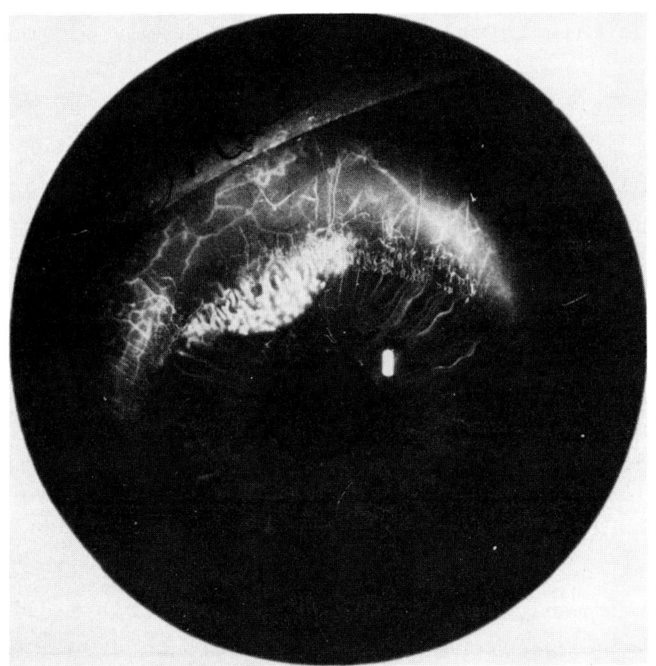

11b

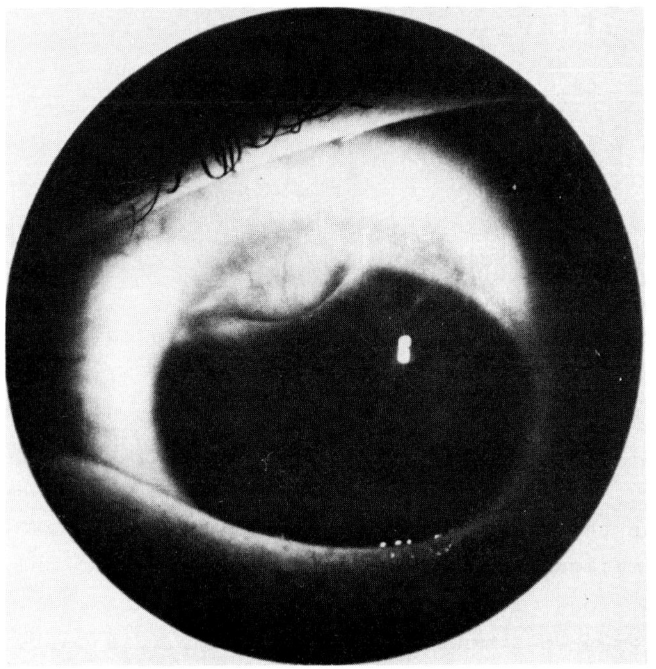

11c

naevi may be pale in colour (Fig. 8) or deeply pigmented (Fig. 9).

The colour of the tumour is also influenced by its vascularity. In extreme cases the tumour can be pink or even red in colour, while in others, vascularity is not at all obvious. The presence of abnormal vessels running to or in a lesion in the iris tends to support the diagnosis of malignant melanoma rather than naevus.

Ectropion uveae is a common sign in melanoma of the iris (Fig. 10) (ten out of seventeen cases where the pupil margin was not obscured by tumour) but naevi also possess actin filaments in their cells and distortion of the pupil margin with ectropion of the pupil may also be seen in iris naevus (one out of eleven cases). Inflammatory signs are characteristically absent in iris naevus, but a flare in the anterior chamber is commonly present in the case of iris melanomas. Very occasionally circum-corneal injection and even KP may be present in patients with malignant melanoma, but the presence of marked inflammatory signs must give rise to the possibility of an inflammatory granuloma as an alternative to a malignant tumour as the likely diagnosis. Congestion of episcleral vessels which is a common sign in ciliary body tumours is also seen in iris tumours. Eleven out of nineteen cases of iris tumour (fifty-eight per cent) showed this feature. Episcleral congestion was not a feature of iris naevus.

As regards investigations, careful clinical examination, photographic recording of the size of the lesion and fluorescein angiography are useful (Cheng et al., 1971; Greitę, 1974; Kottow, 1977; Hodes et al., 1979). On fluorescein angiography the appearance of a melanoma of the iris varies with the degree of pigmentation present. Lightly pigmented malignant melanomas fluoresce early in the dye transit and leak profusely later in the sequence (Fig. 11). Heavily pigmented tumours mask the normal iris pattern in the early frames of the iridogram, but later a halo of fluorescence becomes progressively more marked as fluorescein leaks from the abnormal blood vessels in the tumour (Fig. 12). The appearance is a highly characteristic one. The majority of naevi do not leak fluorescein on angiography, and where the naevus is pigmented, masking of the normal iris pattern is characteristic (Fig. 13). Occasionally lesions which clinically are naevi may fluoresce. There is always the possibility that such lesions are early malignant melanomas, but most ophthalmologists would be reluctant to consider surgery on the basis of fluorescein angiography alone.

Measurements of radioactive phosphorus uptake which are so useful in the case of ciliary body and choroidal tumours are not of value in the diagnosis of iris tumours (Shields, 1978; Hagler et al., 1970; Moseley and Foulds, 1980), as the beta emission of the isotope has low penetrance and physically the measuring probe is of necessity separated from the lesion by the depth of the anterior chamber. This modifies the uptake values unpredictably, making evaluation of the results unreliable.

Ultrasound too is of little practical value in the case of iris tumours, although occasionally useful (Foulds, 1983a) for example, in a patient with an iris melanoma arising posteriorly from an iris naevus and occupying the posterior chamber.

The level of intraocular pressure is an important parameter in the management of iris tumours (Yanoff, 1972). Where the root of the iris is involved and the intraocular pressure elevated the likely explanation is secondary glaucoma due to infiltration of the canal of Schlemm and such eyes are probably inoperable using existing techniques (Foulds and Lee, 1983). Other possible causes of raised intraocular pressure are however occasionally seen and of these the iris naevus syndrome (Scheie and Yanoff, 1975) and melanomalytic glaucoma (Yanoff and Scheie, 1970) are worth considering. In the iris naevus syndrome, for reasons not clearly understood an iris naevus is accompanied by a posterior displacement of Descemet's membrane which comes to overlie the trabecular tissue, interfering with aqueous

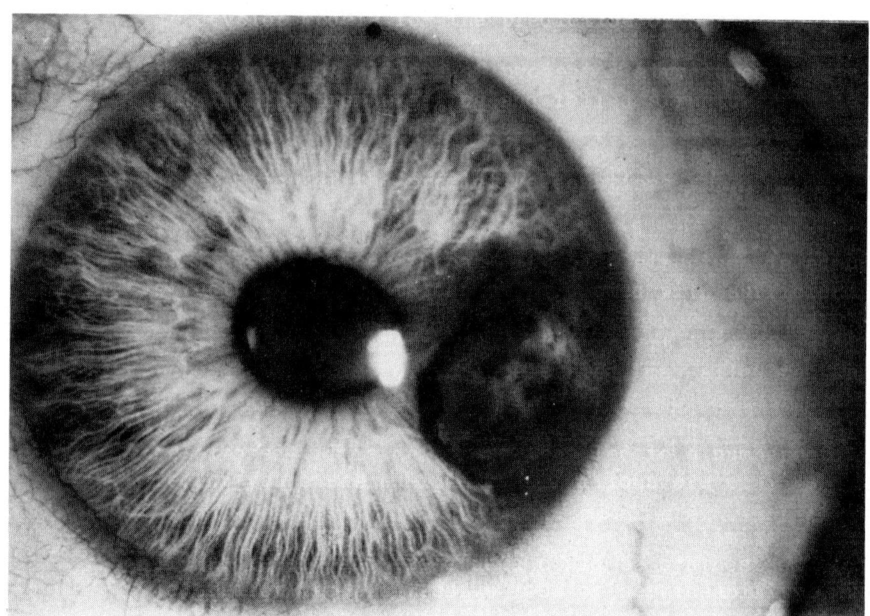

12a

Fig. 12 Fluorescein angiography of a pigmented iris tumour.

a. Clinical photograph.
b. In early frames the tumour masks the iris pattern although punctate staining of the tumour is a feature.
c. In late frames there is a halo of diffusing dye.

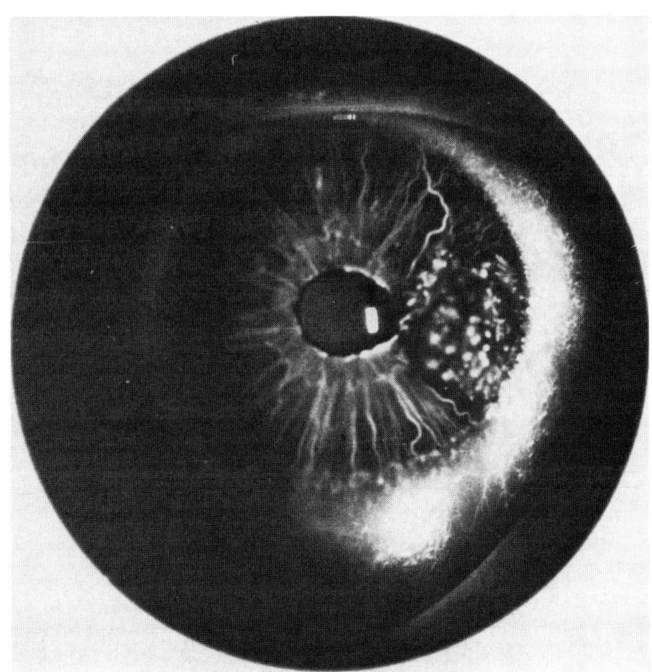

12b

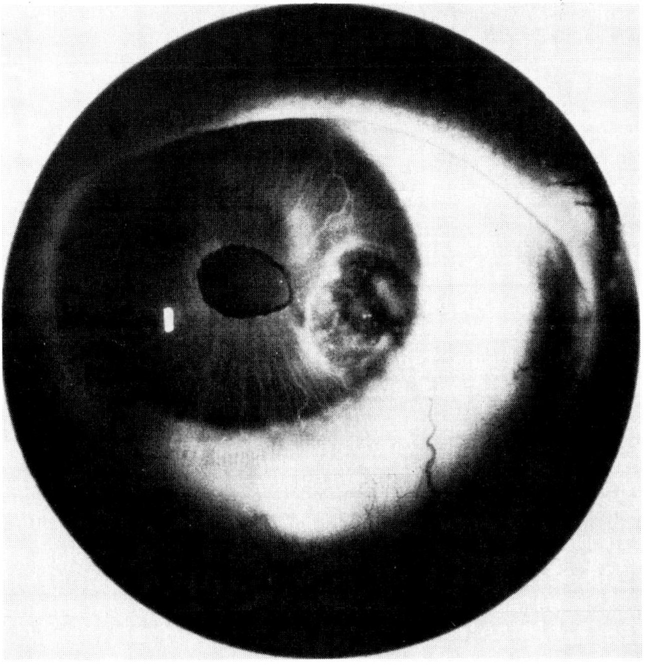

12c

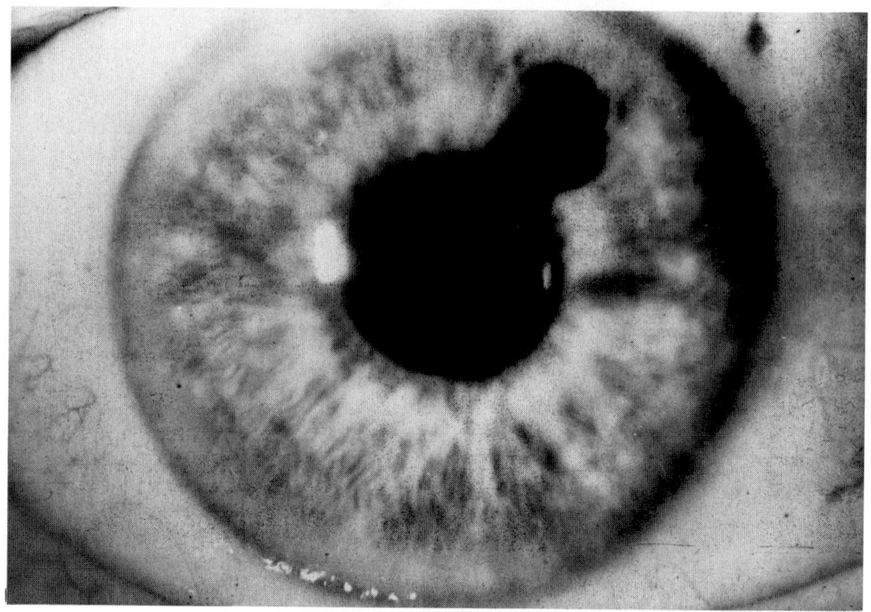

13a

Fig. 13 Fluorescein angiography of a pigmented naevus of the iris.

a. Clinical photograph.
b. Early phase.
c. Late phase. There is masking by the lesion but no leakage.

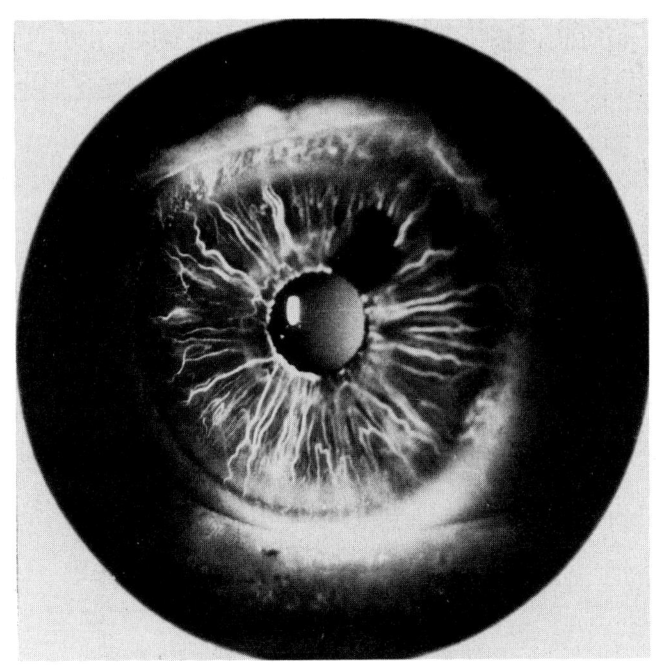

13b

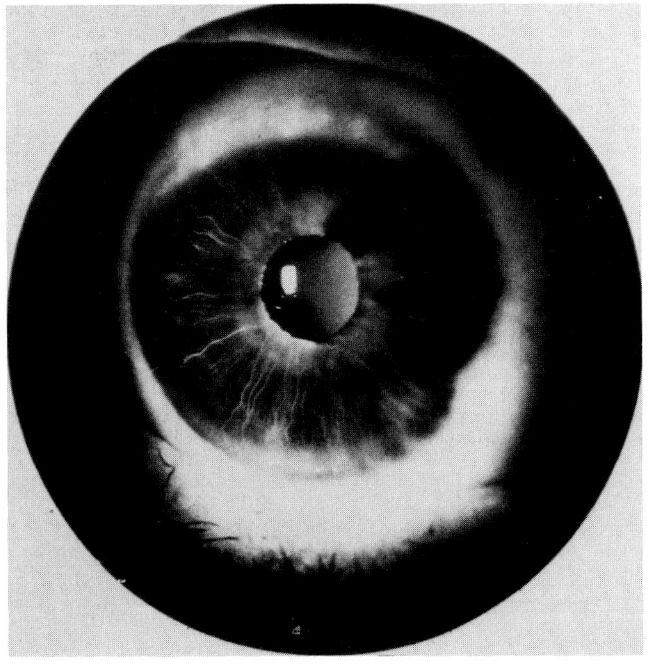

13c

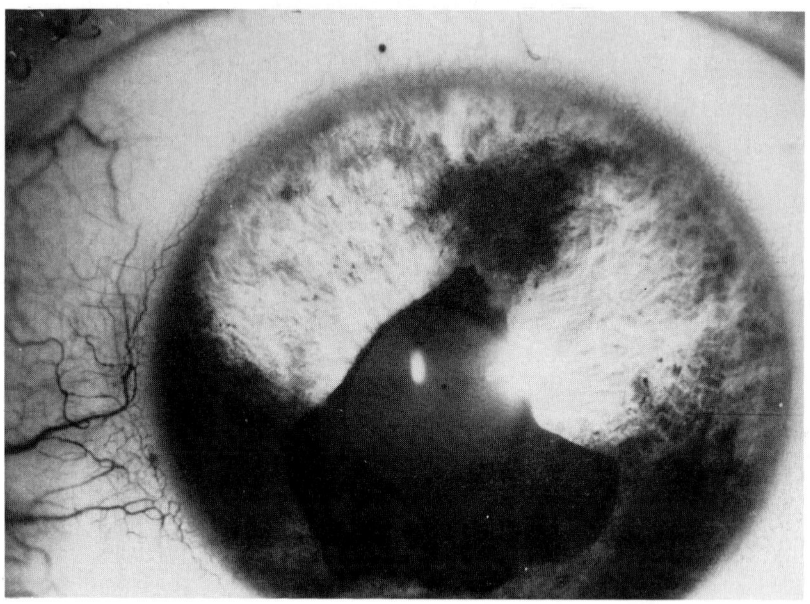

Fig. 14 Patient with an iris naevus and raised intraocular pressure.
The diagnosis was confirmed by histopathological examination of an iridectomy specimen.
(Permission of Trans.Ophthal.Soc.UK).

Fig. 15 Patient with melanolytic glaucoma. ⟶

a. Clinical picture.
b. Pathological features.
In addition to macrophages the trabecular tissue contained some tumour cells.
(Permission of Trans.Ophthal.Soc.UK).

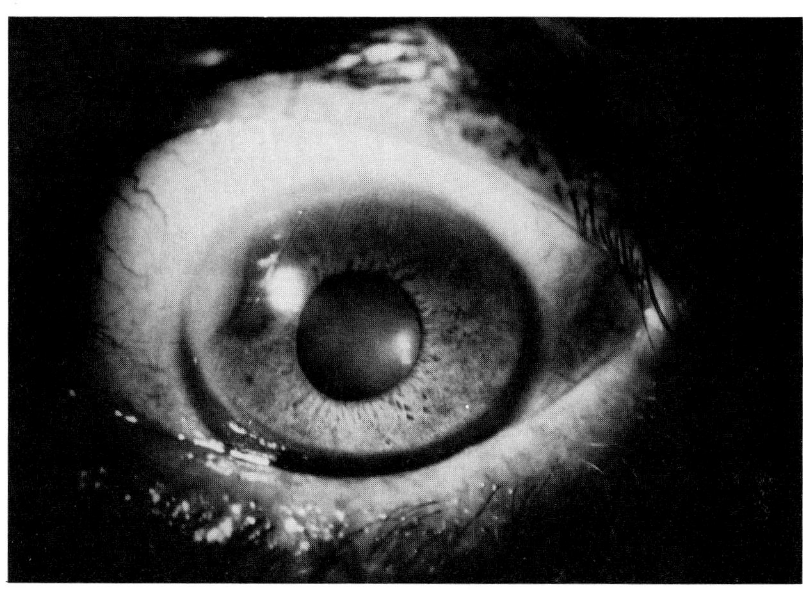

15a

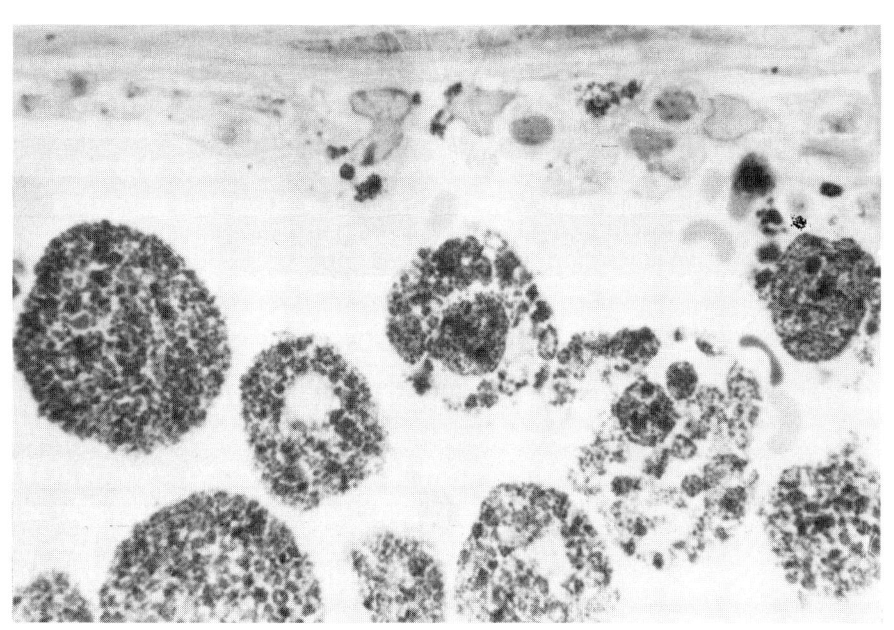

15b

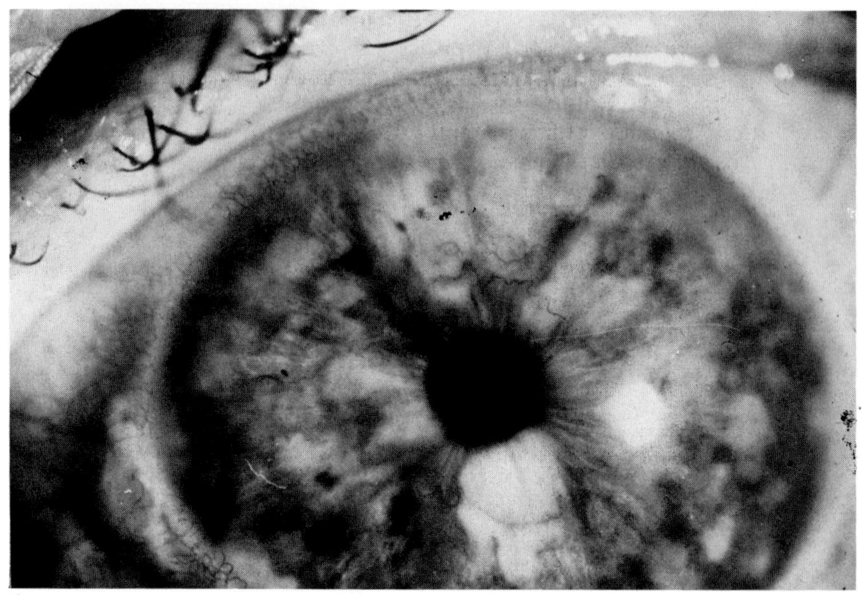

Fig. 16 Iris appearance in a patient with tapioca melanoma.
(Permission of Trans.Ophthal.Soc.UK).

Fig. 17 Fluorescein angiography of a tapioca melanoma.

⟶

a. Early phase to show distortion of iris vasculature.
b. Late phase to show gross dye leakage.

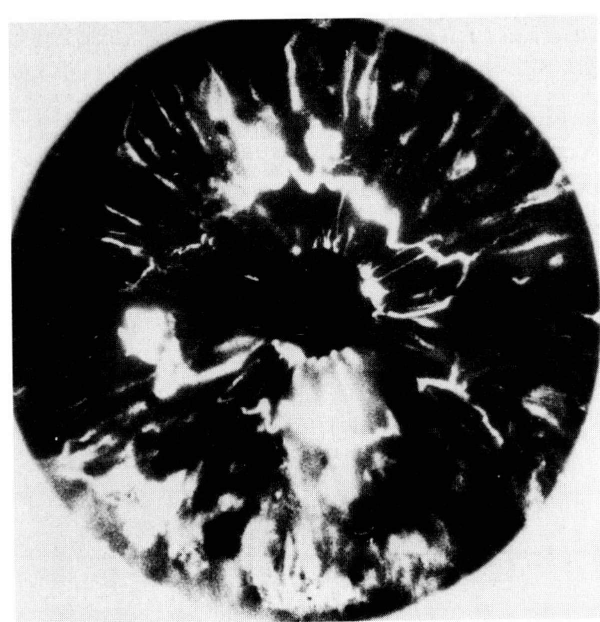

17a

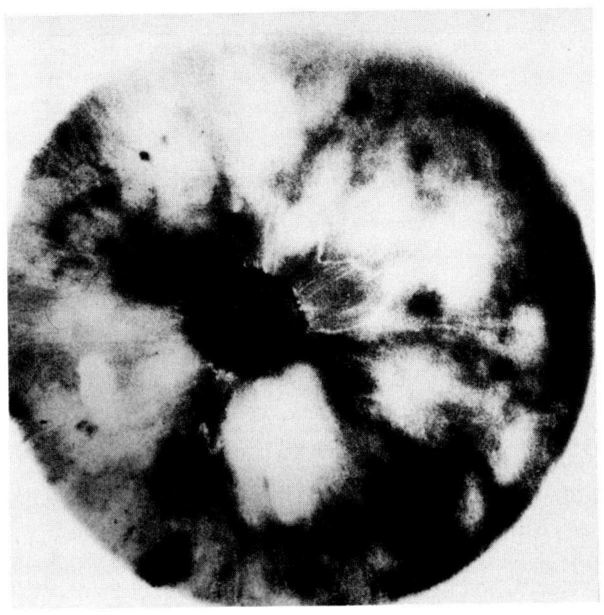

17b

outflow and causing secondary glaucoma. We have seen several examples of this condition in which the intraocular pressure has been controlled and histopathological confirmation of the diagnosis obtained by trabeculectomy (Fig. 14). At least two eyes have retained excellent visual acuity and have shown no progress in the pigmented lesion on the iris over a three and four year follow-up period respectively.

In melanomalytic glaucoma, a tumour in the iris, and it may be quite small, gives rise to a severe macrophagic reaction and these macrophages carrying pigment are scattered throughout the anterior chamber and block the drainage angle (Fig. 15). Local excision of such a tumour may avoid enucleation of the eye and may cure the glaucoma by eliminating the stimulus to macrophagic activity.

Occasionally raised intraocular pressure may present as a complication of a rarer manifestation of iris melanoma such as the tapioca melanoma (Iwamoto et al., 1972). In a case recently seen, the patient had signs of anterior uveitis and raised intraocular pressure, together with numerous pale lesions in the iris stroma (Fig. 16). Fluorescein iridograms showed grossly increased permeability of iris vessels with widespread leakage of fluorescein (Fig. 17). The ophthalmologist who saw the patient queried a granulomatous uveitis and carried out a trabeculectomy operation to control the secondary glaucoma, submitting a biopsy specimen of iris for histopathological examination. Atypical melanoma cells were identified in the specimen, establishing a diagnosis of malignant melanoma. Subsequently, the patient's intraocular pressure remained normal and there has been surprisingly little change in the appearance of the iris over a follow-up period of two and a half years. The eye retains useful vision and the patient is reluctant to consider enucleation.

Thus the diagnosis of malignant melanoma of the iris is usually made on the clinical appearance of the tumour, coupled with for example a history of increasing size of the lesion and possibly a characteristic appearance on fluorescein angiography. Treatment when the iris root is free from

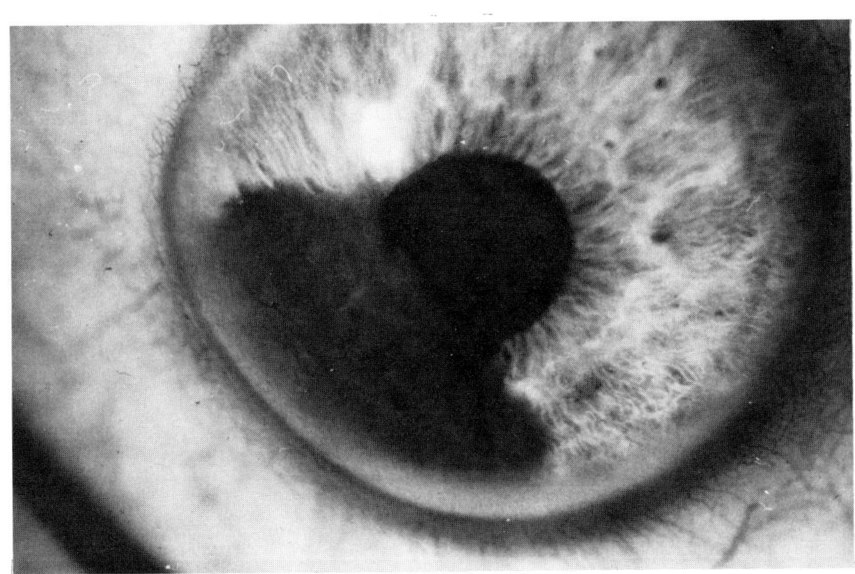

18a

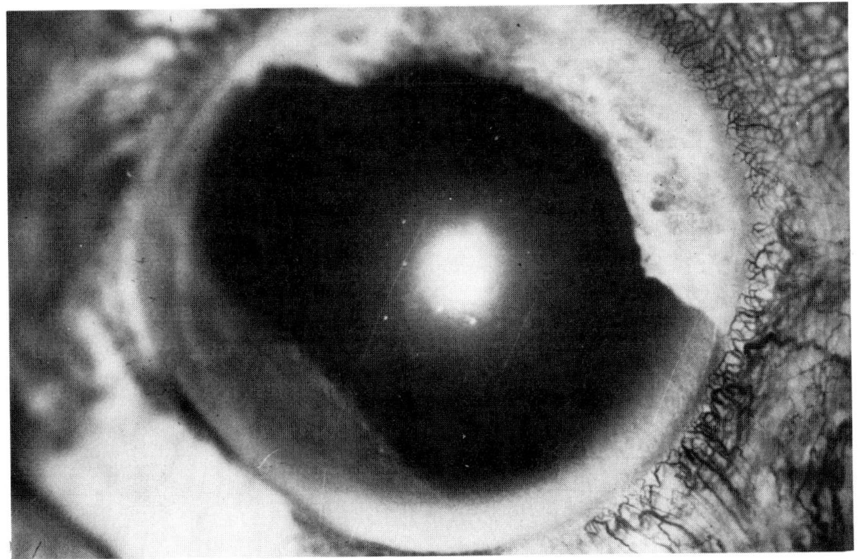

18b

Fig. 18 Malignant melanoma of the iris treated by iridectomy.

a. Pre-operative appearance.
b. Post-operative appearance.

Fig. 19 Recurrence of iris tumour after local resection.

a. Orignal tumour.
b. Post-operative appearance.
c. Recurrence on either side of iridectomy.

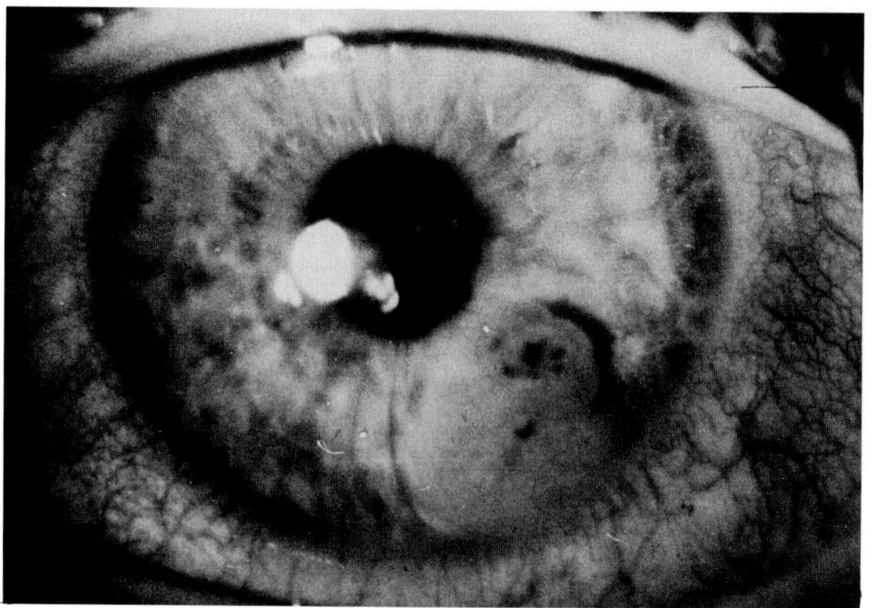

19a

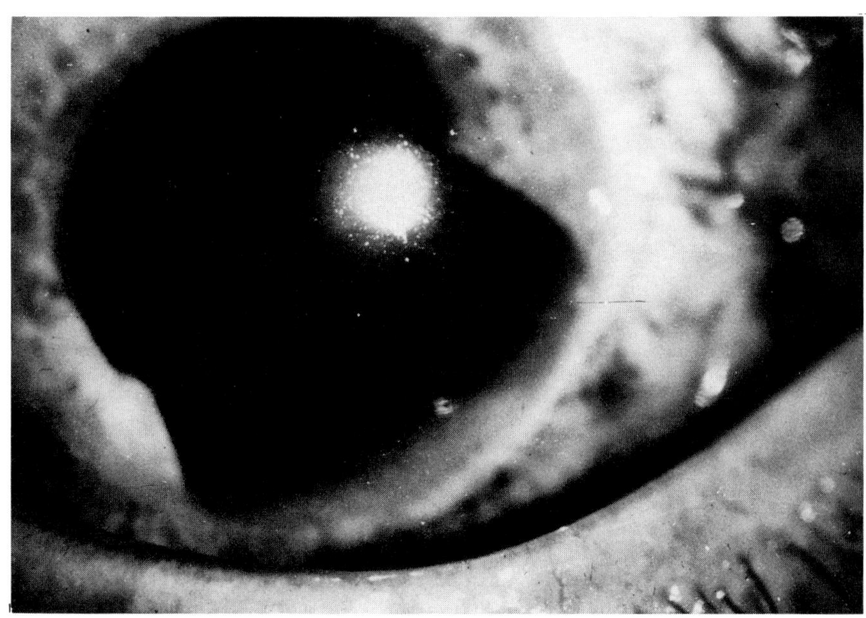

19b

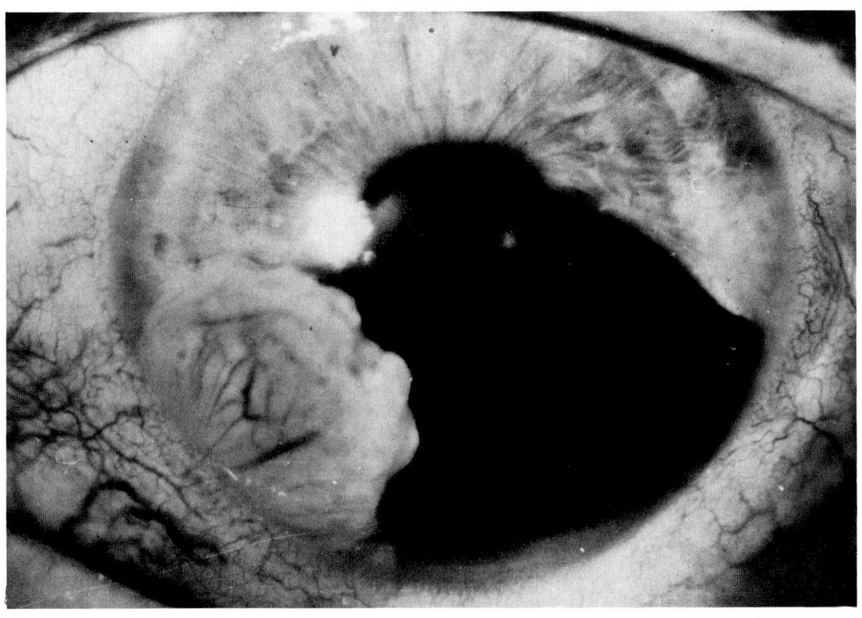

19c

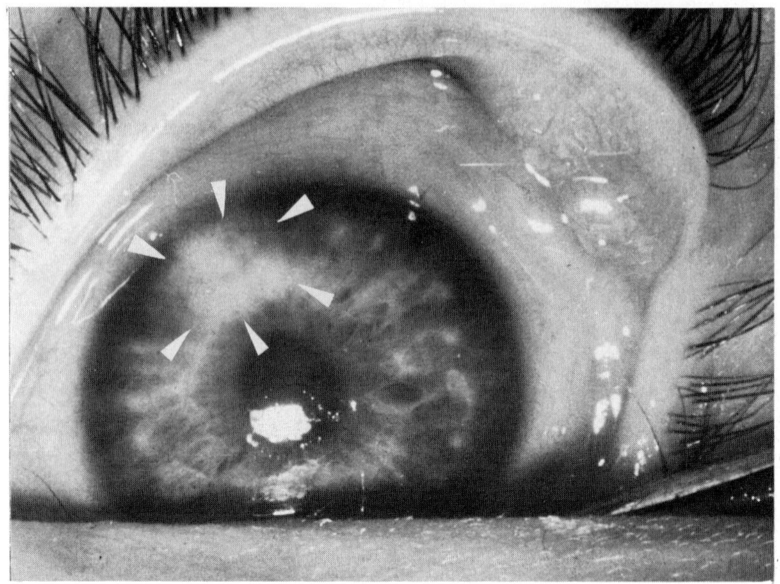

Fig. 20 Xanthogranuloma juvenile which presented with recurrent hyphaema. The lesion responded promtply to treatment with subconjunctival prednisolone.

Fig. 21 Angioma of the iris. ⟶

a. Clinical photograph.
b. Fluorescein iridogram to show vascular abnormality.

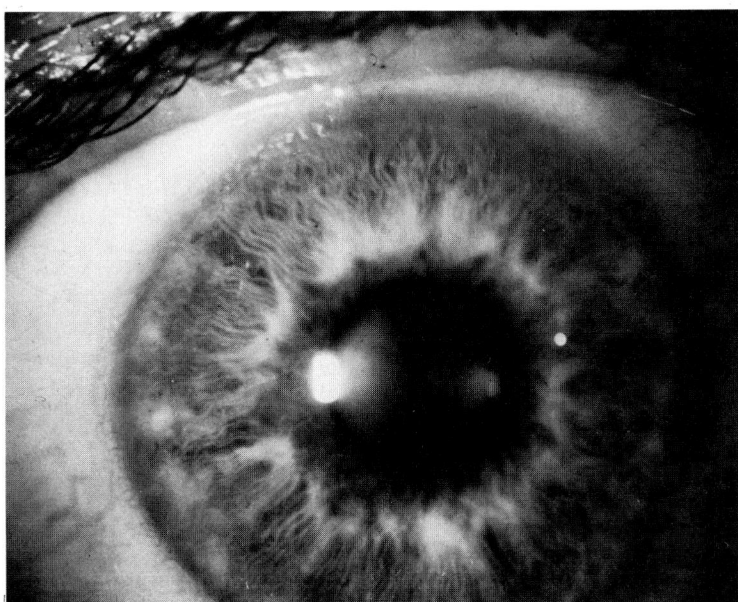

21a

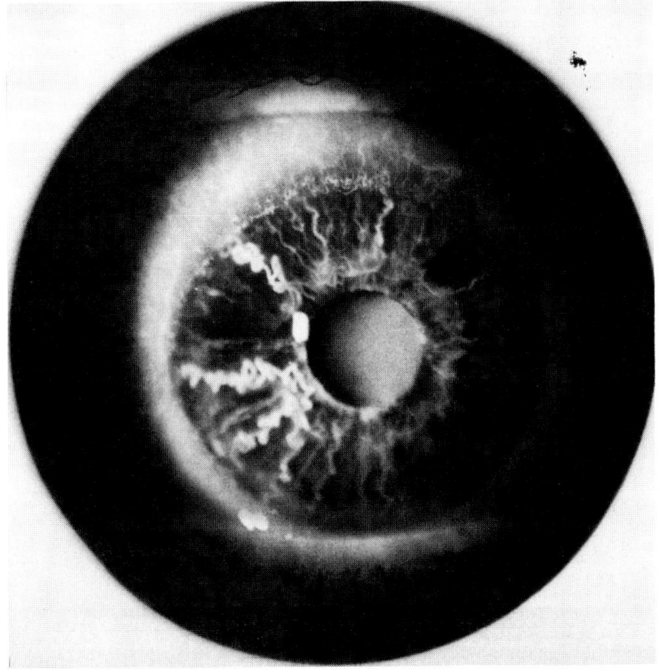

21b

invasion is sector iridectomy with a wide clearance of iris on either side of the tumour (Fig. 18). Where the root of the iris is involved one has to use a technique similar to that employed in cyclectomy and indeed the iridectomy has to be coupled with excision of the anterior ciliary body. It is important in such cases that the tissues of the angle of the anterior chamber are removed with the tumour, either by a full thickness corneoscleral resection and repair with a corneoscleral homotransplant or by a lamellar dissection preserving the superficial layers of cornea and sclera but allowing removal of the deeper layers and tissues of the angle contiguous to the tumour (Foulds, 1978). The results of such surgery are usually excellent in terms of visual acuity and survival, although just occasionally, even where wide excision of the lesion has been practised recurrence of tumour may be a problem, as has happened in one case out of thirteen cases of iris tumour treated surgically (Fig. 19). In this case the anterior ciliary body was involved and recurrence arose from the angle of the anterior chamber on either side of the surgical coloboma.

If one decides to manage a patient by observation one must be certain that adequate follow-up arrangements can be made. We have now seen three patients lost to follow-up who came back after an interval of eight to ten years, two of whom had an inoperable tumour. One of these patients had sight only in the affected eye and he is now totally blind. When seen again after being lost to follow-up for a suspected iris melanoma, vision was still 6/12, but the intraocular pressure was grossly elevated, the disc cupped and the angle of the anterior chamber completely obstructed by tumour infiltration. An attempt to treat the eye by deep X-ray therapy had some temporary benefit, but eventually the eye was lost.

My own view is that if one is in serious doubt as to whether a lesion in the iris is a melanoma or not a diagnostic excision biopsy when the lesion is small is probably the best management. The operation is relatively risk-free and an iridectomy is a small price to pay for the peace of mind

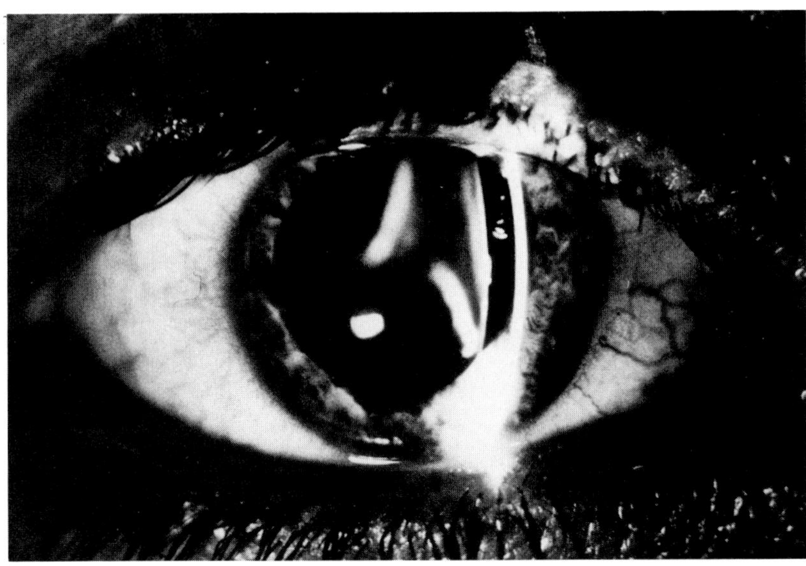

Fig. 22 Indentation of the lens by a ciliary body tumour.

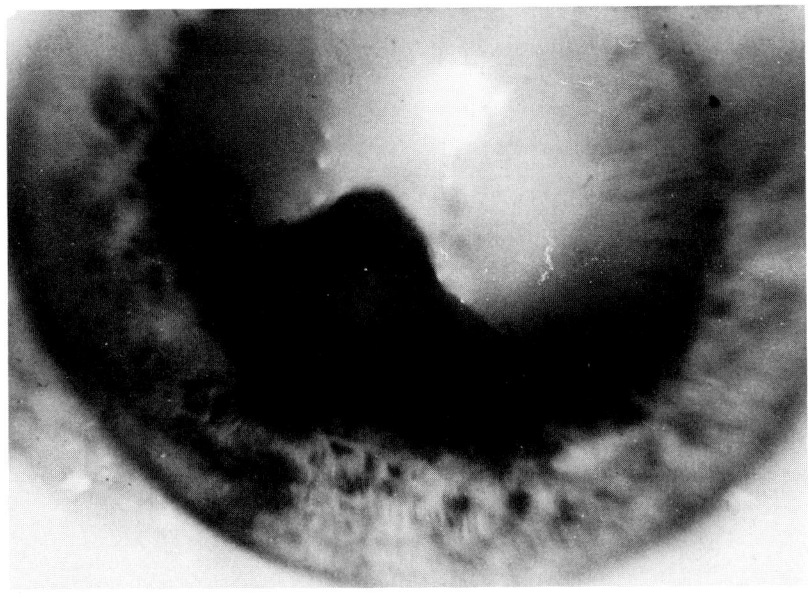

Fig. 23 Localised lens opacity in association with ciliary body tumour.

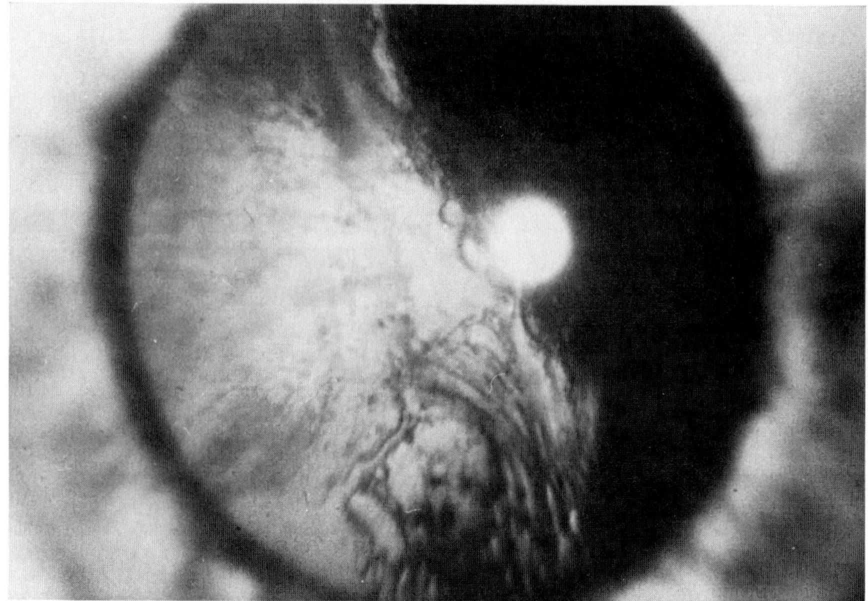

Fig. 24 Generalised lens opacity resulting from ciliary body tumour.

Fig. 25 Bilateral metastatic adenocarcinoma of the ciliary body. ⟶

a. Right eye.
b. Left eye.

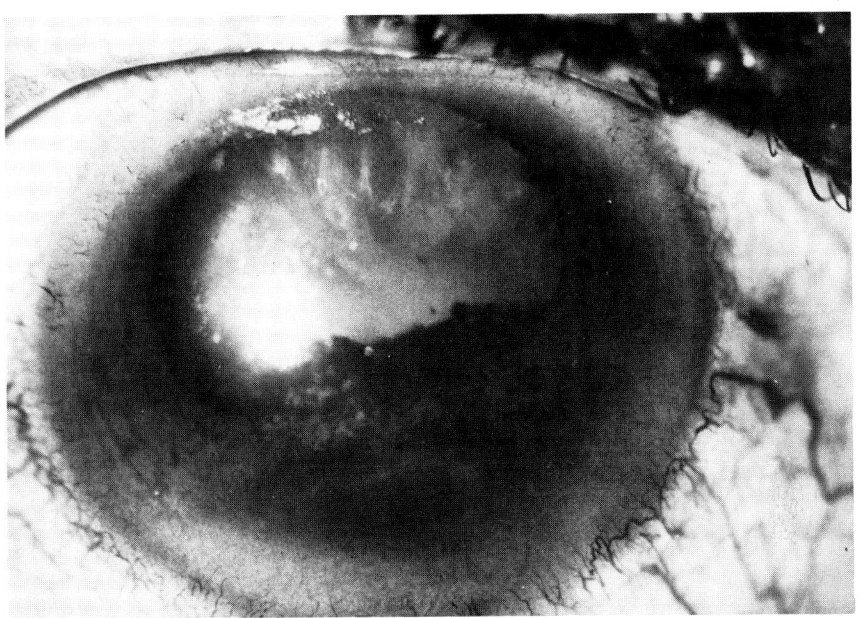

25a

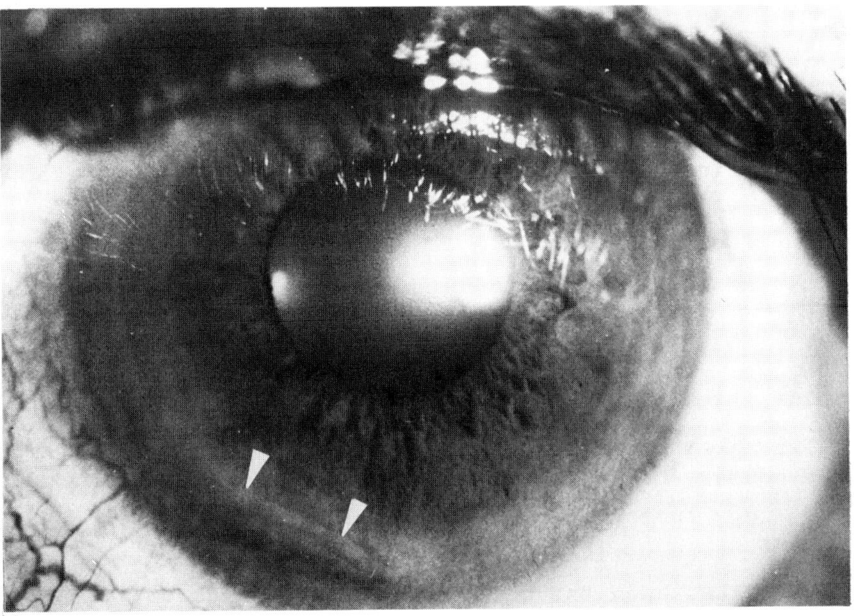

25b

of the patient and the ophthalmologist.

Before leaving tumours of the iris, occasionally one sees a baby with what appears to be a neoplasm in the iris. Rarely this is a retinoblastoma which has seeded forward from the posterior segment and equally rarely the lesion turns out to be xanthogranuloma juvenile (Fig. 20). These latter lesions may occur in the presence or absence of raised serum cholesterol and characteristically respond dramatically to treatment with subconjunctival corticosteroids. Their usual presentation is spontaneous hyphaema. Another rare cause of spontaneous hyphaema is angioma of the iris. This may be part of a Sturge-Weber syndrome or occasionally may present as a solitary abnormality. Fluorescein angiography may show grossly dilated tortuous vessels in the iris (Fig. 21).

Turning now to the consideration of ciliary body tumours, almost half of these appear to originate in the ciliary body, while the remainder involve the ciliary body secondarily by spreading anteriorly from the related choroid or occasionally posteriorly from a tumour originating in the peripheral iris.

Expansion of the ciliary body at an early stage in its development may slacken the pull of the zonule and give rise to an astigmatic error of refraction and blurred vision. Later the tumour may indent the lens or lead to its subluxation (Fig. 22). Cataract is also a common complication. The opacity may be localised and restricted to the area abutting the tumour (Fig. 23), or more generalised, and possibly associated with a disturbance of aqueous production and consequent interference with the metabolism of the lens (Fig. 24).

Blurring of vision related to abnormalities in the lens is the commonest reason for patients to present with tumours of the ciliary body. In a study of thirty-nine cases of ciliary body tumour, cataract or lens dislocation was present in twenty-six (sixty-seven per cent).

By far and away the commonest tumour of the ciliary body is the malignant melanoma. It has however to be distinguished from secondary metastatic tumours and malignant tumours of the ciliary epithelium such as adenocarcinoma.

Benign tumours of the ciliary body include benign adenoma of the ciliary epithelium (Chang et al., 1979), melanocytoma (Bowers, 1964) and in childhood, diktyoma. All of these tumours may be locally destructive, although they may not metastasise. As a rule the true nature of the lesion is only discovered on histopathological examination. From the patient's point of view this pathological diagnosis is better established on a locally excised specimen than on an enucleated globe. A most important differential diagnosis in the case of ciliary body tumours is anterior choroidal detachment and detachment of the ciliary body such as is seen in the uveal effusion syndrome.

The rarely seen diktyoma is an epithelial tumour of the ciliary body with histological features reminiscent of retinoblastoma. It occurs in childhood and is said to be pale in colour and capable of filling the eye with tumour, although not metastasising. To date I have not seen such a case personally.

In the case of secondary tumours, bilaterality is highly suggestive of this diagnosis (Fig. 25). Where a secondary tumour is unilateral there may be no certain way of differentiating it from a primary tumour unless one can identify a primary lesion elsewhere.

In the case of malignant tumours of the ciliary body, important signs are the co-existence of an exudative retinal detachment (Fig. 26) and dilatation and tortuosity of the overlying episcleral vessels, the so-called "sentinel" vessels (Fig. 27). Sentinel vessels were present in twenty-one out of thirty-nine cases of ciliary body tumour which we assessed from this point of view (fifty-four per cent).

Occasionally the presence of visible extraocular extension makes the diagnosis of malignancy inescapable (Fig. 28), although even here there may be difficulty if the ciliary body tumour has arisen in an eye exhibiting congenital melanosis oculi, as was the case in a thirteen year-old girl with a large malignant melanoma of the ciliary body and

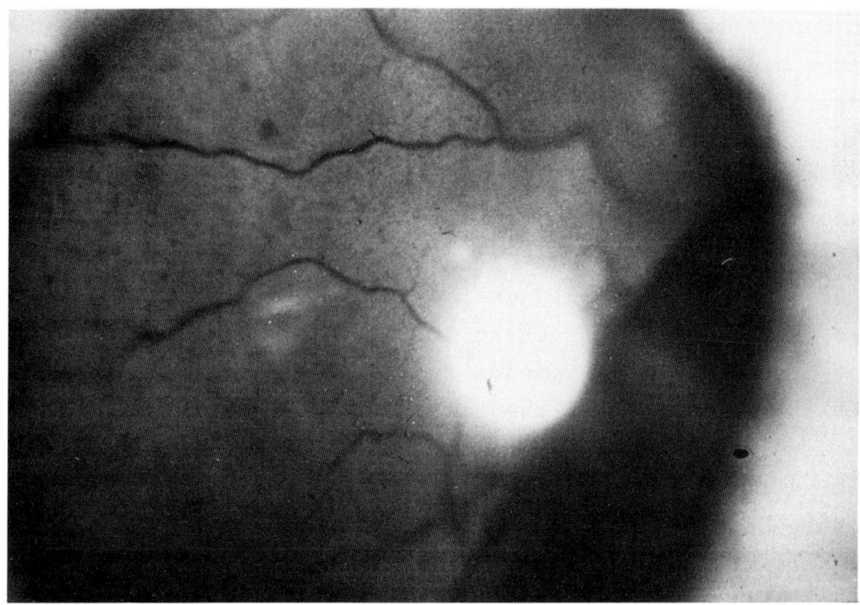

Fig. 26 Retinal detachment complicating ciliary body tumour.

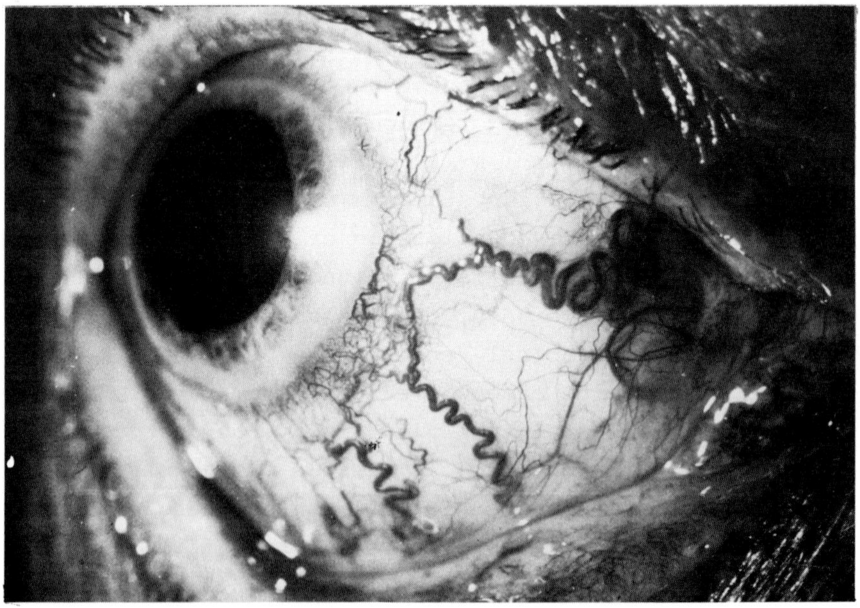

Fig. 27 Dilated episcleral "sentinel" vessels in a patient with a tumour of the ciliary body.

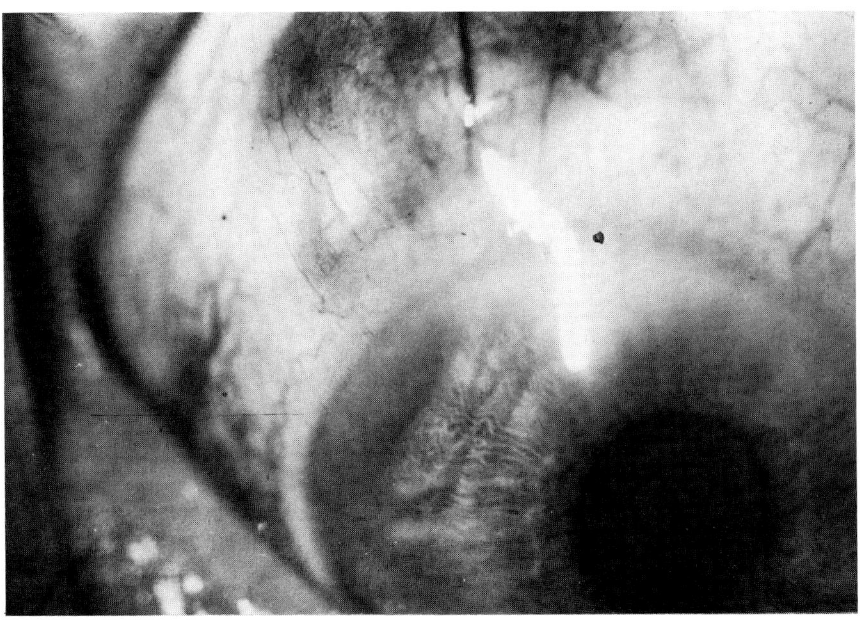

Fig. 28 Visible extraocular extension of ciliary body tumour.

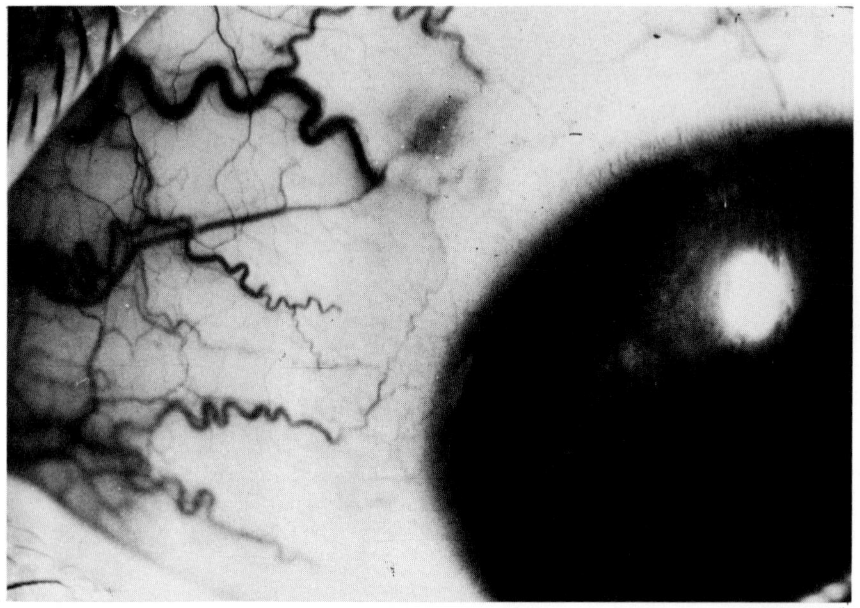

Fig. 29 Presumed extraocular spread of ciliary body tumour in a girl of thirteen years.

Fig. 30 Fluorescein angiography in same patient as in figure 29. →

a. Early filling phase.
b. Late filling phase; the apparent extraocular extension is non-fluorescent.

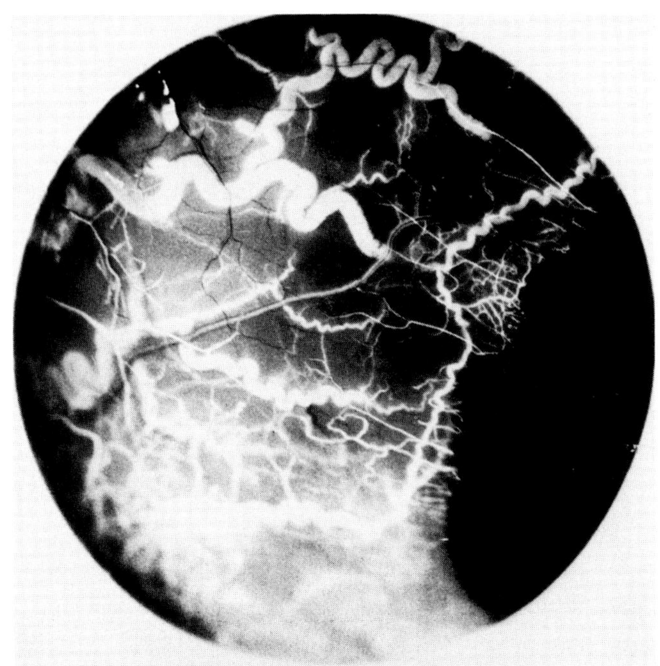

30a

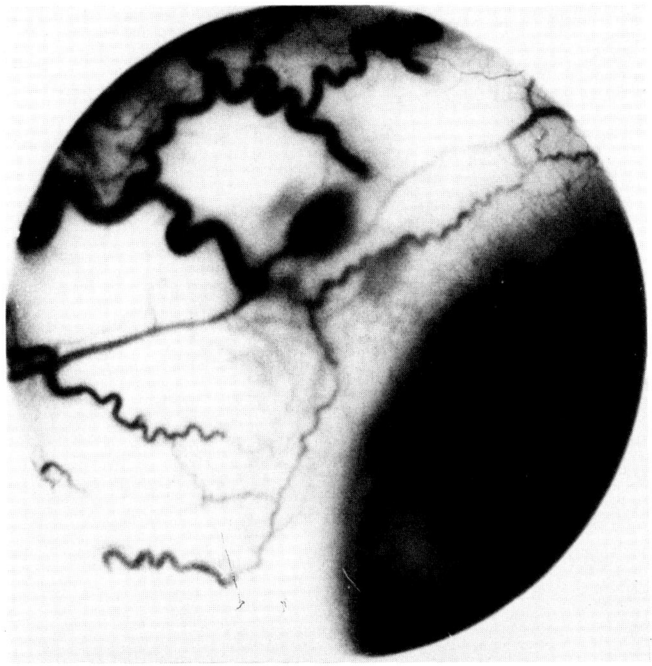

30b

possible extraocular spread (Fig. 29). Fluorescein angiography showed that the scleral lesion did not fluoresce (Fig. 30) and histology of the locally resected specimen confirmed the presence of benign congenital ocular melanosis.

Depending on its position within the ciliary body a tumour may be entirely situated behind the iris so that the angle of the anterior chamber is normal on gonioscopy or the iris may be pushed forwards so that the angle is closed for a variable distance. Occasionally the root of the iris is displaced centrally so that the tumour is easily identified in the anterior chamber (Fig. 31). The pupil in these cases undergoes the same distortion as in traumatic iridodialysis.

In general, tumours of the ciliary body appear dark in colour but often have a mottled greyish-brown appearance with pigment aggregation and dispersion. Frequently the presence of an abnormal vasculature is visible on slit-lamp microscopy and sometimes there is haemorrhage on the surface of the tumour (Fig. 32).

Transillumination is of course positive in the case of tumours in contradistinction to anterior uveal effusion where the lesion transilluminates well. Transillumination can be used in two ways. Firstly, if the transilluminator is placed on the sclera over the tumour the pupil will not light up if the lesion is solid. This is conventional transillumination. Secondly, if a very bright fibre optics transilluminator is applied to the cornea with the pupil dilated a shadow of the tumour may be cast on the sclera, indicating the size of the tumour and helping the decision as to whether or not the lesion is suitable for local resection. Technicallly this is diaphanoscopy.

Fluorescein angiography of tumours of the ciliary body is technically more difficult than iridography or straightforward angiography of lesions of the posterior fundus. Malignant tumours however, whether primary or secondary, show a characteristic mottled hyperfluorescence with late leakage (Fig. 33).

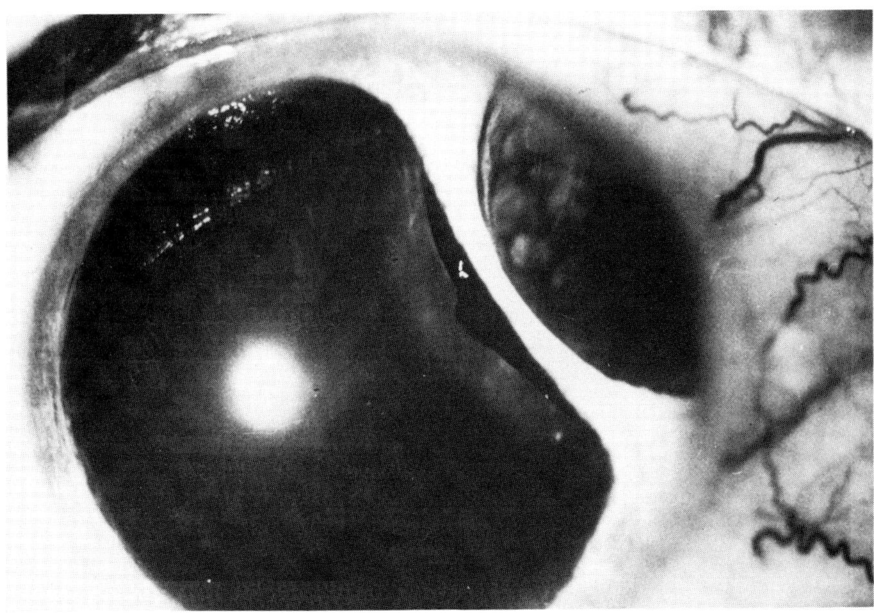

Fig. 31 Displacement of root of iris by large ciliary body melanoma.

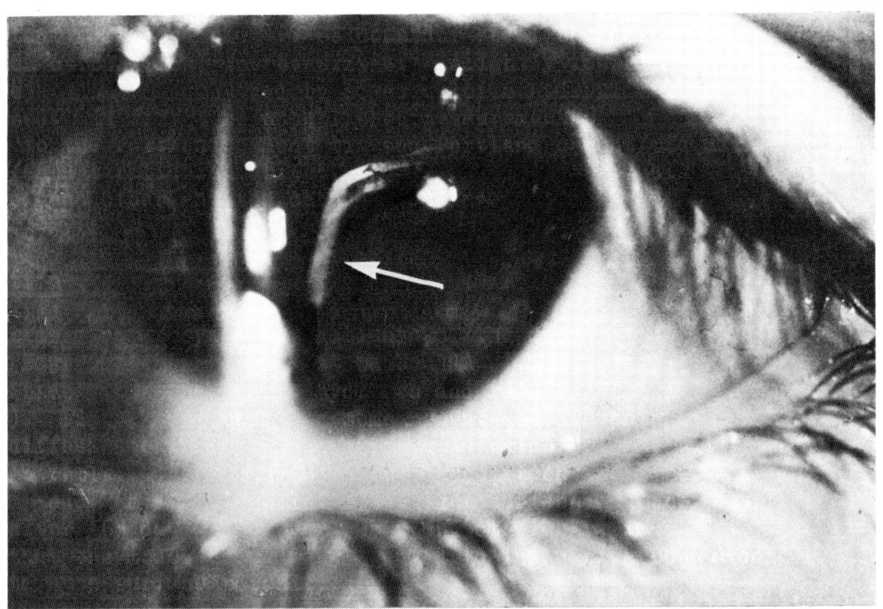

Fig. 32 Slit-lamp appearance of ciliary body tumour showing haemorrhage on its surface.

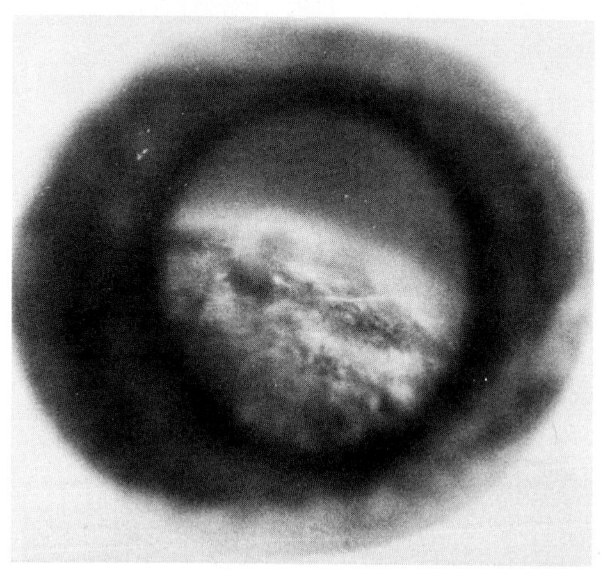

Fig. 33 Fluorescein angiogram of ciliary body tumour showing characteristic mottled staining in late frames.

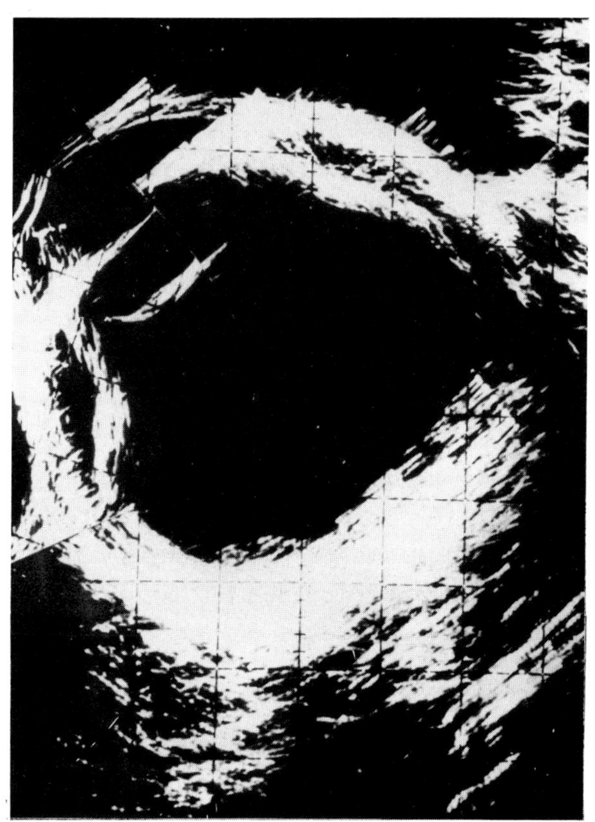

Fig. 34 Ultrasonic appearance of peripheral uveal effusion. The cystic nature of the lesion is easily distinguished from that of a solid tumour.

^{32}P uptake tests are valuable where there is doubt about the diagnosis. In our experience (Moseley and Foulds, 1980) malignant tumours show more than an eighty per cent increase in uptake at forty-eight hours compared to control sites and often the difference is in excess of two hundred per cent. Non-malignant lesions show no significant difference at all or in some conditions including uveal effusion the uptake is increased in the range forty to sixty per cent compared with control values. The diagnosis of ciliary body tumours is rarely in doubt on clinical grounds and we no longer use the ^{32}P test as a routine. It can however give useful supportive evidence if it is clearly negative or strongly positive.

Of all the ancillary investigations, ultrasound is perhaps the most valuable (Foulds, 1983a), not only in confirming the diagnosis of a solid tumour, for the appearances of a cystic lesion, or a peripheral choroidal detachment are easily distinguished (Fig. 34) from a tumour, but in defining its size, and its posterior extent in relation to whether or not it is suitable for local excision (Fig. 35).

For more posteriorly situated tumours, ultrasound may also alert one to the possibility of extraocular extension.

Characteristically, a melanoma, or other solid tumour, shows numerous echoes on B-scan ultrasonography and the highly absorptive nature of the tumour is evidenced by the decreased amplitude of these echoes as the ultrasound beam penetrates the tumour. This leads to the appearance of acoustic shadowing where the sclera may appear to be excavated, an appearance which has to be distinguished from extraocular spread, although this may be difficult in tumours of the ciliary body and anterior choroid where ultrasonic imaging is difficult (Fig. 36).

A case previously reported (Foulds, 1983a) illustrates the value of ultrasound. The patient presented with a dome-shaped mass inferiorly in the ciliary body and anterior choroid with signs of anterior uveitis. Fluorescein angiography showed considerable hyperfluorescence, but no late leakage. Transillumination showed that the lesion was lucent.

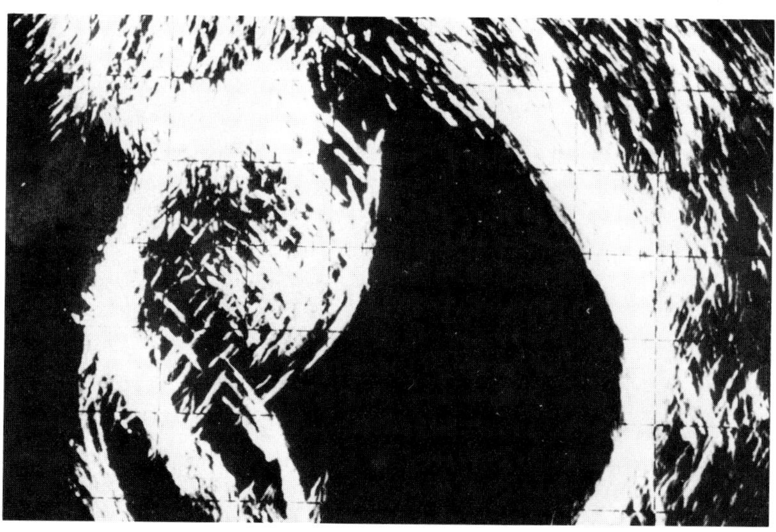

Fig. 35 Ultrasonic appearance of ciliary body tumour. There are numerous intralesional echoes.

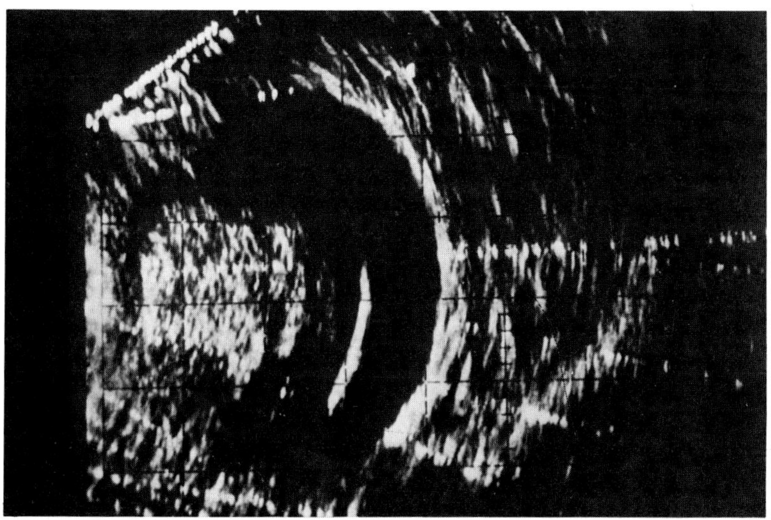

Fig. 36 Acoustic shadowing in a ciliary body and anterior choroidal melanoma which masked an extraocular extension.

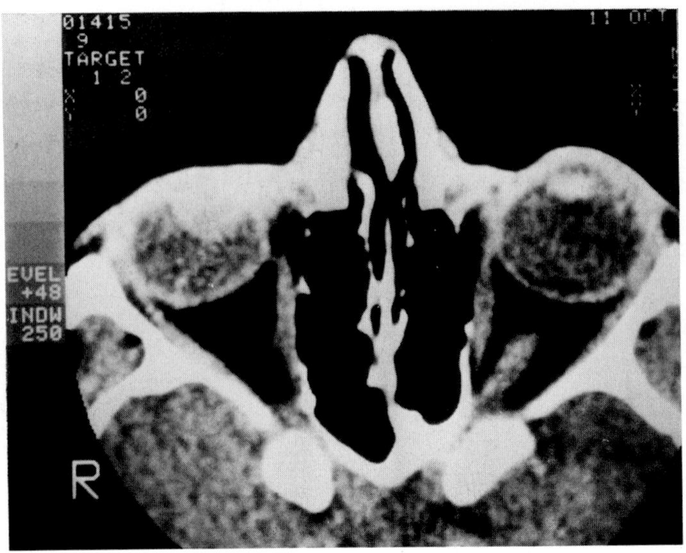

Fig. 37 High resolution CT scan of intraocular tumour involving the ciliary body.

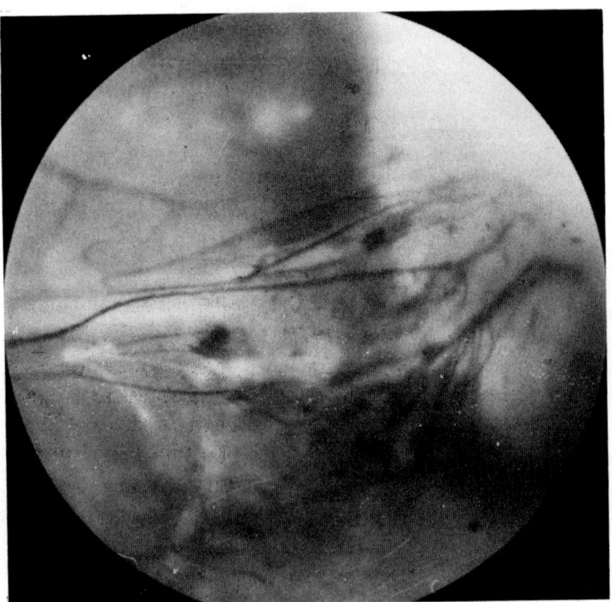

Fig. 38 Traction detachment of retina complicating local resection of a melanoma involving the ciliary body and anterior choroid.

A series of B-scan ultrasonograms however showed that the anterior part of the tumour was cystic but the deeper parts of the lesion contained a solid tumour and on this basis, local resection was carried out and confirmed the presence of an underlying malignant melanoma.

Recently we have been exploring the possibility of using high definition CT scanning in the evaluation of intraocular tumours and certainly the new generation of CT scanners provides sufficient resolution for the identification and determination of the size of such tumours (Fig. 37).

In terms of management of tumours of the ciliary body, the main options lie between local resection of the tumour and enucleation of the eye, with local radiation as a possible alternative in rare cases. In my view the presence of raised intraocular pressure is an absolute contra-indication to local excision, for in ciliary body tumours this almost certainly signifies widespread involvement of the canal of Schlemm. The decision as to whether the tumour is treatable by local resection tends therefore to depend almost entirely on the size of the tumour. From experience based on ninety-one local resections, forty-four of which involved the ciliary body, the maximum amount of ciliary body that can be resected without giving rise to complications such as hypotony or secondary glaucoma is about one third. If a tumour is centred in the ciliary body this means a tumour of about 10 mm in diameter. If however the lesion is in the anterior choroid then a tumour of 13-14 mm in diameter may be resected without sacrificing more than a third of the ciliary body. Occasionally, for example, in the case of an only eye it is justifiable to exceed this limit and recently I excised a 17 x 16 mm tumour involving the anterior choroid and ciliary body in a patient who had severe myopic choroido-retinal degeneration in the other eye. With such large tumours however the outlook in terms of vision and prognosis for survival is much less certain (Foulds, 1983b).

Following cyclectomy there is a high incidence of cataract. In many cases, of course, some degree of cataract is present pre-operatively, but this may progress to a mature cataract during the first or second post-operative year, preventing adequate visualisation of the surgical coloboma. In such cases, cataract extraction is required, both for visual purposes and to aid follow-up, and technically may be difficult in eyes which have previously undergone cyclectomy. Where a large part of the ciliary body and the related angle is removed it is now my practice to remove the lens at the time of the original operation.

The other problem with large cyclectomies is the risk of post-operative bleeding into the vitreous gel, with subsequent development of traction bands and retinal detachment (Fig. 38). All extensive cyclectomies are accompanied by a formal vitrectomy to try to prevent this complication.

Post-operatively, eyes which have had an extensive resection of the ciliary body and anterior choroid, tend to be slower to settle than eyes undergoing posterior choroidectomy, but overall the visual results of local surgery for tumours in these two situations are comparable. In a recent follow-up study (Foulds, 1983b), fifteen out of twenty-six eyes (sixty-nine per cent) undergoing anterior choroidectomy retained a visual acuity within two Snellen lines of the presenting acuity, compared with eighteen out of twenty-eight eyes (sixty-four per cent) undergoing posterior choroidectomy. Not unexpectedly, the visual results in cases of iris tumour or small lesions of the anterior ciliary body are excellent, normal or near-normal vision being retained in most cases.

To summarise, a diagnosis of iris tumour can usually be made on clinical grounds alone, although in doubtful cases, ancillary investigations may be necessary. In the case of iris tumours, if there is doubt about whether or not the lesion is malignant, it is probably reasonable to consider sector iridectomy as a diagnostic and curative procedure, as it may be difficult to maintain adequate longterm follow-up of such patients. In the case of ciliary body tumours, the important differentiation between a malignant tumour and a peripheral choroidal detachment or haemorrhage has always to be borne in mind. We have seen a number of eyes referred to our pathology service which have been excised for simple lesions of this sort, in the mistaken belief that the eye harboured an inoperable ciliary body tumour. In cases of ciliary body tumour, it is important to use the whole range of diagnostic aids which are now available, if tragic mistakes are to be avoided.

Acknowledgements

I wish to thank the many ophthalmologists who have referred cases to me. I am deeply grateful to Mrs. A. Currie for her excellent photographic assistance, and to Miss O.M. Rankin and Mrs J. Murray for secretarial assistance.

References

Ashton, N. Primary tumours of the iris. Brit.J.Ophthal. 48: 650-668, 1964.

Bowers, J.R. Melanocytoma of the ciliary body. Arch. Ophthal. 71: 649-652, 1964.

Chang, M., Shields, J.A. and Watchel, D.L. Adenoma of the pigment epithelium of the ciliary body simulating a malignant melanoma. Amer.J.Ophthal. 88: 40-44, 1979.

Cheng, H., Bron, A.J. and Easty, D. A study of iris masses by fluorescein angiography. Trans.Ophthal.Soc.UK 91: 199-205, 1971.

Font, R.L., Reynolds, A.M. and Zimmerman, L.E. Diffuse malignant melanoma of the iris in the naevus of Ota. Arch.Ophthal. 77: 513-518, 1967.

Foulds, W.S. Techniques for the local excision of ciliary body and choroidal tumours. South African J.Ophthal. 5: 41-47, 1978.

Foulds, W.S. Ultrasound in the management of intraocular tumours. In: Ophthalmic Ultrasonography, Eds. Hillman, J.S. and LeMay, M.M. W. Junk, The Hague, 1983a.

Foulds, W.S. Current options in the management of choroidal melanoma. Trans.Ophthal.Soc.UK 103: 28-34, 1983b.

Foulds, W.S. and Lee, W.R. The significance of glaucoma in the management of the melanomas of the anterior segment. Trans.Ophthal.Soc.UK 103: 59-63, 1983.

Greite, J.H. Fluorography of iris tumors. In: Fluorescein Angiography, Proc.Int.Symp.Fluorescein Angioraphy, Tokyo 1972, ed. K. Shimizu. Igaku Shoin Ltd., Tokyo 1974, pp. 319-331.

Hagler, W.S., Jarrett, W.H. and Humphrey, W.T. The radioactive phosphorus uptake test in the diagnosis of uveal melanoma. Arch.Ophthal. 83: 548-557, 1970.

Hodes, B.L., Gildenhar, M. and Choromokos, E. Fluorescein angiography in pigmented iris tumors. Arch.Ophthal. 97: 1086-1088, 1979.

Iwamoto, T., Reese, A.B. and Mund, M.L. Tapioca melanoma of the iris. Part 2. Electron microscopy of the melanoma cells compared with normal iris melanocytes. Amer.J. Ophthal. 74: 851-861, 1972.

Kottow, M. Fluorescein angiographic behaviour of iris masses. Ophthalmologica (Basel) 174: 217-223, 1977.

Moseley, H. and Foulds, W.S. Observations on the ^{32}P uptake test. Brit.J.Ophthal. 64: 186-190, 1980.

Naumann, G., Yanoff, M. and Zimmerman, L.E. Relation of congenital ocular melanocytosis and neurofibromatosis to uveal melanomas. Arch.Ophthal. 77: 333-336, 1967.

Scheie, H.G. and Yanoff, M. Iris nevus (Cogan-Reese) syndrome. A cause of unilateral glaucoma. Arch.Ophthal. 93: 963-970, 1975.

Shields, J.A. Accuracy and limitations of the ^{32}P test in the diagnosis of ocular tumors. An analysis of 500 cases. Ophthalmology 85: 950-966, 1978.

Yanoff, M. Mechanisms of glaucoma in eyes with uveal malignant melanomas. Int.Ophthal.Clin. 12/1: 51-62, 1972.

Yanoff, M. and Scheie, H.G. Melanolytic glaucoma. Arch.Ophthal. 84: 471-473, 1970.

TREATMENT OF ORBITAL TUMOURS
PRINCIPLES OF ONCOLOGICAL SURGERY

E.A. van Slooten

Some axioms for tumour surgery.

- Cells from all malignant and from some benign tumours can be implanted in any recent wound area and on every serosal surface.
- Several tumours have a specific way of local spread with important technical implications, e.g.

  adenoid cystic carcinoma
  rodent ulcer type of basal cell carcinoma,
  soft tissue sarcoma

  but often the local type of spread can only be ascertained by adequate biopsy.
- Pressure on a tumour may cause local (tissue spaces, serosa etc.) spread and distant (blood borne) dissemination.
- Whenever tumour tissue is apparent at the periphery of a surgical specimen or at the bottom of a rent or inadvertently entered tissue plane, there is a risk of tumour implantation (iatrogenic dissemination).
- No definitive surgery for a possibly malignant lesion should be undertaken without previous morphological examination whenever it is technically possible to obtain representative material.

Space-occupying conditions in the orbit may arise from structures within the orbit or from surrounding structures, skin, bone, mucosa of the nose and sinuses etc. encroaching on the orbital content. We shall limit this discussion to proliferative lesions arising from the content and bony wall of the orbit, the eyelids and conjunctiva.

Oosterhuis, A. (ed.), Ophthalmic tumors.

ISBN 90-6193-528-8. Printed in the Netherlands.

Invasive diagnostic procedures

1. The development of tomography, angiography and ultrasonic echography has provided us with methods to assess the size, localization and often the point of origin as well as the gross nature (solid, cystic, vascular) of space-occupying conditions. This allows exact targeting of all procedures for obtaining morphological material before and also at the time they are being performed.
   Although thin needle aspiration for cytological examination is essentially invasive, the involved tissue damage and risk - if performed by an experienced hand - are so slight, that this method will not be included in "invasive procedures".

Some examples

1.1. When a formal biopsy of an intra-orbital lesion is indicate (inadequate material obtained at repeated cytological aspiration, equivocal result, localization problems) the approach should be planned so as to avoid damage to intra-orbital structures. This is relatively simple in the anterior part of the orbit where a direct approach is usually feasible, but in the posterior part the best way to reach a lesion may be to separate part of the peri-orbita from the bone (as in exenteration, fig.1) and then to incise it where the process is localized.
   When performing the biopsy an attempt should be made to remove material at the border of the lesion, including normal surrounding tissue. This will enable the pathologist to distinguish infiltrative, angio-invasive and other aggressive tumour properties. Furthermore regressive changes are rare at the periphery of a solid tumour.
   Care must be taken not to damage the biopsy material by squeezing or heat. It should be realized that an open biopsy from a possibly malignant lesion must not be performed in this way if it is thought to be amenable to radical surgery by orbital exenteration because the future resection plane will unavoidably be contaminated.

Fig. 1.

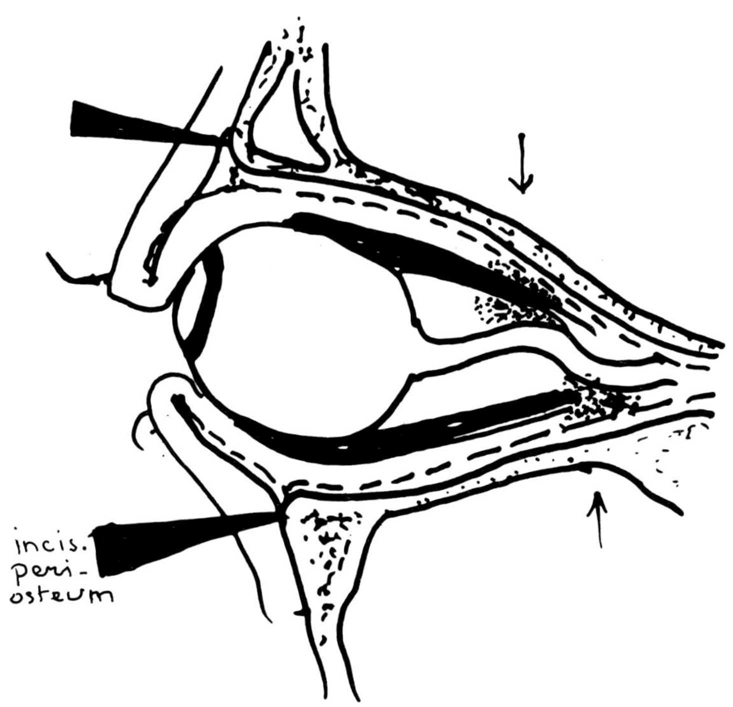

1.2. A biopsy from a lesion probably originating from the bone can often best be obtained with a 2 mm bore trephine bone drill. If performed under X-ray guidance allowing good stereoscopic orientation, nearly every site can be reached with safety except the area immediately surrounding the optic foramen. If performed with care, representative histological material can usually be obtained. Otherwise conventional surgical exploration is indicated.

1.3. For the assessment of local spread of diffusely infiltrating (mainly rodent ulcer type basal cell) carcinoma of the skin, palpation and other non-invasive methods are completely insufficient. Therefore narrow strip biopsies have to be taken in a circle around the centre of the tumour, includi skin and subcutaneous tissue down to the level of the fascia or underlying muscle. These tumours tend to grow parallel to the skin surface in long thin strands. These may easily be missed in punch biopsies. Especially in tumours of the eyelids recurring after radiotherapy, linear 5-7mm biopsies have to be taken including the whole thickness of the eyelid perpendicular to its border on either side of the tumour at least 1 cm from the palpable tumour margins (fig.2). It should be remembered that these

Fig. 2.

Pre-operative assessment of
local spread

Recurrent basal cell carcinoma
after radiotherapy

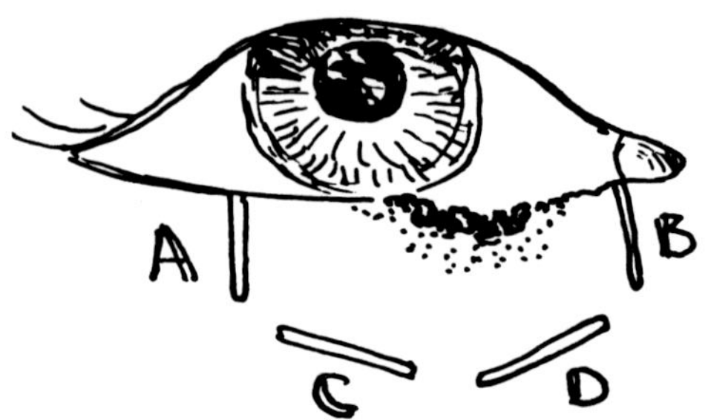

4 Linear biopsies, ± 1 mm thick
A and B. Whole thickness of eyelid.
C and D. Skin + Subcutis down to muscle.

basal cell cancers will grow in the same manner under the conjunctiva and lacrimal duct epithelium. Especially the latter direction of spread may easily be missed, giving rise to large, sometimes intractable recurrences in the lacrimal sac area.

1.4. The spread of proliferative lesions of the conjunctiva such as (pre)malignant melanosis and squamous cell epitheliosis of the verrucous or M.Bowen type is difficult to assess correctly even with the magnifier, although much easier than in similar lesions of the skin. Incipient infiltrative growth, in particular in the scar of a previous excision, easily escapes notice. Therefore even multiple biopsies will never be able to prove that invasive growth has not yet taken place, but narrow strip biopsies will indicate where a safe peripheral resection line may be found. The only way to get a reliable impressic of the nature of such a lesion is to perform a complete excision whenever feasible. Moreover, malignant progression being the rule, there is no point in waiting once the diagnosis is established.

The place for per-operative frozen section examination is extremely limited mainly due to the nature of the tissues that have to be examined (bone, loose areolar-adipose tissue, thin soft skin with very loose subcutaneous tissue etc.). Pre-operative assessment of spread therefore is of vital importance.

2. Curative surgery

2.1. The principles governing malignant tumour surgery are simple and well-known, the most important being:

- Make the exposure as wide as possible, freeing vital structures well away from the tumour boundaries.
- Avoid tumour cell spill by pressure on the tumour, placing toothed hooks on the specimen etc.
- Remove the tumour with an intact margin of healthy

surrounding tissue.

- Place marks on the specimen and corresponding radio-opaque marks in the wound area for anatomic orientation in case post-operative radiotherapy should be indicated at a specific site.

In the very limited space of the orbit the above principles can virtually only be observed in the area of the skin and eyelids and at the site of the lacrimal gland if one attempts to preserve a functioning eye.
Incidentally the great majority of tumours for which radical surgery is the treatment of choice occur in these two areas.
Radical surgery for malignant tumours, e.g. soft tissue sarcoma, at all other sites means orbital exenteration.

2.2. In the region of the eyelids it is important to know beforehand where incisions can be made with safety because immediate reconstruction is a vital factor in the preservation of the eye. Reconstruction in a contaminated area leads to extensive mutilation, complicated combined treatment and sometimes to intractable recurrence.

2.3. Tumours of the lacrimal gland can only be adequately treated after removing the latero-superior wall of the orbit and even then post-operative radiotherapy is usually indicated, the majority of malignant tumours belonging to the adenoid cystic carcinoma type with extensive growth along pre-existing structures, mainly nerves.

2.4. Melanoma, cancer of the glands of Meibom and squamous cell carcinoma of the conjunctiva should always be treated according to the rules of tumour surgery even if this entails loss of the eye. Recurrence is often intractable and may be accompanied by distant metastasis.
From the onset of treatment the pre-auricular and submandibular lymph nodes should be frequently and painstaking

examined because regional metastatic spread often occurs and may still be treated with curative intent.

3. Combined treatment

Due to the limited space, the importance of preserving the eye and also the nature of most tumours and potentially malignant proliferative conditions occurring in the orbit, in many cases combined treatment is indicated.

Some examples:

3.1. Childhood rhabdomyosarcoma.
Initial treatment with a combination of cytostatic agents followed by excision of residual tumour and another short course of chemotherapy.

3.2. Melanosis of the conjunctiva with local infiltrating melanoma.
Excision of the melanoma followed by brachytherapy.

3.3. Lacrimal gland tumour.
Wide local excision followed by a combination of an A.P. oblique megavolt radiotherapy field sparing the cornea and lens and a lateral electron beam field limited to a small segment of the eyeball.

Conclusion

Tumour surgery in the orbit should never be lightly undertaken. Even minor inaccuracies may lead to the loss of an eye or greater disfigurement.
Recurrence is often concurrent with distant metastasis. There may be a causal relationship.

MANAGEMENT OF MALIGNANT ORBITAL TUMOURS

J. E. WRIGHT

INTRODUCTION

Primary cancers of the orbit are relatively uncommon, some are indolent and locally symptomatic, others have a marked propensity for local destruction often accompanied by widespread distant metastases.

New diagnostic techniques and methods of treatment which have been introduced in recent years have had a dramatic impact upon the diagnosis and methods of management, of tumours affecting the orbit. Computerised tomography has enabled the clinician to define the position and extent of tumours within the orbit and NMR, potentially can provide information about the metabolism of different types of tumour tissue. The management of lacrimal gland tumours is now carried out by a multidisciplinary team including ophthalmologists, head and neck surgeons, neurosurgeons and plastic and reconstructive surgeons to ensure both adequate resection of tumours and reconstruction of the orbit. Most dramatic, however, has been the introduction of a combination of chemotherapy and radiation therapy in the management of rhabdomyosarcomas. Whereas formerly these tumours had a high mortality rate despite a combination of treatment with radiotherapy and exenteration, modern methods of treatment have resulted in extremely long disease-free intervals, and high rates of cure.

Rhabdomyosarcoma

This is a tumour of children and adolescents occurring from infancy up to the age of about 16 years. The most frequent age of onset is between 6 and 8 years. Although rare in adults, the neoplasm has been observed in all age groups including several patients in their eighth decade. Rhabdomyosarcoma occurs more often in males than females (ratio 3:2).

Oosterhuis, A. (ed.), Ophthalmic tumors.

ISBN 90-6193-528-8. Printed in the Netherlands.

The tumour usually grows rapidly and causes a marked local response, the signs and symptoms depend on the site of origin of the neoplasm. Anteriorly situated lesions produce localised swelling and redness of the eyelids often associated with chemosis. Children with this swelling are frequently regarded as having orbital cellulitis and are initially treated with antibiotics. However, the diagnosis soon becomes obvious for despite antibiotic therapy the mass continues to expand and there is no elevation of the white cell count. Lesions further back in the orbit will produce generalised swelling and proptosis often accompanied by oedema of the optic disc and poor vision caused by pressure of the tumour on the optic nerve. Radiographs and CT scans of the skull and orbit should be obtained and the mass biopsied at the earliest opportunity.

The tumour is usually diffuse and friable; occasionally, there is a good capsule and the inexperienced surgeon may think he is dealing with an odd dermoid cyst. However, in the majori of cases the lesion is diffuse, white or grey, and bleeds readi when sectioned. The histological features of these tumours are somewhat variable. The more differentiated lesions are termed pleomorphic whereas the more undifferentiated lesions are calle embryonal; the latter are the most common. It is important tha the diagnosis is supported by the recognition of cross striations in the cytoplasm in some of the cells. However, in some of the highly undifferentiated embryonal tumours this can be extremely difficult and may require electron-microscopy of fresh specimens so that primitive myofilamentous cells and more differentiated myofibrilorhabdomyoblasts can be recognised. The histological type does not appear to influence the prognosi What does undoubtedly influence the prognosis is early recognition and treatment.

Once the diagnosis has been made the patient should be admitted to an oncology unit for a multidisciplinary approach to the problem. In addition to the initial investigations bone scans and bone marrow aspiration studies are necessary. In the past orbital exenteration or radiotherapy was thought th best treatment for this condition.

However, over 50% of patients treated by surgery or radiotherapy alone, succumb to the disease, some with local recurrence, but the majority with distant metastases. The prognosis was particularly bad for children below the age of six. The addition of chemotherapy has markedly improved the early prognosis so that the two year survival rate has now risen to over 80%. The tumours of younger children are particularly chemosensitive so that the poorer results in the younger children are no longer seen. It is too early to know the long-term survival and complication rates of patients treated with combined chemotherapy and radiotherapy but there is as yet no evidence of later recurrences or increased morbidity.

The most effective drugs are Actinomycin D, Doxorubicin (Adriamycin), Vincristine, and Cyclophosphamide (Cytoxan). The following scheme is recommended for those patients in whom investigations show no evidence of blood borne metastases: Vincristine 1.5 mg/m^2; Actinomycin D 1.0 mg/m^2 and Cyclophosphamide 300 mg/m^2. These drugs can be given intravenously on the first day of chemotherapy and repeated seven days later. After a further seven days radiotherapy is begun and a 5,000 rads. tumour dose is administered in five to six weeks. During radiotherapy Vincristine 1.5 mg/m^2 and Cyclophosphamide 200 mg/m^2 are administered intravenously once a week. Two weeks after the end of radiotherapy Vincristine 1.5 mg/m^2, Doxorubicin 40 mg/m^2 and Cyclophosphamide 400 mg/m^2 are administered once every three weeks until the total dose of Doxorubicin reaches 400 mg. at which time Actinomycin D 1.0 mg/m^2 is substituted for Doxorubicin. This regime is continued until one year has elapsed after the start of drug treatment.

More aggressive chemotherapy is recommended for patients with evidence of distant metastases at presentation; the regime consists of the following: Vincristine 1.5 mg/m^2, Doxorubicin 40 mg/m^2, Cyclophosphamide 300 mg/m^2 administered weekly for six weeks provided the bone marrow will tolerate this. Radiotherapy is started as soon as possible during this period of intensive chemotherapy. During radiotherapy weekly injections of Vincristin and Cyclophosphamide are given as above.

If a complete remission of the disease is obtained Vincristine, Doxorubicin and Cyclophosphamide are given until the total dose of Doxorubicin reaches 400 mg/m^2 at which time Actinomycin D 1.0 mg/m^2 is substituted. This regime is continued for at least 18 months.

Exenteration of the orbit should be reserved for those patients in whom there is a recurrence of the tumour or obvious failure of the combined chemotherapy and radiotherapy to control growth of the tumour. This procedure is highly disfiguring. The initial incision is down to the orbital margin through 360° using cutting diathermy. Once the orbital margin has been reached the periosteum of the orbit can be elevated, the nasolacrimal duct cauterised, and the anterior and posterior ethmoidal arteries diathermied and the whole of the orbital contents removed. Following transection of the structures in the orbit it is essential that the orbit be thoroughly cleaned so that no tissue remains in the orbital apex. The orbit can be left to granulate but it is preferable to use a split skin graft and apply it to the bare bone of the orbital walls. In the majority of patients there is a 90% take of this type of skin graft which speeds the healing process considerably.

Lymphoma

The orbit may be the site of a primary lymphoma or the presenting site of a generalised lymphoma. It is most common in the middle aged and elderly. In children the Burkitt's lymphoma predominates; whereas in the elderly the well-differentiated lymphocytic form is the most common. Sex incidence is approximately equal except in the elderly among whom the disease is more common in females. Lymphomatous tumours within the orbit vary from well differentiated lymphocytic types of lesions, sometimes called reactive lymphoid hyperplasia through frank malignancy. Histologic interpretation of orbital biopsy material can be very difficult. Many specimens show a lymphocytic lesion in which there are no clear features of benign hyperplasia or of malignancy and are reported as lymphocytic tumours of indeterminate nature.[1] In recent surface markers have been used to determine whether the cell population is monoclonal or polyclonal in an attempt to further differentiate this group.[2] The value of these observations is still under review.

50% of patients with a histologically definite malignant lymphoma but with no evidence of dissemination developed systemic lymphoma within five years. The remainder appear to be cured by local radiotherapy alone. Chemotherapy is not needed unless or until there is dissemination. The malignant types of lymphomatous disease are often seen in the orbit as part of the generalised disease process. In a high proportion of patients in whom the biopsy shows frank malignancy evidence of systemic lymphoma is found at the time of presentation or subsequently. On the other hand, disseminated lymphoma or chronic lymphatic leukaemia occurs in only 25% of patients whose biopsy specimens are reported as indeterminate lymphocytic lesions.

The majority of lymphomatous lesions occur in the anterior part of the orbit. In most cases the mass is noticed by the patient at an early stage. There is usually a swelling of the eyelid with or without displacement of the eye. A rubbery mass which has a characteristic reddish pink appearance is usually palpable and visible beneath the conjunctiva. Pain or signs of an inflammatory reaction are usually absent, a most important point in distinguishing this type of lesion from a pseudo tumour. Tissue diagnosis is essential and a biopsy can be readily obtained either by a trans-conjunctival or trans-septal approach. It is advisable to perform full investigations for evidence of systemic spread regardless of the histological appearances. An exception can be made in the case of an elderly patient with an indeterminate tumour or a well differentiated lymphocytic lymphoma since the results of investigations are rarely positive.

Those patients discovered to have systemic lymphoma are treated with a combination of chemotherapy and radiotherapy. In the majority of patients, however, investigations are negative and these patients are treated by radiotherapy. A

A tumour dose of up to 3,000 rads. in three weeks achieves virtually 100% local control regardless of the histological type of tumour. Rapid regression occurs and there are rarely any local complications of treatment. The prognosis depends on the histologic type. The majority of well differentiated lymphocytic lymphomata and indeterminate lymphocytic tumours do not disseminate; those that do, often run a protracted and relatively benign course as chronic lymphatic leukaemia or cutaneous lymphoma.

Lacrimal Gland Tumours

Tumours arising from the lacrimal gland are relatively uncommon but the ophthalmologist who initially sees the patient can materially alter the prognosis by his decisions about management. Treatment of these lesions was thought to be uniformly poor until 1948 when Godtfredsen[3] showed that benign tumours, if totally excised, had a good prognosis whereas malignant tumours did not. He based his histological classification on that used by Ringertz[4] for salivary gland tumours. Since then other authors using the classification devised by Foote and Frazel[5] have confirmed these findings. It is important to recognise benign mixed cell tumours on clinical grounds so that a biopsy can be avoided and the tumour, together with the whole of the lacrimal gland, is removed in toto. Font and Gammell[6] analysed a large series of lacrimal tumour specimens referred to the A.F.I.P. from a large number of centres. They noted an incidence of recurrence within five years of 32% if the tumour underwent biopsy before excision, but only 3% if it was excised totally without prior biopsy, they also found that there was a 70% chance of a second recurrence within 15 years. Using an actuarial method of analysing their statistics they forecast that after 20 years 10% of those patients with recurrent tumour had undergone malignant change and 20% after 30 years. These forecasts referred, however, to patients treated in a large number of centres with varying degrees of expertise and success. The overall recurrent rate for benign mixed cell tumours in their series was 13% after five years, and 30% after 15 years, a reflection of the large proportion of patients who must have undergone either a biopsy or incomplete excision as their primary treatment.

It is essential when dealing with lesions of the lacrimal gland that a neoplasm arising from the epithelium of the gland is recognised as soon as possible.[7] Carcinomas of the lacrimal gland cannot be distinguished from other rapidly expanding lesions in this region other than by histologic examination. However, benign mixed tumours can be readily recognised on clinical grounds. They present in patients who are in their late 20s to early 60s as a slowly progressive, painless, upper lid swelling without inflammatory symptoms or signs. There is often a palpable mass in the outer temporal quadrant of the orbit. A careful, detailed history will reveal that the duration of symptoms is usually longer than 12 months. Radiographs often show enlargement of the lacrimal fossa without invasion of overlying bone. The importance of recognising this tumour cannot be over emphasised, any temptation to biopsy the lesion should be resisted and total removal of the whole of the lacrimal gland and the tumour through a lateral orbitotomy undertaken.

Rupture of the capsule of a benign mixed tumour affects the prognosis adversely, because tumour cells are seeded into the surrounding tissues. A recurrence is thus inevitable. In most cases the cell picture remains that of a pleomorphic adenoma but malignant change can occur. In patients in whom the recurrences remain benign the prognosis is often indistinguishable from that seen in a true carcinoma. The tumour cells invade the apex of the orbit as well as the surrounding bone. Following a painful and lingering course, death ensues for in most cases the tumour spreads beyond the line of surgical resection and although radiotherapy may be used as a palliative measure, benign mixed tumours are relatively radio-resistant.

The modified lateral orbitotomy approach offers the only way to achieve adequate removal of a benign mixed tumour for the whole of the gland together with the overlying periosteum together with the palpebral lobe must be carefully dissected out using an operating microscope. The capsule is not touched and the tumour together with the normal parts of the lacrimal gland are totally removed. A trans-cranial, anterior orbitotomy or the Burke lateral orbitotomy make it extremely difficult or impossible to avoid a sub-total piecemeal removal of the gland and tumour.

Using these techniques the author has not encountered any recurrent tumour in 30 patients managed in this manner. In particular, there have been no recurrences in any of the 12 patients whose lacrimal gland was totally removed at least five years previously.[8]

Malignant tumours arising from the lacrimal gland have two characteristic features; a short history with a rapidly worsening course and pain. Radiographic findings may be helpful in distinguishing between the malignant and benign lacrimal tumour. Carcinomatous lesions often enlarge so rapidly that radiographs in the early stages are normal. Later enlargement of the lacrimal fossa with or without demonstrable invasion of bone may be seen. Occasionally, calcification within the malignant tumour can be demonstrated. The presence of calcification within a tumour is diagnostic of malignancy. In patients with such tumours, it is important that both axial and coronal CT scans are obtained so that the structure of the bone in relation to the tumour can be examined in some detail. Other lesions affecting the lacrimal fossa must be considered in the differential diagnosis. Acute dacryoadenitis, unless caused by a viral infection, usually responds to systemic antibiotic therapy. However, if there is a failure to respond to antibiotics over a period of two weeks a tissue diagnosis should be made. Unfortunately, a good proportion of carcinomas involving the lacrimal gland are initially treated as cases of acute dacroadenitis refractory to antibiotic therapy. Inflammatory pseudo tumours are relatively uncommon as are lymphomatous lesions, the latter is particularly common in patients over 65 years old. Again, tissue must be obtained so that the appropriate treatment can be instigated. All these patients have a short history of lacrimal fossa swelling with or without associated inflammatory signs. In all these patients a biospy should be obtained through a trans-septal incision. The extra-periosteal approach should never be used, because the integrity of the periosteal barrier must be maintained to prevent possible seeding of the extra-periosteal space by malignant cells.

Patients found to have malignant epithelial neoplasms should be evaluated to determine the extent of the tumour. When there is evidence of restriction of the tumour mass within the periosteal barrier, without involvement of the orbital apex, a radical resection of the area can be undertaken. The skills of a neurosurgeon, head and neck surgeon, and plastic surgeon, as well as that of an ophthalmic surgeon should be united for such a surgical approach. Surgical resection in these cases should include portions of the lateral and superior orbital walls as well as the removal of lids and orbital contents. Seven patients have been treated in this manner by the author. Five of these patients have now survived beyond five years without evidence of recurrent tumour. Radiotherapy and chemotherapy may be considered for those cases in which spread has occurred beyond even these wide surgical margins. The outlook for these patients is extremely poor. Death occurs from invasion of adjacent structures, the middle cranial fossa is particularly vulnerable and there is often considerable pain and distress prior to death.

Orbital Metastases

The orbit is an uncommon but well recognised site for metastasis from malignancy arising elsewhere in the body. Frequently such tumours arise from the breast, lung, prostate or gastro-intestinal tract. In some cases the metastasis expands rapidly and causes pain, chemosis and displacement of the globe. A schirrous carcinoma from the breast does, however, result in a fibrotic mass within the orbit, this produces retraction of the globe and a relative enophthalmos with restriction of movement and double vision.

A female patient with no history of trauma, and normal radiographs who experiences double vision accompanied by enophthalmos, invariable has a primary schirrous carcinoma of the breast. A tissue biopsy should be obtained from all these patients before starting treatment.

An uncommon but well recognised metastasis encountered in infants and young children is a neuroblastoma. These tumours originate in the sympathetic nervous system, usually the primary tumour is well advanced and there is evidence of metastasis to other sites, but occasionally the orbital tumour is the first sign of the disease. The child is noticed to have swellings of the eyelids, chemosis, and proptosis, with rapid progression of these signs often with an associated inflammator reaction within the orbit and widespread subcutaneous haemorrha Tissue should be obtained from the orbit in those cases in whic the diagnosis is in doubt so that radiotherapy and chemotherapy can be started.

The prognosis for patients with orbital metastasis is grave Few survive more than a few years. Nevertheless, palliative treatment is indicated to relieve symptoms and maintain morale. Nearly all cases respond to radiotherapy with regression of the tumour leading to relief of pain if present, and preservation of the remaining useful vision in the affected eye. In a few cases, there can be quite marked improvement of vision. When there are bilateral lesions treatment can be given by a single, lateral field or by opposed lateral fields, taking care to avoid both lenses. A fairly high dose should be given to avoid re-growth of the tumour during the patient's remaining lifespan, a 3,500 rad. to 4,000 rad. tumour dose for three weeks is recommended.

When a patient has a secondary tumour arising from a prostatic carcinoma, treatment with Oestrogen will often produce a quite dramatic resolution of the primary and secondary tumours, but apart from these cases the outlook for patients with orbital metastases is uniformly poor and efforts should be directed towards palliative treatment and the control of pain.

REFERENCES

1. Morgan G, Harry J:Lymphocytic tumours of indeterminate nature: a 5 year follow-up of 98 conjunctival and orbital lesions. Br. J. Ophthalmol 1978; 62:381-385.

2. Garner A, Rahi AHS, Wright JE: Lymphoproliferative disorders of the orbit: an immunological approach to diagnosis and pathogenesis. Br. J. Ophthalmol. 1983; 67, No.9:561-569.

3. Godtfredsen E: Pathology of mucous and salivary gland tumours in the lacrimal gland and the relation to extra-orbital mucous and salivary gland tumours (studies on orbital tumours). Br. J. Ophthalmol. 1948; 32:171-179.

4. Ringerts N: Pathology of malignant tumours arising in the nasal and paranasal cavities and maxilla. Acta Otolaryngol [Suppl] (Stockh) 1938; 27.

5. Foote AW, Frazell EL: Tumours of the major salivary glands. Cancer 1953; 6:1065-1133.

6. Font RL, Gammel JW: Epithelial tumours of the lacrimal gland. An analysis of 265 cases. In Jakobiec FA: Ocular and Adnexal Tumors, Aesculapius, Birmingham, Ala, 1978: 787-805.

7. Wright JE, Stewart WB, Krohel GB: Clinical presentation and management of lacrimal gland tumours. Br. J. Ophthalmol 1979; 63:600-606.

8. Wright JE, Factors affecting the survival of patients with lacrimal gland tumours. Can.J.Ophthalmol. 1982; 17:3-9.

9. Font RL, Ferry AP, Carcinoma metastatic to the eye and orbit. Cancer 1976; 38:1326-1335.

MALIGNANT ENT TUMOURS AND THE ORBIT

E.N. Brons

Incidence

Most malignant tumours of the nasal cavity and paranasal sinuses occur between the 5th and 7th decade (10,19,25). The male : female ratio is from 1.5-2.0 : 1 (10,19,22,25). The incidence rate is 0.3 to 1.0 cases per 100,000 persons a year in most countries (26). High rates are found in Japan - 2.4 for males and 1.3 for females (22). Carcinomas of the nasal cavity and accessory sinuses account for 0.2-0.8% of all human malignancies (5).

Histology

The vast majority (55-75%)(12,18,19,25) are squamous cell carcinomas, including its histological variations of undifferentiated carcinoma and transitional cell carcinoma, followed by 10-15% adenocarcinomas (including adenoid cystic carcinoma), 0-15% sarcomas and 0-5% melanomas.

This article will deal only with carcinomas because most of the ENT tumours with orbital invastion potency are carcinomas of the maxillary and ethmoid sinuses.

Aetiology

There is a significant relationship between adenocarcinoma of the nasal cavity and accessory sinuses and woodworkers in the furniture industry (1) and workers in the boot and shoe industry (2), also a definite relation between squamous cell carcinoma and workers in the nickel industry (22,23). Smoking and drinking do not appear to be contributory (12,26).

Oosterhuis, A. (ed.), Ophthalmic tumors.

ISBN 90-6193-528-8. Printed in the Netherlands.

Origin

The primary is in 55-65% of the cases located in the maxillary sinus, in 15-30% in the ethmoid sinus, and in 15-20% in the nasal cavity (12,18,19,25). Origin in the sphenoid and frontal sinus is rare.

Symptoms and signs

The most frequent as well as earliest symptoms are nasal obstruction, dull pain, and sanguineous (sometimes purulent fetid) discharge.

Cancer of the sinuses is encountered only rarely while confined within the cavity (silent bony cage area), and almost without exception presents itself as an extended disease.

"Sinusitis", neurologic or dental complaints may be the first sign of a tumour of the paranasal sinuses.

Ocular symptoms arise from an upward extension from the maxillary sinus or a lateral extension from the ethmoid sinus into the orbit, whereby exophthalmos, diplopia, epiphora, protrusion of lids and inner canthus area, paraesthesia along the course of the infraorbital nerve, and visual impairment develop.

Extension by the lymphatics occurs late and by the blood stream even later.

Screening programme

1. Investigation by an otolaryngologist, ophthalmologist, neurologist, dental surgeron and internist.
2. Tympanometry (Eustachian tube function).
3. X-ray studies of the sinuses and skull base.
4. CT scan.
5. Nasendo-, antro- and nasopharyngoscopy with biopsies (histological diagnosis and extension of the lesion).

Treatment

The clinical stage is of more importance to prognosis and potential curability of the disease than the histologic type of the tumour (5,12,19). It is generally accepted that the therapy of choice is a combination of radical surgery and radiotherapy of 6,000 rads (4,10,11,17,19,32,33). This is also true for adenoid cystic carcinoma (9,20) where irradiation therapy is an important adjuvant in treatment. New means of therapy for carcinoma of the nasal cavity and paranasal sinuses, in which limited surgery is combined with other treatment modalities such as (topical) chemotherapy, immunotherapy, radiotherapy, and cryosurgery seem promising (16,27). Tey still need further evaluation.

The issue of the timing of irradiation seems undecided. Some authors favour preoperative irradiation therapy (7,17,32,33), others prefer postoperative irradiation (4,11,13,19).

Limitations to operability (10,15,34)

1. Involvement of the nasopharynx.
2. Bilateral involvement of the orbital periosteum.
3. Regional and generalized metastases.
4. Advanced age with associated senility.
5. Poor general condition.

Invasion of the base of the anterior cranial fossa is not considered to be a contraindication(6,14,15,29,30), neither is invasion of the more lateral aspect of the base of the middle cranial fossa (9,35).

The mean 5-year survival rates after radical surgery and irradiation therapy are: maxillary sinus carcinomas 75% T3-lesions and 33.3% T4-lesions (4), 54% (11), 38% (NED survival) (17), squamous cell carcinomas 43% (19), and adenocarcinomas 0% (19).

Orbital exenteration combined with maxillectomy results in a significant functional loss and cosmetic deformity. Consequently many surgeons are reluctant to accept orbital exenteration when the indications are not very stringent and preserve the orbital contents when there is no involvement of the orbital periosteum (3,11,15,24,28,30,31,34). This surgical procedure is called a partial maxillectomy (21,24,28,30,31,33). Konno et al.(16) resects the involved orbital periosteum (sometimes with orbital fat exposing the inferior and medial rectus muscles) and covers the orbital contents with a fascia lata graft.

If orbital exenteration is necessary, the technique of a cheek-eyelid-conjunctiva flap allows for immediate reconstruction of the eye socket and the fitting of a prosthesis in selected cases (8).

References

1. Acheson, E.D., Cowdill, R.H., Hadfield, E. et al. 1968. Nasal cancer in woodworkers in the furniture industry. Brit.Med.J. 2:587.
2. Acheson, E.D., Cowdill, R.H. and Jolles, B. 1970. Nasal cancer in the Northhamptonshire boot and shoe industry. Brit.Med.J. 1:385.
3. Adkins, W.Y. Jr. 1976. Maxillectomy with preservation of orbital function. Surg.Forum 27:548.
4. Ahmad, K., Cordoba, R.B. and Fayos, J.V. 1981. Squamous cell carcinoma of the maxillary sinus. Arch.Otolaryngol. 107:48.
5. Batsakis, J.G., Rice, D.H. and Solomon, A.R. 1980. The pathology of head and neck tumors: squamous and mucous-gland carcinomas of the nasal cavity, paranasal sinuses, and larynx, part 6. Head & Neck Surg. 2: 497.
6. Bridger, G.P. 1980. Radical surgery for ethmoid cancer. Arch.Otolaryngol. 106:630.
7. Cheng, V.S.T. and Wang, C.C. 1977. Carcinoma of the paranasal sinuses. Cancer 40:3038.
8. Conley, J. and Baker, D.C. 1979. Management of the eye socket in cancer of the paranasal sinuses. Arch.Otolaryngol. 105:702.
9. Goepfert, H., Luna, M.A., Lindberg, R.D. and White, A.K. 1983. Malignant salivary gland tumors of the paranasal sinuses and nasal cavity. Arch.Otolaryngol. 109:662.
10. Hendrick, J.W. 1958. Treatment of cancer of the paranasal sinuses and nasal fossa. Arch.Otolaryngol. 68:604.
11. Hordijk, G.J. and Brons, E.N. 1984. Carcinomas of the maxillary sinus (a retrospective study). In preparation, Clin.Otolaryngol.
12. Jackson, R.T., Fitz-Hugh, G.S. and Constable, W.C. 1977. Malignant neoplasms of the nasal cavities and paranasal sinuses. The Laryngoscope 87:726.
13. Jesse, R.H., Goepfert, H. and Lindberg, R.D. 1975. Carcinoma of the sinuses: a review of treatment. In: Cancer of the head and neck. Eds Chambers, R.G., Janssen de Limpens, A.M.P., Jacques, D.A. et al. Amsterdam, Excerpta Medica, p. 153.
14. Ketcham, A.S., Wilkins, R.H., Van Buren, J.M. and Smith, R.R. 1963. A combined intracranial facial approach to the paranasal sinuses. Amer.J.Surg. 106:698.

15. Ketcham, A.S., Chretien, P.B., Van Buren, J.M. et al. 1973. The ethmoid sinuses: a re-evaluation of surgical resection. Amer.J.Surg. 126:469.
16. Konno, A., Togawa, K. and Inoue, S. 1980. Analysis of the results of our combined therapy for maxillary cancer. Acta Otolaryngol. suppl. 372.
17. Lee, F. and Ogura, J.H. 1981. Maxillary sinus carcinoma. The Laryngoscope 91:133.
18. Majumdar, B. and Kent, S. 1983. Malignant neoplasms of the nose and paranasal sinuses. A survey of cases treated in a regional centre. Clin.Otolaryngol. 8:97.
19. Mann, W. and Schuler-Voith, C. 1983. Tumors of the paranasal sinuses and the nose - a retrospective study in 136 patients. Rhinology 21:173.
20. Miller, R.H. and Calcaterra, T.C. 1980. Adenoid cystic carcinoma of the nose, paranasal sinuses, and palate. Arch.Otolaryngol. 106:424.
21. Montgomery, W.W. 1971. Surgery of the upper respiratory system. Philadelphia, Lea & Febiger, vol. 1.
22. Muir, C.S. and Nectoux, J. 1980. Descriptive epidemiology of malignant neoplasms of nose, nasal cavities, middle ear and accessory sinuses. Clin.Otolaryngol. 5:195.
23. Pedersen, E.A., Høgetveit, A.C. and Andersen, A. 1973. Cancer of the respiratory organs among workers at a nickel refinery in Norway. Int.J.Cancer 12:32.
24. Pope, T.H. 1978. Surgical approach to tumors of the nasal cavity. The Laryngoscope 88:1743.
25. Robin, P.E., Powell, D.J. and Stansbie, J.M. 1979. Carcinoma of the nasal cavity and paranasal sinuses: incidence and presentation of different histological types. Clin. Otolaryngol. 4:431.
26. Roush, G.C. 1979. Epidemiology of cancer of the nose and paranasal sinuses: current concepts. Head & Neck Surg. 2:3.
27. Sakai, S., Murata, M., Sasaki, R. et al. 1983. Combined therapy for maxillary sinus carcinoma with special reference to cryosurgery. Rhinology 21:179.
28. Schramm, V.L. and Myers, E.N. 1978. How I do it - lateral rhinotomy. The Laryngoscope 88:1042.
29. Schramm, V.L., Myers, E.N. and Maroon, J.C. 1979. Anterior skull base surgery for benign and malignant disease. The Laryngoscope 89:1077.
30. Sessions, R.B. and Larson, D.L. 1977. En bloc ethmoidectomy and medial maxillectomy. Arch.Otolaryngol. 103:195.
31. Sessions, R.B. and Humphreys, D.H. 1983. Technical modifications of the medial maxillectomy. Arch.Otolaryngol. 109:575.
32. Sisson, G.A. 1970. Symposium III - Treatment of malignancies of paranasal sinuses (discussion and summary). The Laryngoscope 80:945.
33. Som, M.L. 1974. Surgical management of carcinoma of the maxilla. Arch.Otolaryngol. 99:270.
34. Weymuller, E.A.V. Jr., Reardon, E.J. and Nash, D. 1980. A comparison of treatment modalities in carcinoma of the maxillary antrum. Arch.Otolaryngol. 106:625.
35. Cheesman, A.D. Personal communication.

VASCULAR DISORDERS IN THE ORBIT AND IN THE ORBITAL REGION

R.J.W. de Keizer

Endocrine exophthalmos, (pseudo-)tumours, bone fractures and vascular diseases are the most frequent lesions in patients with orbital disorders (Wright, 1981) (Table I). On comparison of data of various centres the distributions of vascular lesions show a remarkable difference. In the series of Wright for instance the most frequent lesions are varices. In our series, however, they are the carotid-cavernous fistulae (Table II).

A difficulty in the comparison of diagnostic material of various centres is the lack of a uniform classification. Henderson (1980) for instance differentiates between vascular neoplasms and vascular malformations. Reese (1976) on the other hand divided orbital tumours into polymorphous and monomorphous tumours. The following classification is based on their principles but more adapted to clinical use.

1) Clinically recognizable vascular disorders like capillary haemangioma, lymphangioma, traumatic and non-traumatic carotid-cavernous fistula and varix.
2) Primary tumours of the orbit like cavernous haemangioma, local partially thrombosed arteriovenous malformations, blood cysts and aneurysms of the ophthalmic artery.
3) Vascular disorders detectable by their neuro-ophthalmological signs and symptoms, such as the Tolosa-Hunt syndrome, the orbital apex and fissure syndromes, and arterial or venous thrombosis in the orbit or in the peri-orbital region.
4) Phakomatoses like the Wyburn-Mason, the Von Hippel-

Oosterhuis, A. (ed.), Ophthalmic tumors.

ISBN 90-6193-528-8. Printed in the Netherlands.

Table I. Frequency of orbital disorders of the Leiden University Eye Clinic 1982-1983.

dysthyroidism	36	fibrous connective tissue tumour	2
enthyroid Graves	7	tumour of adipose tissue and muscle	1
vascular	18	cyst	2
pseudotumour	14	fractures	26
inflammation	10	Wegener	1
meningioma	12	haematoma	4
neurofibromatosis	2	pseudoproptosis	6
glioma	2	idiopathic	2
E.N.T. neoplasm	11	granulomatosis	1
neurosurgical entities	3	metastatic carcinoma	6
bone tumour	8	other	4
non-Hodgkin lymphoma	8		
	131		55

Total = 186

Table II. Vascular anomalies of the orbital centres of Amsterdam (1976-1981) and Leiden (1982-193) seen by the author.

capillary haemangioma	4	haemangiopericytoma	1
venous malformation	3	vascular meningioma	-
orbital varix	5	vascular leiomyoma	-
carotid cavernous fistulas		naevus flammeus Sturge-Weber	4
- spontaneous	28	aneurysm	-
- traumatic	20	Tolosa-Hunt	3
arteriovenous malformations		granulomatosis	1
- Wyburn-Mason	3	venous thrombosis	5
- local in the orbit	2	idiopathic secondary vascular glaucoma	6
- other	4	blood cyst	-
cavernous haemangioma	10		
lymphangioma	2		
haemangioblastoma	2		
haemangio-endothelioma	2		

Lindau and the Sturge-Weber syndromes.

5) Benign or malignant vascular neoplasms like the haemangio-endothelioma and the haemangiopericytoma.

Clinically recognizable vascular disorders

Capillary haemangioma

Facial capillary haemangioma can easily be recognized. In the post-natal days it will grow rapidly. After the first year it usually recedes spontaneously (Peeters & Bleeker, 1975). Histopathologically the tumour is a proliferation of endothelial cells and pericytes (capillaries). The ectatic capillary channels are characteristic. Staining of reticuline easily demonstrates the proliferation of endothelial cells as they are outlined by the reticulum sheath (Haik et al., 1979; Reese, 1976). The capillary haemangioma has to be differentiated from cavernous haemangioma and arteriovenous malformations. Capillary haemangiomas in and under the skin turn blue upon congestion of the face and become white under pressure of a palpating finger (Haik et al., 1979). They are sometimes accompanied by haemangiomas elsewhere in the body. Extension into the orbit must be suspected if proptosis is present.

The therapy is as a rule conservative. One has to focus on the prevention of amblyopia either by eyelid closure or astigmatism induced by tumour pressure (Plessner-Rasmussen et al., 1983). Frequent ophthalmic examination is imperative and orthoptic treatment may be required. Sometimes one has to resort to radiotherapy or surgery or even to steroids. Side-effects of these therapies are wellknown. Irradiation may result in facial deformity and asymmetry. Infectious or metabolic disorders may result from steroid administration. Surgery may be associated with complications and may lead to deformity due to scar formation. Plessner-Rasmussen et al. (1983) advocate a low dosis of radiotherapy (1-3 times 300-500 rad).

Lymphangioma

Lymphangiomas are cyst-like structures of the conjunctiva, eyelid or orbit. The vascular spaces contain a clear fluid and sometimes a haemorrhage. Wright (1981) classified lymphangiomas among the haemangiomas. Jacobiec and Jones (1982) considered them as a separate entity. Histopathologically a capillary cavernous type and a cystic type can be distinguished in correspondence with the clinical picture of lymph structures of the eye and orbital region. The vascular spaces are lined with flattened endothelial cells. The stroma between the spaces is loose and hypocellular with foci of lymphoid cells. Sometimes hyperplasia is seen when a patient has caught a viral upper respiratory infection (Reese, 1976).

Motility disturbances and serious cosmetic problems may necessitate surgical intervention. Of our two patients with lymphangioma one was treated with local excision and a conjunctival graft but in the other one the extension in the orbit and adnexa was so extensive and the visual acuity so low that exenteration was the only possible treatment.

Traumatic carotid-cavernous fistula (CCF)

The traumatic direct CCF is a direct communication between the internal carotid artery and the cavernous sinus. Clinically it is characterized by a symptomless post-traumatic period and subsequent pulsating exophthalmos and intraorbital murmur, which show a strong tendency to progress (Henderson, 1980; De Keizer, 1981[a,b]). These clinical signs are so characteristic that the diagnosis can be made instantly. Carotid angiography reveals the nature of the shunt and its leakage into the venous system and enables us to plan the therapeutic intervention.

The traumatic CCF has to be distinguished from other lesions causing pulsating exophthalmos, such as neurofibromatosis, orbital varix, or a defective orbital roof. Doppler blood velocity measurements (haematotachography) may contribute to the diagnosis (De Keizer, 1982; De Keizer et al., 1984).

Table III. Results of therapy in 20 patients with a traumatic carotid-cavernous fistula.

	total number	cured	±	failure	†
conservative	3	1	1		1
embolization					
- spontaneously	1	1			
- balloon	10	9		1	
"Hamby"	5*	5			
other methods	2	1			1

* This number includes the patient unsuccessfully treated with a balloon.

Table IV. Results of therapy in 28 patients with a spontaneous carotid-cavernous fistula (type: direct, internal dural or external dural).

	total number	cured	±	failure	no follow-up
conservative	26	19	3	1	3
embolization					
- balloon	2	2			
- gelfoam	1*	1			
other methods	-	-			

* This is the patient in whom conservative treatment had ben unsuccessful.

Typical Doppler patterns of the direct CCF as registered in one of our patients are given in figure 1.

In direct CCF balloon embolization is preferable to carotid occlusion by muscle emboli as advocated by Hamby (1966). Balloons close the shunt specifically in the cavernous sinus but leave the circulation of the internal carotid artery unimpaired (Peeters and Van der Werf, 1980). In 11 of our series of 20 patients embolization treatment with one or more balloons was carried out. Eight of them were cured, in one patient this was only possible by carotid obstruction by the balloon, in another patient the shunt was closed simply by the usual manipulation with the catheter; one patient got postoperative problems by collapse of the balloon but the fistula could be closed by the Hamby technique (Table III) (De Keizer, 1981[b]; De Keizer et al., 1984).

Spontaneous carotid-cavernous fistula (CCF)

Spontaneous CCF is characterized by specific loops of the epibulbar vessels in the limbal area (Fig. 2), a slight proptosis and a distinct tendency to develop glaucoma, which we found in 73% of 31 patients (De Keizer, 1981[a]; De Keizer et al., 1984). Motility disturbances are not specific in spontaneous CCF. Spontaneous CCF can be divided into dural and direct fistulas (Fig. 3) and real orbital arteriovenous fistulas. The latter are very rare but in our series of 31 spontaneous CCF they were diagnosed four times. Doppler velocity measurements can be helpful to differentiate between the direct and dural type of fistula (Fig. 4) (De Keizer, 1982). It can be useful to measure the episcleral venous pressure and to use biomicroscopy to study the direction of blood flow from the ciliary vein to an anterior conjunctival vein (De Keizer, 1981[b]). In most cases pretreatment carotid angiography is not necessary since in 75% of the cases the fistula closes spontaneously in the course of time. Progression of the lesion is usually seen in direct CCF resulting from a rupture of an intracavernous aneurysm (Fig. 3). Gelfoam embolization was successful in one of our patients (Table IV).

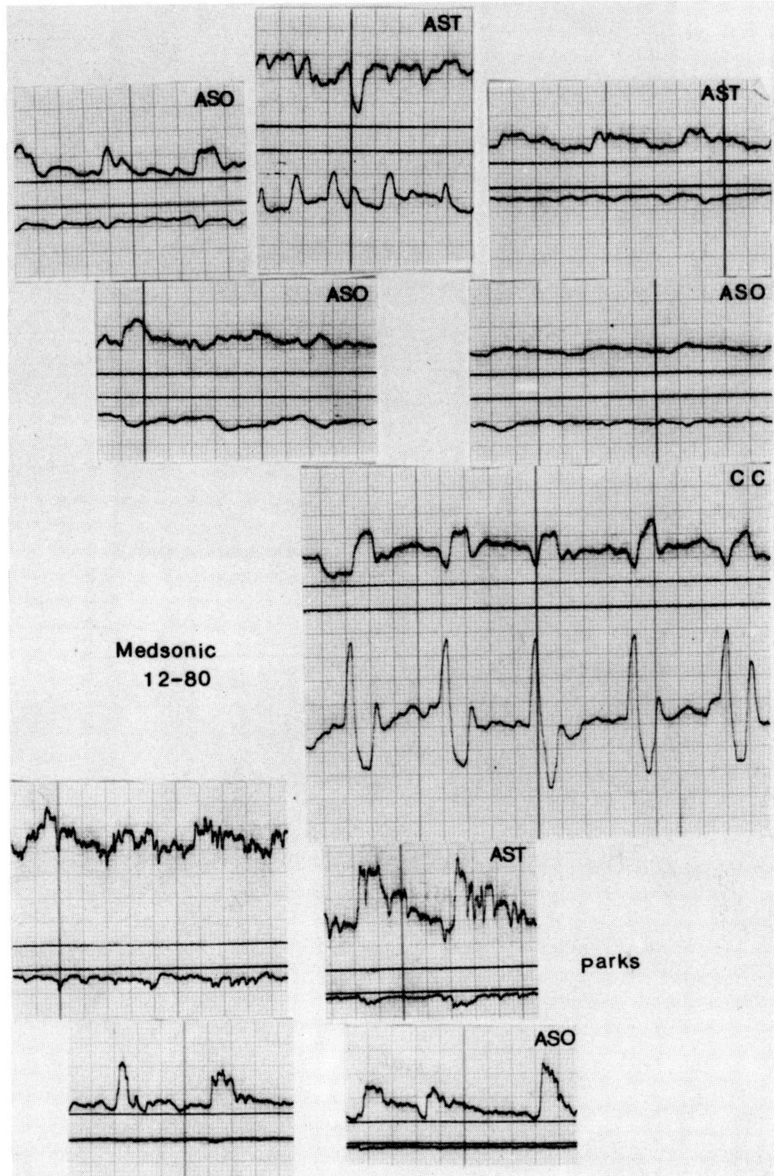

Fig. 1a Typical Doppler pattern in the common carotid artery and the superior ophthalmic vein with high blood velocities in a 72 years old patient with a traumatic direct carotid-cavernous fistula. Bottom right: ASO blood flow without and with augmentation.

ASO: localization of supraorbital artery.
AST: localization of supratrochlear artery.
cc: common carotid artery.

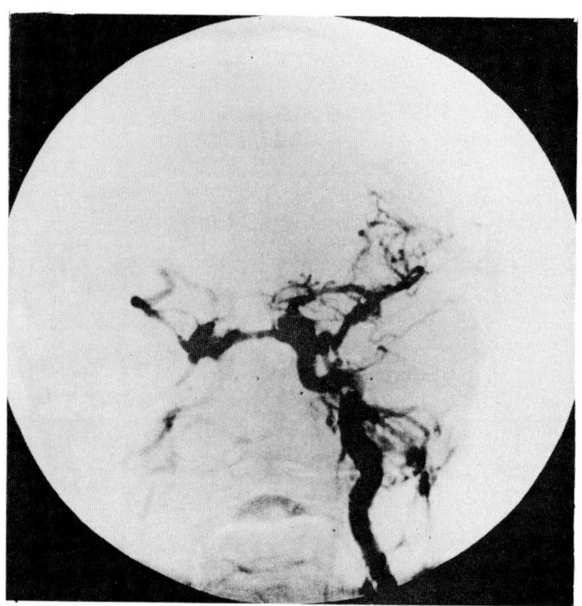

Fig. 1b Angiography of the same patient shows the arterio-venous blood flow via both orbits.

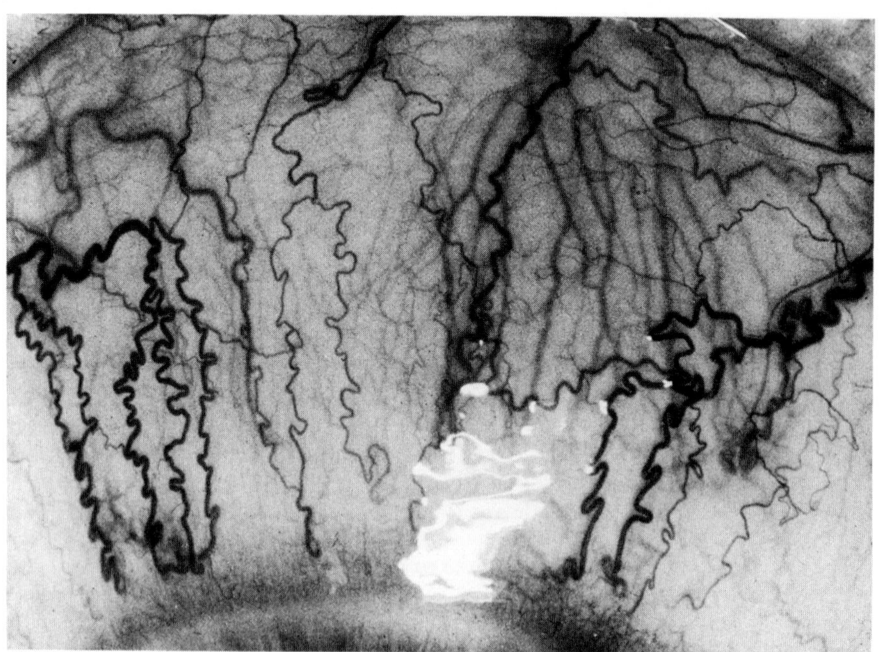

Fig. 2 Typical arterialized venous loops on the eye in spontaneous carotid-cavernous fistula. The anterior ciliary vein, the anterior and the posterior conjunctival vein are interconnected.

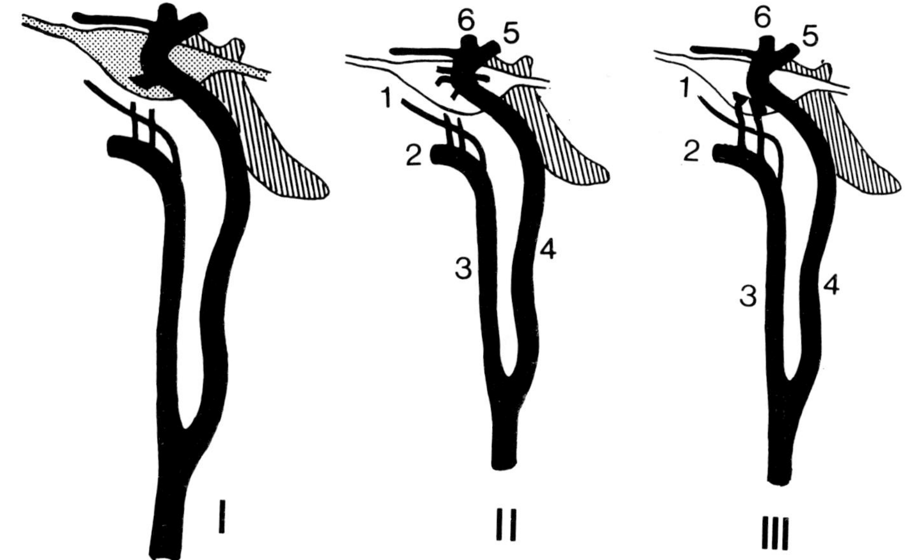

Fig. 3 I Direct carotid-cavernous fistula (traumatic or spontaneous) of the internal carotid artery.
II Spontaneous carotid-cavernous fistula of the dural type between the internal carotid artery and the cavernous sinus.
III Spontaneous carotid-cavernous fistula of the dural type between the external carotid artery and the cavernous sinus.
1 = middle meningeal artery
2 = internal maxillary artery
3 = external carotid artery
4 = internal carotid artery
5 = middle cerebral artery
6 = anterior cerebral artery

By courtesy of Professor F.L.M. Peeters.

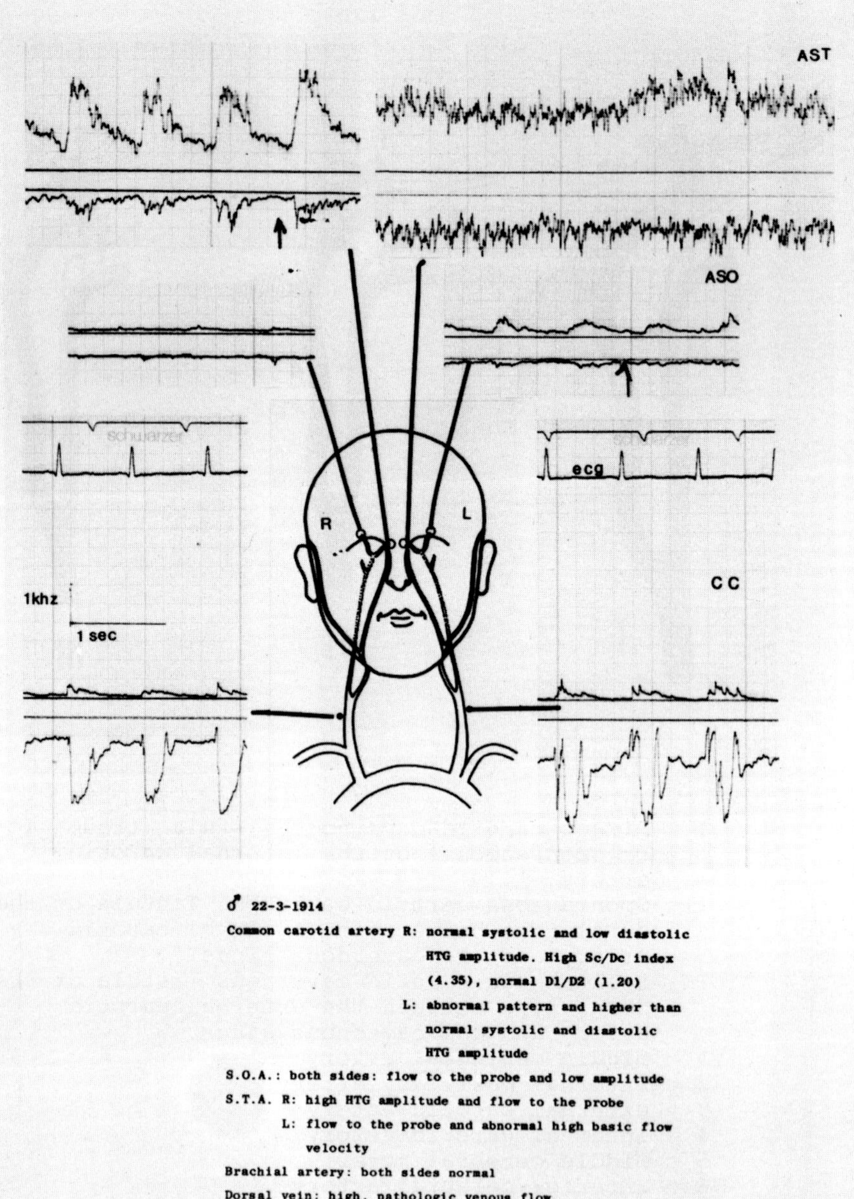

Fig. 4 Doppler blood velocity measurement in a 65 years old man with a spontaneous dural internal carotid-cavernous fistula and typical "arteriovenous" pattern of the orbital vessels.

Orbital varices and venous malformations

Orbital varices are characterized by intermittent exophthalmos. Several patients have a blue translucent tumour with or without proptosis. Elevation of the venous pressure during the Valsalva manoeuvre or during coughing or stooping increases the exophthalmos because the veins in the head and neck have no valves. Accordingly, blood will accumulate in the large spaces of the varices, which are drained only slowly (Fig. 5ab). Phlebography of the orbit may clearly demonstrate these varices (Fig. 5c). Conventional X-ray photography sometimes reveals phlebolites to support the diagnosis (Fig. 6).

Orbital varices must be differentiated from cerebral malformations (Iraci et al. (1979) and from collateral circulation consequent to congenital cerebral disorders and venous thrombosis, respectively (De Keizer, 1984).

The therapy of choice for orbital varices is conservative. The patient has to avoid all actions that produce congestion of the head. Sometimes, however, it is advisable to remove one or more of the larger venous channels. The injection of sclerosing fluids is dangerous because of the risk of orbital inflammation and visual loss. Moreover, it is very difficult to restrict the therapeutic effect to the affected vessels.

Primary orbital tumours

Cavernous haemangioma

This is the most frequently observed primary orbital tumour. It is a well delineated tumour that usually becomes manifest in the second or third decade of life. It has a slight tendency to progress. In many cases it is located inferotemporally in the muscle cone (Moseley and Sanders, 1982). Sometimes it causes choroidal folds, papilloedema or motility disturbances. Ultrasonography demonstrates a cyst-like structure on the B-scan and acoustical interfaces at the anterior and posterior border of the cyst on the A-scan. Changes in position of the optic nerve and eye muscles in different directions of gaze, which rule out significant

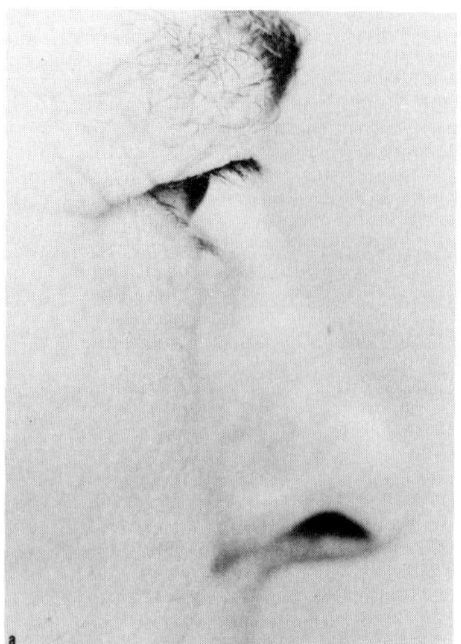

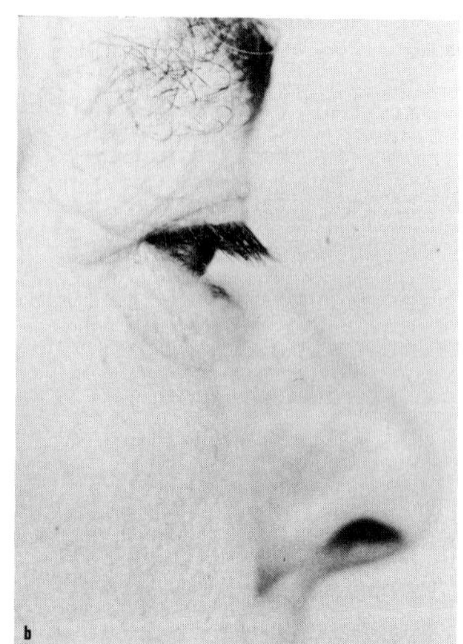

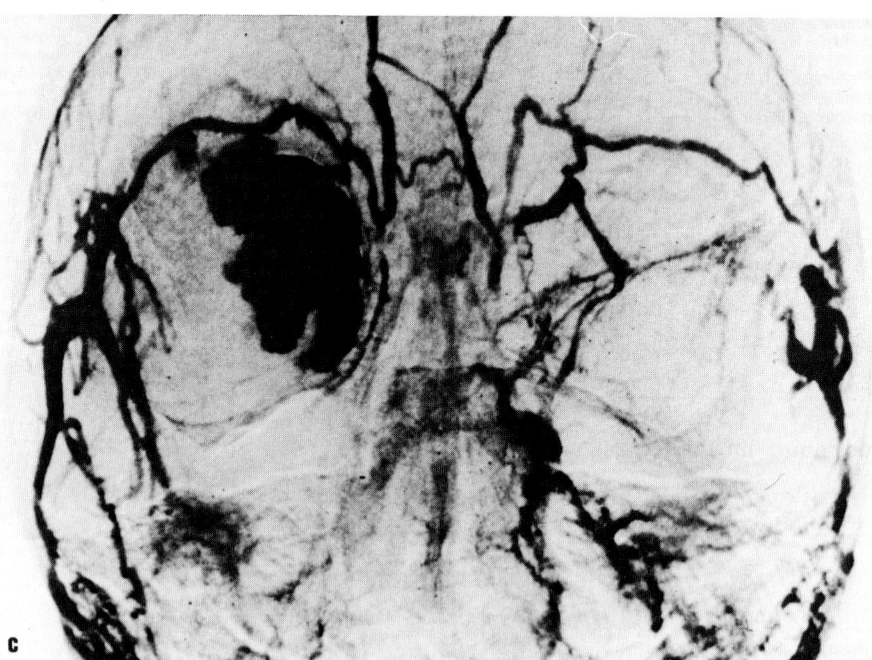

Fig. 5 A 66 years old woman with an orbital varix and intermittent exophthalmos.

a. increase in exophthalmos induced by Valsalva manoeuvre.

b. regression of exophthalmos after Valsalva manoeuvre.

c. phlebogram showing large orbital varix.

tumour attachments, can be demonstrated by CT-scan (Unsöld et al, 1979; Moseley and Sanders, 1982).

Depending upon the localization of the tumour it can be operated by a lateral Krönlein approach or by the anterior orbital approach. Histopathologically the cavernous haemangioma is well encapsulated but the cavernous spaces are lined with flat endothelial cells together with muscle cells in the stroma. It is always remarkable that despite the large cavernous spaces the afferent and efferent vessels are always of modest dimensions. Accordingly, the size of a cavernous haemangioma does not respond to pressure or suction.

An example of localization within the muscle cone is given in a patient with choroidal folds and a visual acuity of 0.6. The CT-scan revealed a tumour in the muscle cone close to the optic nerve, which gave the impression of a meningioma of the optic nerve sheath (Fig. 7). Subtraction angiography demonstrated small abnormal arteries feeding the tumour. After excision histopathology revealed a cavernous haemangioma.

An example of a haemangioma outside the muscle cone is given in a patient with a slowly progressive proptosis existing for 20 years. The clinical diagnosis was Graves' ophthalmopathy and this was sustained by endocrinological investigation. In a later stage this diagnosis proved to be incorrect since the symptoms turned out to be caused by the use of oral contraceptives. However, a special vascular loop on the external rectus muscle was detected, which induced us to perform further investigation. The coronal sections of the CT revealed a haemangioma.

Arteriovenous malformations

In two patients suspected of an orbital tumour the histopathological diagnosis was thrombosed arteriovenous malformation. Pre-operatively the CT-scan had shown a well demarcated tumour. Orbital phlebography and arteriography showed only some displacement of vessels.

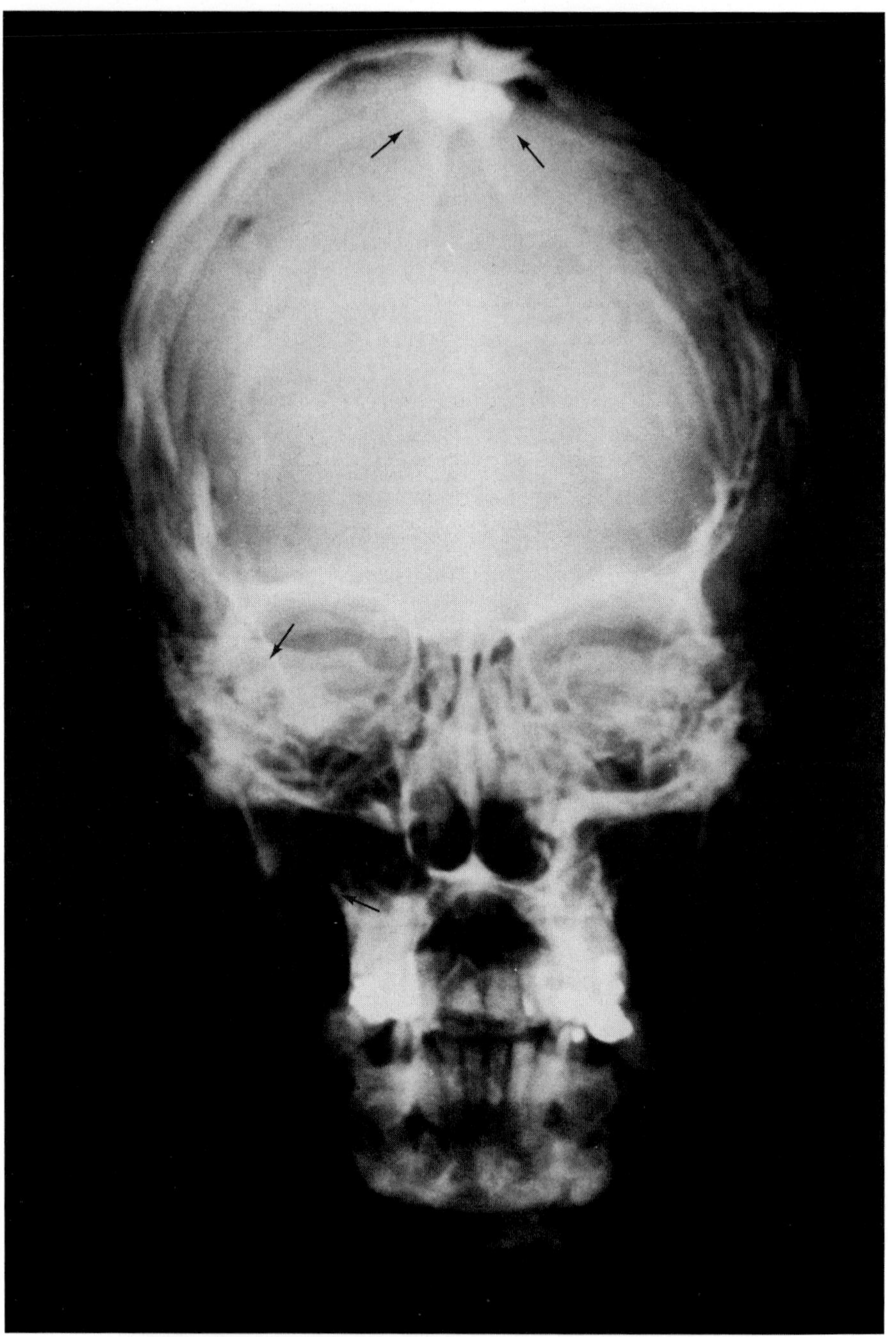

Fig. 6 X-ray photograph of a patient with Sturge-Weber syndrome showing phlebolite (arrow) and cerebral calcified angioma (2 arrows).

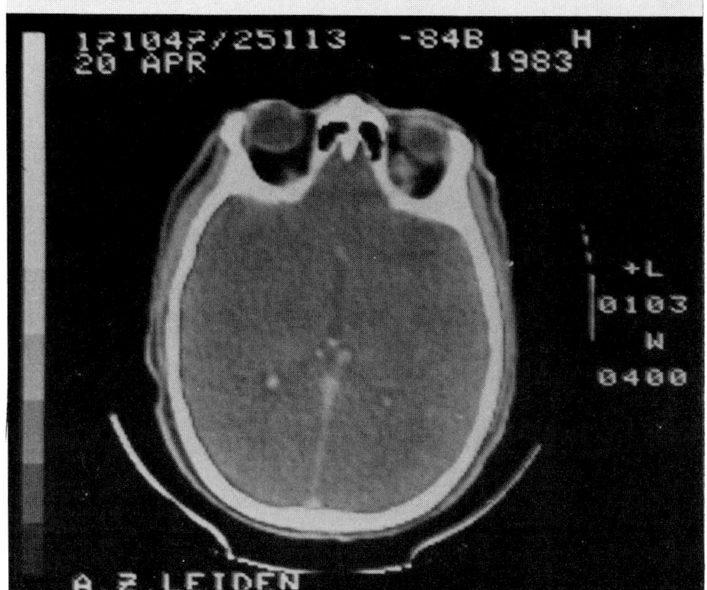

Fig. 7 Axial CT scan of an orbital tumour in a 72 years old man. On CT scan and angiography the diagnosis seemed to be a meningioma; a cavernous haemangioma was extirpated.

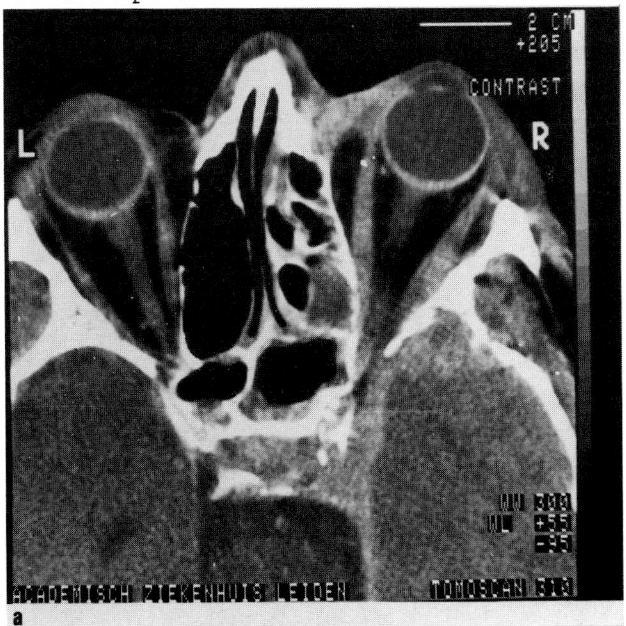

Fig. 8 Patient with exophthalmos, enlarged muscles and dilated superior ophthalmic vein. The clinical picture and the CT scan showed a superior fissure syndrome.
a. Exophthalmos and enlarged muscles.

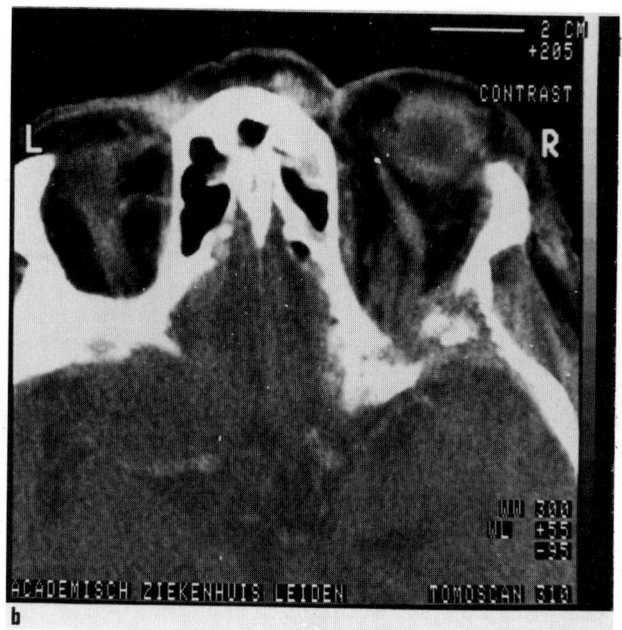

b. Dilated superior ophthalmic vein and tumour in lateral orbital wall.

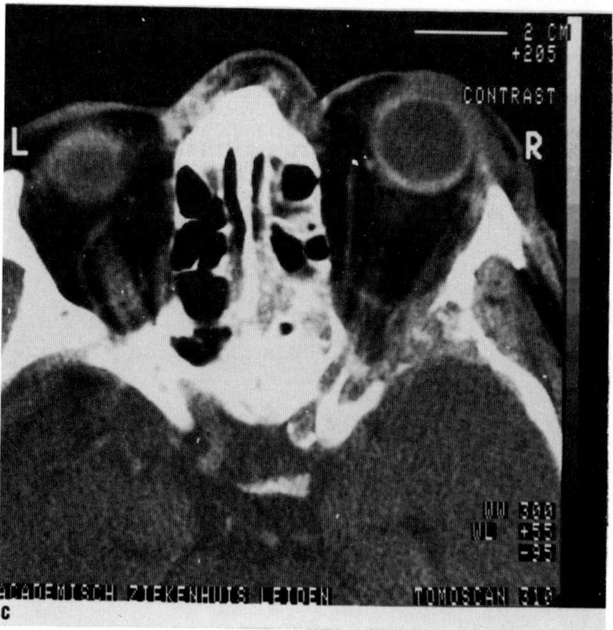

c. Nasopharyngeal carcinoma extending into the orbit and middle cranial fossa.

Blood cysts and aneurysms of the ophthalmic artery

In our series we did not encounter these disorders. Aneurysms of the ophthalmic artery are very rare. Huber and Yasargil (1983) described visual problems and even an acute haemorrhage. Blood cysts are equally rare. They are filled with old blood originating from rupture of a varix after trauma or from blood dyscrasia (Lloyd, 1982).

Vascular disorders detectable by neuro-ophthalmological signs and symptoms

Painful ophthalmoplegia or the Tolosa-Hunt syndrome

This syndrome consists of a total ophthalmoplegia together with excruciating pain and sometimes with exophthalmos. The syndrome is consequent to a granulomatous inflammation in the cavernous sinus which sometimes extends into the superior ophthalmic vein.

Steroid therapy is effective within a couple of hours. The response is so prompt that it can be used as a diagnostic test.

Syndromes of the orbital apex and of the orbital fissure

These syndromes may arise from granulomatous lesions, orbital tumours or macroaneurysms of the mid-cranial fossa. It is important to differentiate from carcinoma of the nasopharynx (Fig. 8). CT-scan, orbital phlebography, arteriography, and the effect of steroid therapy are of great importance for assessment of the proper diagnosis.

Arterial or venous thrombosis

Vasculopathy - this term is used for arterial or venous thrombosis - in vessels of the eye may be combined with orbital and sometimes even cerebral thrombosis (Brismar and Brismar, 1978; De Keizer, 1984). The condition is sometimes hard to recognize. In six of our patients with strange disturbances a vasculopathy was finally identified as the cause:

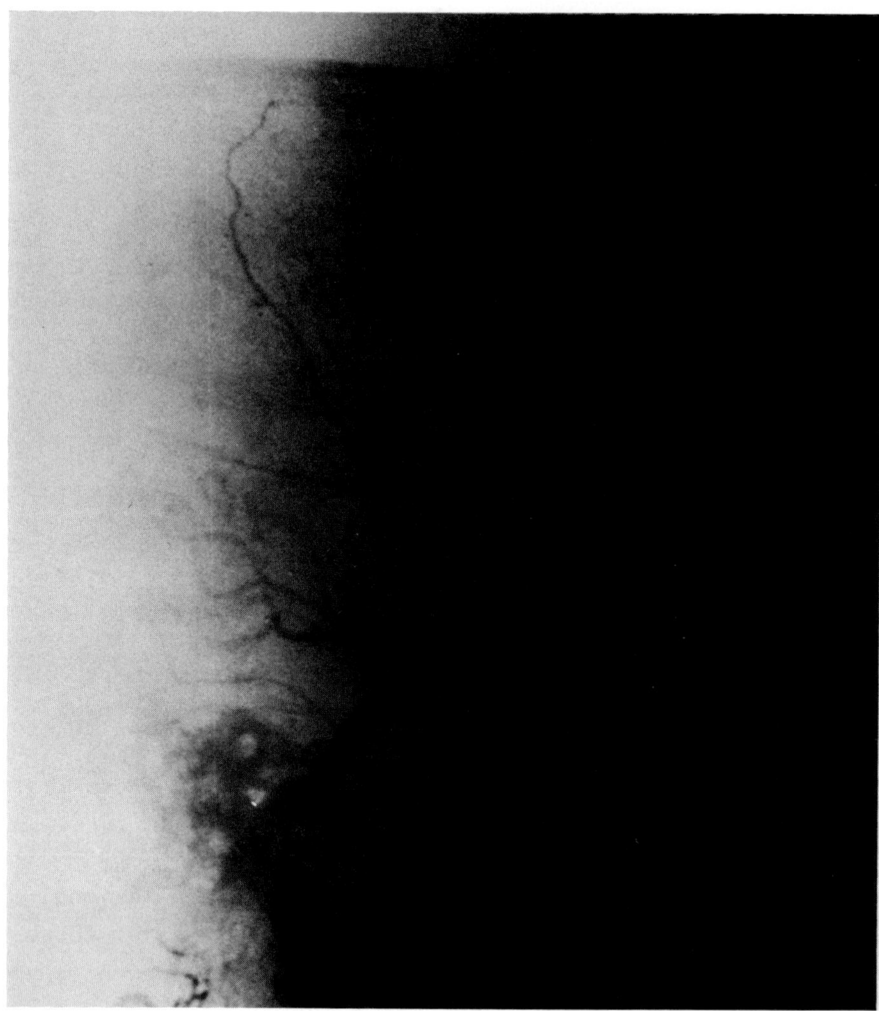

Fig. 9 Patient with bilateral exophthalmos, high ESR, venous loops on the eyeball, and thrombosis of the superior ophthalmic vein and the ophthalmic artery; only the latter is visible in the figures.

three had a haemolytic uraemic syndrome, two had a thrombosis of the superior sagittal sinus and one had a thrombosis consequent to a granulomatous lesion localized in the midcranial fossa. Three other patients showed the typical Tolosa-Hunt syndrome.

Phakomatoses

Wyburn-Mason syndrome

This syndrome, characterized by facial, retinal and cerebral arteriovenous malformations, was found in three patients of our series. Two other patients showed only arteriovenous malformation of the retina and one patient showed facial and orbital arteriovenous malformations. Patients with the Wyburn-Mason syndrome run the risk of haemorrhage within the cerebral arteriovenous malformation. The retinal malformation (Fig. 10) does seldom decompensate and therapy is not necessary but the facial malformation (Fig. 11) may require treatment.

This kind of arteriovenous malformation shows the so-called grow phenomenon (French, 1977), meaning that the normal vessels in the direct surroundings of the tumour will be involved in the process, at first haemodynamically and later on anatomically.

Embolization of the big afferent branches of the external carotid artery is often successful. Secondary cosmetic surgery is sometimes necessary (De Keizer and Van Dalen, 1981); this was done in two of our patients.

Von Hippel-Lindau syndrome

This syndrome, a combination of haemangioblastoma of retina and cerebellum, is dominantly hereditary. In one of our patients optic atrophy was initially considered to be of traumatic origin until angiography revealed a haemangioblastoma. Histologically the tumour consists of spaces with thin walls covered by polygonal cells with swollen foamy cytoplasm and lipid deposits.

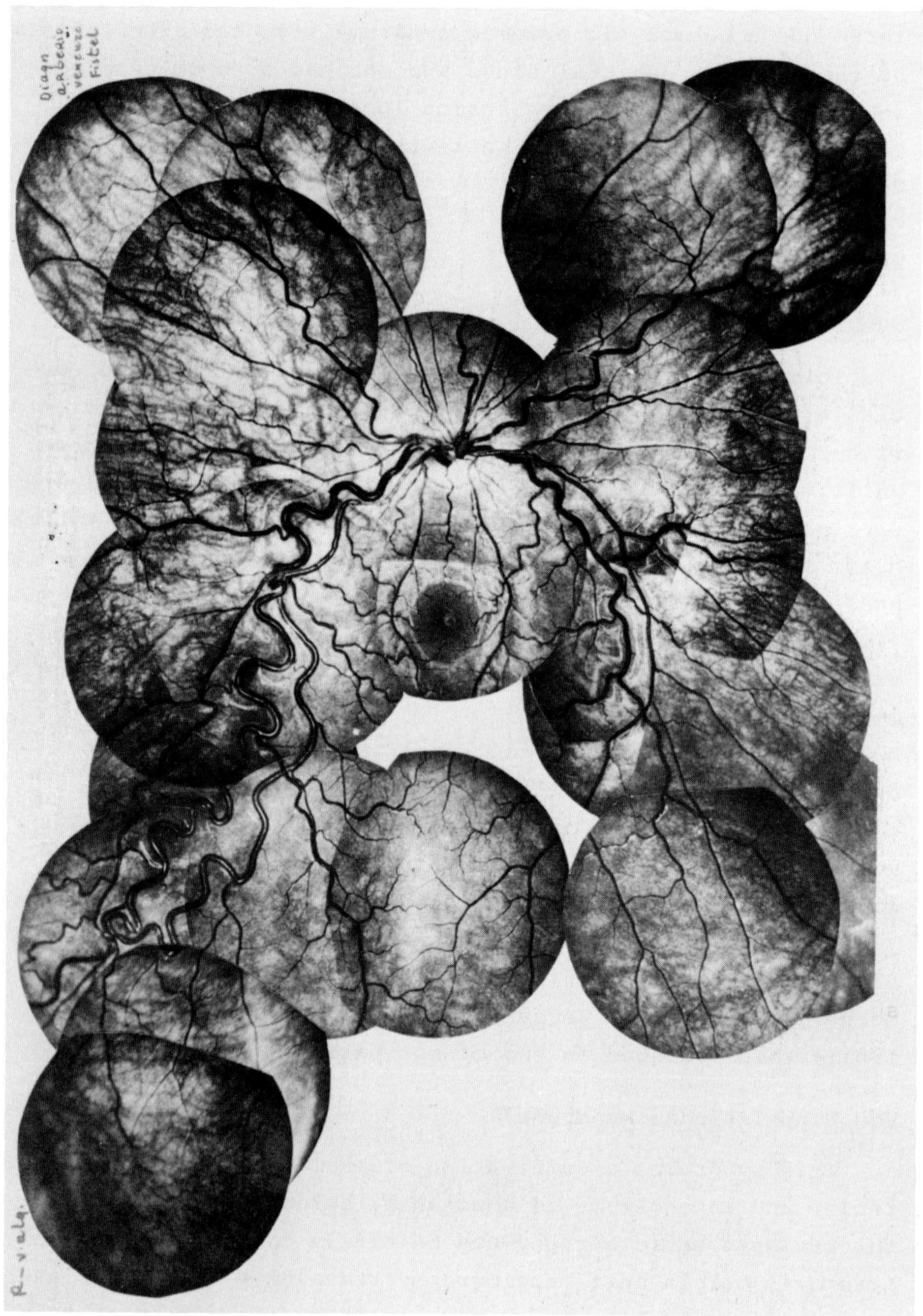

Fig. 10 Retinal arteriovenous malformation.

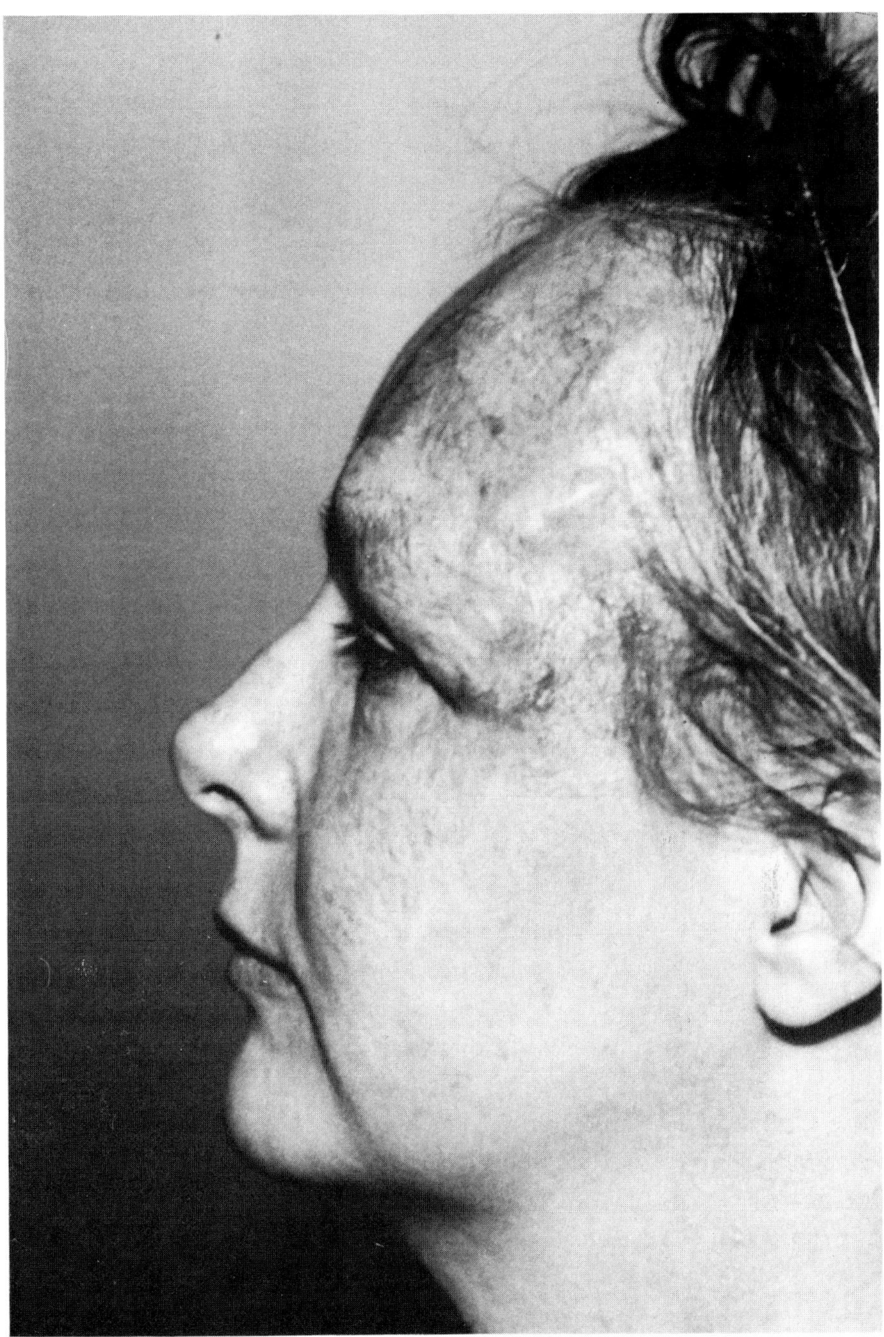

Fig. 11 Facial arteriovenous malformation.

Sturge-Weber syndrome

The syndrome is characterized by a portwine haemangioma in the region of the trigeminal nerve, sometimes accompanied by a buphthalmos or juvenile glaucoma secondary to a high episcleral venous pressure (Phelps, 1978; De Keizer, 1981[b]. The patients often have epileptic seizures caused by cerebral haemangiomas, the so-called angiodysplasia of the leptomeninges (Moseley and Sanders, 1982).

The portwine haemangioma or naevus flammeus or teleangiectatic haemangioma of Reese is a variety of the capillary haemangioma. It is violet but its colour does not change on pressure and the tumour does not recede. In case of intracranial localization calcified double lined gyriform shadows on the X-ray photographs may point to the diagnosis. Angio-osteohypertrophy or the Klippel-Trenaunay syndrome is a combination of these lesions with varicose veins and haemangiomas of the upper and lower extremities and hypertrophy of bone and soft tissue (Lindauer, 1971).

We observed 4 patients with Sturge-Weber syndrome; three came from the out-patient department because of glaucoma, the other one complained of orbital pain.

Vascular neoplasms

These rare tumours, haemangio-endothelioma which we saw only twice, and haemangiopericytoma, which we saw only once, can be either benign or malignant (Sugar et al., 1970). The diagnosis is usually made by the histopathologist. Histological classification of the tumours is as follows: grade 1 is a benign endothelial proliferation within the reticulum sheath of the vessel wall; grade 2 is a transition to grade 3; grade 3 is characterized by abundant mitoses, undifferentiated spindle cells, and angioblastic cells with large nuclei and marked pleomorphism (Friendly et al., 1982).

References

Brismar, G. and Brismar, J.: Aseptic venous thrombosis or Tolosa-Hunt syndrome. Proc. 3rd Int.Symp.Orbital Disorders, Amsterdam, 1977. Dr. W. Junk Publ., The Hague, 1978, pp 392-397.

De Keizer, R.J.W.: Spontaneous carotid cavernous fistulas. Neuro-Ophthalmology 2: 35-46, 1981a.

De Keizer, R.J.W.: Spontane carotico-caverneuze fistels. Thesis, Schipper-Drukwerk, Zaandijk, 1981b.

De Keizer, R.J.W.: A Doppler haematotachographic investigation in patients with ocular and orbital symptoms due to a carotid cavernous fistula. Docum.Ophthal. 52: 297-307, 1982.

De Keizer, R.J.W.: Unusual vascular lesions (a vasculopathy) in the ocular and orbital regions. Ophthalmologica 188: 183, 1984.

De Keizer, R.J.W. and Van Dalen, J.T.W.: Wyburn-Mason syndrome. Subcutaneous angioma extirpation after preliminary embolisation. Docum.Ophthal. 50: 263-273, 1981.

De Keizer, R.J.W., Peeters, F.L.M. and Veenhuijzen, H.B.: Diagnostic and therapeutic considerations in carotid-cavernous fistulas as a cause of exophthalmos. Orbit 3: 153-169, 1984.

French, L.A.: Surgical treatment of arteriovenous malformations. Clin.Neurosurg. 24: 22-33, 1977.

Friendly, D.S., Font, R.L. and Milhoral, T.H.: Hemangioendothelioma of frontal bone. Amer.J.Ophthal. 93: 482-490, 1982.

Haik, B.G., Jakobiec, F.A., Ellsworth, R.M. and Jones, I.S.: Capillary hemangioma of the lids and orbit. Ophthalmology 86: 760-789, 1979.

Hamby, W.B.: Carotid cavernous fistula. C.C. Thomas, Springfield USA, 1966.

Henderson, J.W.: Orbital tumors. W.B. Saunders Co., Philadelphia USA, 1980, pp 154-176.

Huber, A. and Yasargil, M.G.: Die Aneurysmen der Arteria ophthalmica. Klin.Mbl.f.Augenheilk. 182: 537-543, 1983.

Iraci, G., Galligioni, F., Gerosa, M., Fiore, N., Andrioli, G., Pardatscher, K., Salar, G. and Marin, G.: Intracerebral venous angiomas as a cause of exophthalmos. Ann. Ophthal. 11: 603-612, 1979.

Jacobiec, F.A. and Jones, I.S.: Vascular tumors, malformations, and degenerations. Clinical Ophthalmology vol. 2, chapter 37, ed. T.D. Duane. Harper & Row, Philadelphia, 1982.

Lindauer, S.M.: The Klippel - Trenaunay syndrome. Ann.Surg. 174: 248-263, 1971.

Lloyd, G.A.S.: Vascular anomalies in the orbit. Orbit 1: 45-54, 1982.

Moseley, I.F. and Sanders, M.D.: Computerized tomography in neuro-ophthalmology. Chapman & Hall, London, 1982, pp 53 and 264.

Peeters, H.J.F. and Bleeker, G.M.: Orbital haemangioma in children. Proc. 2nd Int.Symp.Orbital Disorders, Amsterdam, 1973. Modern Probl.Ophthal. 14: 398-401, 1975.

Peeters, F.L.M. and Van der Werf, A.M.J.: Detachable balloon technique in the treatment of direct carotid-cavernous fistulas. Surg.Neurol. 14: 11-19, 1980.

Phelps, C.D.: The pathogenesis of glaucoma in Sturge-Weber syndrome. Ophthalmology 85: 276-286, 1978.

Plessner-Rasmussen, H.-J., Marushak, D. and Goldschmidt, E.: Capillary haemangiomas of the eyelids and orbit. A review of 5 children. Acta Ophthal. 61: 645-654, 1983.

Reese, A.B.: Angiomatous tumors. In: Tumors of the Eye, 3rd ed., Harper & Row, New York, 1976, pp 264-294.

Sugar, H.S., Fishman, G.R., Kobernick, S. and Goodman, P.: Orbital hemangiopericytoma or vascular meningioma? Amer.J.Ophthal. 70: 103-108, 1970.

Unsöld, R., Hoyt, W.F. and Newton, T.H.: Die computertomographischen Merkmale des kavernösen Hämangioms und ihre Bedeutung für die Differentialdiagnose im Muskeltrichter gelegener Tumoren der Orbita. Klin.Mbl.f.Augenheilk. 175: 773-785, 1979.

Wright, J.E.: The role of ultrasound in the investigation and management of orbital disease. Docum.Ophthal.Proc. Series 29: 273-276. Dr. W. Junk Publ., The Hague, 1981.

THE OTORHINOLARYNGEAL ASPECTS OF THE TREATMENT OF BENIGN ORBITAL DISORDERS

J.P.A. Gillissen

The orbit is surrounded by the territory of the ENT-specialist. The orbital walls are the demarcation of the orbit, the sphere of interest of the ophthalmic surgeon. It is not surprising that interdisciplinary consultation is frequently necessary in case of lesions in and around the orbit. This is particularly true for a number of benign orbital disorders. For instance, the Orbital Centre of the University of Amsterdam has needed ENT-assistance in 320 cases during the last two years. In order of frequency these were:

meningioma	81
haemangioma	71
mucocele	52
dermoid cyst	41
neurofibroma and neurinoma	32
fibrous dysplasia	14
osteoma	13
lipogranuloma	6
eosinophilic granuloma	2

In the present paper I will explain where and how the ENT-surgeon can assist the ophthalmologist in orbital surgery, sometimes in co-operation with the neurosurgeon.

Meningioma

In our material of 61 females and 20 males the disorder had become manifest in females in about the 4th decade while in males there was no prevalence of a certain age. Jakobiec reported that in his material 25% of the meningiomas were seen in the first decade. This is entirely different from

Oosterhuis, A. (ed.), Ophthalmic tumors.

ISBN 90-6193-528-8. Printed in the Netherlands.

our records.

If a meningioma primarily originates from the nerve sheath of the optic nerve and if the tumour does not extend beyond the optic foramen, surgery is usually performed by the ophthalmologist without assistance of a neurosurgeon or and ENT-specialist. The majority of the orbital meningiomas, however, develop from the sphenoid bone or from the basal frontal region. In these cases the ophthalmologist needs the co-operation of other disciplines.

Patients with meningioma of the orbit usually consult an ophthalmologist because of exophthalmus and sometimes loss of vision. X-ray photographs and CT-scans delineate the expansion of the tumour and sometimes reveal its pathology as well, for instance if the lesion is marked with positive contrast on the CT-scan. The bone is thickened and becomes more dense. In case of a primary meningioma of the optic nerve the optic canal may be enlarged.

Depending on the localization of the tumour other disciplines may be consulted. In first instance it has to be decided whether surgical intervention is necessary or can be postponed, since orbital meningiomas usually are very benign and grow slowly. Many neurosurgeons are of opinion that surgery stimulates growth of the meningioma. Since it is as a rule impossible to remove a meningioma completely, the stimulation of growth is a strong argument in favour of postponement. On the other hand, postponement entails the risk that enormous tumours will have to be removed because of cosmetic disturbances and danger to vision in old people but may have become inoperable. In addition the mental burden of the horrible cosmetic aspect during the second half of the patient's life should not be neglected as a strong argument for early intervention. Accordingly, it is nowadays agreed that orbital meningioma should be operated before it causes cosmetic malformation or visual disturbances.

It may be of interest that in one family among our patients there was a clear-cut hereditary meningioma. Five members had during their lifetime one or even several of these tumours, often with different localizations. For instance, one woman first developed a meningioma in the cranial vault and some years later a meningioma of the spinal column. Combinations with acoustic neuroma were sometimes seen. One of them concerns a girl of 16 years who has such a neuroma bilaterally. Combinations with neurofibroma are not frequently seen. The variety in localization of orbital meningiomas once more emphasizes the need for co-operation of ophthalmologist, ENT-specialist and neurosurgeon.

Haemangioma

The differentiation between capillary haemangioma and cavernous haemangioma is not always very marked. During the last 10 years 8 newborn children, 6 girls and 2 boys, with capillary haemangiomas were presented at our clinic. Capillary haemangioma in the very young child has a tendency to regress spontaneously after the sixth month of life. The only reason to operate haemangioma in young children is the danger of amblyopia if the tumour obscures the visual axis. Under these circumstances one has to keep in mind that operating a haemangioma is not without risk, in particular when the tumour extends far into the orbit.

Cavernous haemangioma was seen in 63 patients, 38 of which (60%) were female. The disorder becomes manifest at all ages but there are two peaks: one in the first and one in about the fourth decade. Cavernous haemangioma is often situated within the muscle cone and easily gives rise to visual disturbances and folds in the ocular fundus. Exophthalmos and motility disturbances may complete the picture. Consultation of the ENT-specialist is advisable when the haemangioma is situated against the orbital wall. Erosion of the bone or even a complete defect may open the door to complications in the surrounding sinuses and other tissues.

Estimation of the extension of the tumour from X-ray photographs, or even better from NMR pictures, should be subjected to the opinion of the ENT-discipline. The larger the tumour becomes, the greater the risk of complications during the operation, and therefore total extirpation at short notice is advocated.

Mucocele

Although mucoceles manifest themselves in the orbit by exophthalmos and diplopia, this disorder is typically the responsibility of the otolaryngologist. Among the records of the last ten years we met mucoceles in 52 patients. There was a slight prevalence of females and patients above the age of 40 years. In 46 of the patients the mucocele originated from the frontal sinus. In the remaining 6 patients the ethmoid sinus was primarily affected. We never encountered mucoceles from the maxillary sinus. Probably, mucoceles in this location cause other symptoms before they invade the orbit and are not presented at the Orbital Centre.

Mucoceles invade the orbit very slowly and are recognized only when they have become fairly substantial. Although exophthalmos is always present, the patients seldom complain of diplopia. The diagnosis is easily made on palpation. The tumour feels like a table tennis ball. X-rays reveal a cloudy shadow and absence of part of the orbital wall. CT-scans demonstrate the mucocele even more easily. A warning must be given with regard to the combination of mucocele and infection. One of our patients lost vision within 24 hours due to this inflammation. As soon as infection is suspected a mucocele should be operated instantly under cover of antibiotics. During surgery one must always be careful with the trochlea. Sometimes it is not possible to keep it intact, which may result in diplopia after surgery. Fortunately, this diplopia disappears spontaneously within a few days. In 3 patients however we had to perform secondary muscle surgery to obtain a satisfactory result.

The walls of mucoceles are very thin. Therefore it is often very difficult to remove the mucocele in toto. If this is not possible, it is necessary to treat the lining of the mucocele with alcohol in order to prevent recurrence. This denaturation is contraindicated if the dura mater is exposed. Despite this precaution we had a recidive in 4 out of 51 patients. These recurrences should be operated as soon as possible.

Dermoid cyst

These cysts have an epidermal lining and contain a mixture of keratine, hair and sometimes dental elements. They originate from developmental abnormality as the orbit takes shape in early foetal life. It is a typical tumour of childhood. In our series we have 41 dermoid cysts, without sex predilection but in the males the cysts had developed later, above the age of thirty years. The localization of dermoid cysts is mainly in the upper temporal region near the lacrimal gland. In most cases they cause a displacement of the eye in forward direction. They are attached to the bony wall and by erosion they can protrude into the temporal fossa. These sand-hour-like tumours have a characteristic elastic feeling.

The treatment of choice is total extirpation. Not only should the cysts be removed but, since dermoids do not infrequently have a tail into the apex of the orbit, also this tail should be removed to prevent recurrence. The sand-hour-shaped dermoid cysts in particular should be subjected to combined effort of ophthalmologist and otolaryngologist.

Neurofibroma and neurinoma

Both are of neural origin. Neurofibroma develops from the Schwann cells of the sheath around the nerves. Tumours like these are not encapsulated. The nerve itself is hard to identify at its course through the tumour. In the orbit neurofibromas are usually situated in the upper quadrants. Exophthalmos and diplopia are the first complaints. The diagnosis can be made from the very typical soft-elastic feeling of the overlying skin. The CT-scan easily indicates the diffuse growth of a plexiform neurofibroma in the orbit. Histopathologically, the disease shows a meshwork of interwoven fibres of Schwann cells and surrounding fibres. Café-au-lait spots are nearly always found somewhere in the skin. Surgery of plexiform neurofibroma is rarely radical because of its diffuse spreading.

In our series we have 32 patients with neurofibroma, 19 males and 13 females. In order to confirm the diagnosis surgery was done in all our patients, with very little benefit to the patients however. In the plexiform neurofibroma in particular, ptosis due to lesion of the levator muscle or its supplying nerve occurred in 6 patients, 3 of them needing additional cosmetic surgery afterwards. Operation of a recidive should only be performed in case of severe complaints as some authors are of opinion that surgery of a plexiform neurofibroma will stimulate growth of the remaining rest, as in case of meningioma. From our small material no conclusions are allowed.

The neurinomas in our series usually resulted from a trauma or from surgery. The growth of a neurinoma is extremely expansive. Pain is the main complaint and extirpation is the treatment of choice. In spite of operation 2 of our patients kept complaining of serious pain; neurosurgery was needed in both cases.

Fibrous dysplasia

This is another example of a lesion developing inside and outside the orbit. It is part of a general disease and can occur polyostotically as well as localized around the orbit. In our series we have 14 patients with fibrous dysplasia; about 2/3 of them were females. X-ray photographs usually are suggestive of the true nature of the tumour. Surgical exploration is necessary to confirm the diagnosis. Without treatment the disease will usually recede spontaneously. Surgery is only needed in case of severe cosmetic malformation or in case vision is threatened.

Osteoma

Osteoma can be divided into 3 types: bony osteoma, ripe osteoma and fibrous osteoma. Osteoma of the frontal bone is the main primary location. Sometimes the primary lesion is situated in the ethmoid cells. Osteoma may cause displacement of the eye as well as disturbances of vision if it protrudes into the orbit. If it obstructs the paranasal sinus, sinusitis or mucoceles may be the result. In the last 10 years we have met 13 patients with osteoma in and around the orbit; there was no sex or age preference. Surgery is necessary when the tumour causes cosmetic or functional complaints. In one of our patients the tumour had extended so much that secondary neurosurgical treatment was necessary.

Lipogranuloma

We have 6 patients with a lipogranuloma of the orbit. This disease is also known as chocolate cyst of the orbit. So far only 20 patients with this disorder have been described in literature. The clinical picture is dominated by swelling and pain in the region lateral to and above the orbit. X-ray photographs reveal a sharply defined defect in the bone. On surgical exploration one finds a cavity filled with a brown fluid and slush-like material. In this slush there are extracellular crystals. There are foam cells and giant cells with more than one nucleolus.

Surgical removal of the cyst and curetting of the cavity usually leads to complete healing without recurrence.

Eosinophylic granuloma

Eosinophylic granuloma is a non-malignant deposition of histiocytes in the connective tissue and even in the bone; it is part of histiocytosis X. The granuloma is exclusively seen in childhood, often combined with anaemia, thrombopenia and leucopenia, and may be part of the classic Hand-Schüller-Christian disease with insipid diabetes, exophthalmos and impaired bone formation.

In our material we have two cases of eosinophylic granuloma. The disease has a clear-cut tendency to heal spontaneously. Recovery can be speeded up by local infiltration with corticosteroids.

Eosinophylic granuloma as part of histiocytosis X is a typical example of an orbital disorder associated with a general disease. Not only the otolaryngologist and neurosurgeon but also the paediatrician should be consulted, as kidney trouble for instance often accompanies histiocytosis X.

CHEMOTHERAPY OF ORBITAL TUMOURS

F.J. Cleton

Most orbital tumours will be treated by surgery or radiotherapy. Only a few tumours will metastasize and as a consequence be considered for chemotherapy. Medical oncologists therefore have a limited experience in the treatment of such tumours. This is a good reason to concentrate patients with orbital tumours in centres, where surgeons, radiotherapists, pathologists and medical oncologists can combine their efforts to provide optimal treatment. A similar situation exists for several other rare tumours, where the multidisciplinary approach has led to better results.

The main objective of chemotherapy is the destruction of tumour cells by interfering in their metabolism. The advantage over surgery and radiotherapy is that the effect is systemic and covers the whole body. This also implies the major limitation of chemotherapy, which is the lack of specificity. Biochemical differences between normal cells and tumour cells are minor and only quantitative, which means that side effects are always associated with this form of treatment. The second limitation is the development of resistance by the tumour cells through mutation. The chance of a mutation increases with the tumour mass and the number of cells. Therefore chemotherapy is most successful in a small tumour mass. In practice this rarely happens, because any visible tumour will number more than 10^8 cells, which in terms of biology already constitutes a considerable mass. For this reason chemotherapy is often combined with either surgery or radiotherapy. Timing appears to be very important in such combinations. In general chemotherapy is most

Oosterhuis, A. (ed.), Ophthalmic tumors.

ISBN 90-6193-528-8. Printed in the Netherlands.

effective when given prior to one of the other modalities.

When the indications for chemotherapy are considered, several properties of the tumour should be known. The growth rate, the tendency to infiltrate neighbouring tissues and to spread via the circulating blood are of importance. Usually only tumours which metastasize are considered for chemotherapy. In the orbit several tumours which can cause local problems have a low grade of malignancy. These tumours are poor candidates for chemotherapy. Another factor concerns the sensitivity of the tumour to cytostatic drugs. Lymphomas are usually sensitive, whereas melanomas are relatively insensitive tumours. Finally there should be a measurable criterium for tumour response. Because of the lack of specificity we should also consider the tolerance of the patient of cytostatic drugs. Depending on the type of chemotherapy and the drugs used, the function of certain tissues such as the kidneys, the liver and the bone marrow, can be a limiting factor. Drugs like methotrexate[R] and cisplatinum cannot be given to patients with an impaired renal function. In elderly patients the capacity of the bone marrow is often insufficient and only low dosages of cytostatics are tolerated. The life expectancy of the patient and his quality of life shall also determine our choice of treatment. Modern chemotherapy is an intensive treatment, which usually lasts long and requires careful control.

In our choice of treatment, the inhibition of skeletal growth in children by radiotherapy or the mutilation by surgery can pose important problems.

From experimental work in chemotherapy it is known that cytostatic drugs can best be given in a combination at the highest tolerated dose. For most drugs the dose-response curve is steep. In a combination of 3 to 4 drugs, each single drug can be given in the same full dosages as employed when given as a single agent. Most therapeutic regimens consist of short courses with an interval of 3-6 weeks. Treatment usually implies the use of infusion pumps for administration of large quantities of fluid to inhibit renal toxicity. The patients should be carefully monitored, preferably in special oncological wards. The patient's tolerance, in terms of blood counts, liver-, kidney- and heart function, should be constantly monitored. The response of the tumour should be measured before each treatment. The response is expressed as a complete remission when no tumour rest can be found. A partial remission is defined as more than 50% decrease in tumour mass and no change is less than 25% decrease in tumour mass. Any increase in tumour mass or appearance of new lesions is considered progression.

Although orbital tumours are rare, some can be managed by chemotherapy. In children the main candidate is embryonal rhabdomyosarcoma. This tumour is sensitive to combination chemotherapy with Vincristine, Actinomycin-D and Cyclophosphamide or Iphosphamide. Often the tumour can be excised after several courses of chemotherapy without severe mutilation of the face by radical surgery or radiotherapy. The other primary tumours of the orbit include malignant lymphoma, osteosarcoma and Ewing sarcoma, which are all more or less sensitive to chemotherapy. In most cases chemotherapy shall be complemented by radiotherapy or surgery. Melanoma of the eye is little sensitive to chemotherapy and will only be considered after systemic spread. Obviously surgery and radiotherapy are the best treatment modalities for this tumour.

Localizations of some pediatric tumours (for instance neuroblastoma) and leukaemia in the orbit can be a reason for chemotherapy. Neuroblastoma is sensitive to the OPEC regimen, including Oncovin^{R}, Platinum, Etiposide^{R} and Cyclophosphamide. In adults the malignant lymphomas and the soft tissue sarcomas are the main indication for chemotherapy. The diagnosis of malignant lymphoma in the orbit can be very difficult and the help of a competent experienced pathologist is always required. Pseudolymphoma and reactive hyperplasia of lymphoid tissue should be recognized. They should not be treated with cytostatic drugs, but will occasionally react well to corticosteroids. The non-Hodgkin lymphoma can be separated in a low grade malignancy and a high grade malignancy type. The high grade type with an unfavourable prognosis is usually disseminated and requires intensive chemotherapy, often combined with irradiation of the largest bulk of tumour. The lymphoblastic type of lymphoma often spreads to the brain. A small percentage of patients with these highly malignant lymphomas can be cured, but the majority does not survive more than a year.

Surprisingly, the low grade malignant types of lymphoma cause much discussion. These tumours are usually disseminated to the bone marrow, the spleen, the liver and many lymph nodes. They can often easily be brought into a complete remission, but always relapse. The life expectancy of the patients is often over 10 years. Intensive chemotherapy has not resulted in improving this survival. The patients are therefore only treated when the tumour causes distressing symptoms. Local radiotherapy is also a good alternative, especially in elderly patients.

Soft tissue sarcoma of the orbit in adults will always primarily be treated by the surgeon. Chemotherapy can provide a temporary palliation but never results in a cure. In disseminated soft tissue sarcoma the CyVaDic regimen, consisting of Cyclophosphamide, Vincristine, Adriamycin and DTIC, can induce a complete or partial remission in 30-40% of patients.

The medical oncologist will probably be confronted most with metastases of solid tumours, such as breast cancer or lung cancer, in the orbit or in the retina. The usual choice of treatment is radiation, which causes a good palliative effect.

In the treatment of tumours of the appendices, such as the eye lids or the lacrimal glands, there is as yet no place for chemotherapy.

The medical oncologist dislikes to treat non-malignant conditions with cytostatic drugs, especially because of the late (carcinogenic) effects. When certain diseases have a distinctly malignant course, this may form an exception. For most oncologists a progressive orbital localization of Wegener's granulomatosis will be an exception. This disease is sensitive to treatment with a combination of Cyclophosphamide, Vincristine and Prednisone. Some dramatic effects have been observed on lesions in the orbit, in the lungs and in the kidneys.

REFERENCES

Henk JM, Wright JE and Sandland MR. 1982. Eye and Orbit. In: Treatment of Cancer. (K.E. Hainan, ed.) Hammersmith Hospital, London.

Voûte PA and Kraker de J. 1977. Medical treatment of malignant orbital tumours in children. Proceedings 3rd Int. Symposium on Orbital disorders. Amsterdam.

Voûte PA, Vos A., Kraker de J and Behrendt H. 1979. Rhabdomyosarcomas: chemotherapy and limited supplementary treatment program to avoid mutilation. National Cancer Institute Monograph no. 56.

Haynes BF, Fishman ML, Fanci AS and Wolff SM. 1977. The ocular manifestations of Wegener's granulomatosis. The Am J of Med 63: 131.

RADIOTHERAPY OF TUMOURS OF THE ORBIT AND OCULAR ADNEXA

H.A. van Peperzeel

The role of radiotherapy in malignant tumours of the orbit and the ocular adnexa is limited. In most cases there is a preference for surgical treatment.

In a number of cases, however, the radiotherapist is consulted for the treatment of this type of tumours because ophthalmologists shrank from decisions such as enucleation of the eye or exenteration of the orbit. Of course, these surgical procedures are mutilating but the mutilation is not greater than by amputation or exarticulation of a limb. If life can be preserved by timely surgical intervention, that means in a period of the disease when the chance of distant metastases is low, it is an error to omit surgery and to let the critical time expire in which life can be preserved.

Therefore, it is of great importance that also ophthalmologists take part in oncologic teams in which oncologic surgeons, radiotherapists and medical oncologists discuss together which possibilities each discipline can contribute in the treatment of a special type of tumour in an individual patient. In the discussion the pathologist is indispensable and the experience of the oncologists in the natural history of the tumour is essential in the choice of treatment.

Not only can a curative therapy be started in time, also senseless mutilations can be prevented and a correct palliative treatment can be started.

For the following tumours of the orbit and adnexa the radiotherapist has to be consulted:

- m.Hodgkin and non-Hodgkin lymphoma
- basal cell carcinoma and squamous cell carcinoma of the eyelid and conjunctiva

Oosterhuis, A. (ed.), Ophthalmic tumors.

ISBN 90-6193-528-8. Printed in the Netherlands.

- adenocarcinoma of the lacrimal gland
- embryonal rhabdomyosarcoma in children
- metastases of malignant tumours elsewhere in the body.

In each case it should be decided if radiotherapy can make a curative or palliative contribution in the treatment. In the decision the likelyhood of a favourable response of the tumour has to be weighed against the complications of the therapy.

Irradiation is aimed at killing the tumour with as less damage as possible to the surrounding healthy tissues. The risk of radiation damage depends on:

- the tolerance of the irradiated healthy tissue, e.g. skin, conjunctiva, cornea, lens, retina;
- the quality of the irradiation beam;
- the use of advanced radiation techniques;
- the experience in the radiotherapeutic centre.

From this summing up it is already clear that for most orbital tumours centralisation of the treatment in a radiotherapy department of an oncologic centre is indicated. Not only is consultation among oncologic surgeon, radiotherapist and medical oncologist then possible, also advanced techniques and different beam qualities are available which, together with the experience of the radiotherapist in the treatment of these not frequently occurring tumours, is required for obtaining optimal results.

The complications that may occur are:

- atrophy of the skin with fibrosis and retraction of the eyelids
- loss of eyelashes
- transient conjunctivitis
- reduction of tear secretion, with dehydration of conjunctiva and cornea
- cataract
- retinopathy

The complications depend on the dose given and the risk of complications becomes greater as the dosage increases. Now let us see what radiotherapy can attain in the cases mentioned.

M. Hodgkin and non-Hodgkin lymphoma

In this systemic disease localisation in an organ is in most cases the manifestation of an advanced stage of the disease (stage IV). Less frequently it is an extranodal localization , mostly stage IE. Therefore in all cases the following is necessary:

- histological diagnosis
- complete staging of the disease
- in case of stage IV polychemotherapy as therapy of choice; radiotherapy has only a supplementary place in the treatment;
- in case of stage IE radiotherapy with megavoltage photons in a dose of 40 Gy in 4 weeks; irradiation damage hardly occurs in this dose scheme and the local results are very good;
- accurate follow-up for years.

In cases of non-Hodgkin disease stage IE after radiotherapy the local results are even better than in the nodal stage I (IE = involvement of a single extralymphatic organ or site; I = involvement of a single lymph node region). This is due to the fact that not all cases IE of the non-Hodgkin lymphomas become systemic - especially not the cases with histologically low grade malignancy -, which makes the nodal forms of non-Hodgkin lymphomas so notorious. In histologically high grade malignancies a stage IE can advance rapidly, but even then polychemotherapy can result in a 5 years' survival of about 40%. An accurate follow-up of the patient is therefore required.

Basal cell carcinoma and squamous cell carcinoma of the eyelids

In my opinion, radiotherapy is the therapy of choice, especially with regard to the cosmetic aspect. In comparison with surgery the percentage of complete response is the same. With special techniques and skill also in those regions complicated by folds and not easily reachable corners the results can be the same as in those cancers in the skin which are easily reachable. The 5 years tumour-free survival is 90-95%.

Of importance in these carcinomas are the pathological criteria:

- histology
- the spiky way of growth
- the depth of infiltration
- the size of the lesion
- the presence of lymph node metastases in case of squamous cell carcinoma.

The depth of infiltration is the most important factor in the prognosis; the size of the lesion is especially important for the cosmetic effect. Attention has to be paid to:

- a sufficiently great radiation field, especially in spikily growing basal cell carcinoma;
- the radiation dose has to be calculated on the tumour bed and not on the surface of the tumour;
- a dose equivalent of about 50 Gy in 10 fractions in 2 weeks overall time is needed with Roentgen contact therapy (50 kV) or with electrons of 2-4 MeV;
- an individually made mould surrounds the lesion widely and the eye itself is shielded in order to prevent conjunctivitis and cataract;
- a follow-up of at least 5 years is needed to collect information on recurrences, new localisations and, in case of squamous cell carcinoma, lymph node metastases.

Complications are rare but loss of eyelashes may occur. In case of a recurrence after radiotherapy surgery is possible with good results, whereas radiotherapy after irradical surgery has disappointing results. Especially when after irradical removal a reconstruction is made, postoperative radiotherapy has to be given over a great field, which limits the dose and badly influences the cosmetic results.

A special case is the squamous cell carcinoma of the conjunctiva. When the lesion is superficial, radiotherapy can be considered as a substitute for surgery. Strontium 90 applications or irradiation with low energy electrons can give good results, especially in the case of carcinoma in situ. Conjunctivitis with photophobia may occur, but this disappears spontaneously some weeks or months after the irradiation. Late damage is not observed and the risk of radiation cataract is minimal.

In cases of deep infiltration surgical procedures are always needed and enucleation or exenteration may be necessary.

Adenocarcinoma of the lacrimal gland

These tumours are not radiosensitive. Surgery is the only procedure with a chance of eliminating the malignancy. In case of incomplete excision re-operation is necessary until the tumour has been completely removed.

Radiotherapy is considered as palliative treatment for fighting pain in inoperable cases or recurrences that infiltrate into the orbital bone.

Rhabdomyosarcoma

The therapy of choice is surgery, but in children radiotherapy can be contributory; 75% of the rhabdomysarcomas in the orbital area in children are of the embryonal type and only 25% are of the alveolar type.

This tumour needs a combination treatment in which the surgeon, the medical oncologist, and the radiotherapist participate, and because the tumour is rare and the therapy still in an experimental stage, treatment in a controlled clinical trial is recommended.

The tumour is notorious for meningeal infiltration; in the past extensive surgery has been done followed by radiotherapy in high doses; even polychemotherapy has been given. The prognosis, which has been very bad, has improved in the last 10 years. Surgery nowadays is less extensive and polychemotherapy is given postoperatively in high doses. The local dose of radiotherapy can be lower or can even be omitted. Survival rates of 25-75% have been mentioned in literature, showing that results differ greatly between centres.

When the tumour is limited to the orbit, after exenteration megavoltage photon therapy up to a dose of 50 Gy in 5 weeks is given; 90% local cure is reached and adjuvant chemotherapy has not further improved the results.

The radiation therapy can cause severe deformation in young children owing to the inhibition of bone growth. Maxillofacial reconstruction may be needed when the child is about 15 years old. Also difficulties with the teeth may occur, for which regulation gives no solution; the problem has to wait until the maxillofacial reconstruction can be performed.

A problem which becomes more frequent and which asks for adequate radiotherapy are the orbital metastases from malignancies elsewhere in the body. Intensive chemotherapy lengthens the lifespan of patients with general metastases and therefore these secondaries are found in sites where in the past they were only rarely seen because most patients had already died from their primary tumour or by metastases in the lungs or the liver.

In adults the orbital metastases originate from mammary or lung carcinoma, in children from neuroblastoma, Wilms' tumour or Ewing sarcoma.

In all primary tumours it is imperative to confirm the diagnosis histologically. In metastasis this is not always possible or meaningful. However, the site of the primary tumour elsewhere in the body should be looked for.

Excellent palliative results are reached with megavoltage photon therapy in a dose of 30 Gy in 2 weeks. Vision remains good or improves. The irradiation is given in the same way as in case of a retinoblastoma. Cataract is rare and other complications are not seen in such low dosis radiotherapy. Recurrences of these metastases are not frequent since most patients have advanced metastatic disease with short survival times. Therefore, in those cases radiotherapy is an excellent palliative treatment.

Concluding we see that radiotherapy plays only a modest but beneficial role in the treatment of malignant tumours of the orbit and adnexa. In more than 90% of all cases the treatment can be given to the patients as "out-patients". It must be strongly emphasized that radiotherapy for orbital tumours has to be centralized so that the treatment can be given by an oncological team with advanced radiotherapy techniques and sufficient experience in tumour radiotherapy and its complications.

DIAGNOSTIC FEATURES OF EYELID TUMOURS WITH SPECIAL EMPHASIS ON EPITHELIAL TUMOURS

E. Scheffer and W.A. van Vloten

This chapter deals with the clinical and histological differential diagnosis of a number of selected eyelid tumours. Briefly, the management of these tumours will be discussed.

Tumours of the eyelid may occur as primary growths originating in one of the constituent lid tissues; they may occur as an extension of a tumour in adjoining skin, eye or orbit; they may represent metastatic growth secondary to a primary tumour elsewhere or they may be part of a generalized process, e.g. malignant lymphoma or leukaemia. They have to be differentiated from pseudo-malignant tumours and reactive processes (Henkind & Friedman, 1976).

All tumours which may occur elsewhere in the skin may occur also in the eyelids (Apple & Naumann, 1980; Yanoff & Fine, 1975; Hogan & Zimmerman, 1962). The eyelids are a predilection site of sebaceous carcinomas (Rao et al., 1982) and of the mucinous adenocarcinoma of eccrine origin (Wright & Font, 1979). Phakomatous choristoma (a congenital tumour of lens epithelium) is a benign tumour, unique for the eyelid (Zimmerman, 1971; MacMahon et al., 1976).

Malignant tumours

Basal cell carcinoma is by far the most common malignant tumour affecting the eyelids (Hogan & Zimmerman, 1962; Aurora & Blodi, 1970; Apple & Naumann, 1980). The tumour is found predominantly in older patients; it takes about a year before they seek medical attention. More than 60% of the basal cell carcinomas occur in the lower eyelids. Symptoms mentioned by the patients are irritation, mass of growth, ulceration, bleeding.

Oosterhuis, A. (ed.), Ophthalmic tumors.

ISBN 90-6193-528-8. Printed in the Netherlands.

A typical basal cell carcinoma appears as a small elevated nodule, sometimes with an ulcerated centre, raised translucent pearly borders and fine teleangiectatic vessels (Fig. 1a). Several clinical types can be distinguished as nodular, ulcerative, morphea-like, and superficial types. Although basal cell carcinomas do not metastasize in general, they may cause extensive local destruction and tend to recur after inadequate treatment. Especially medial canthal tumours can spread deeply into the orbit. Therefore, cosmesis should be a secondary concern regarding therapy.

The best way to treat basal cell carcinomas is still a matter of debate; size, shape and histological pattern must be considered. Modalities are surgical excision, radiation or cryosurgery (Biro et al., 1982; Albright, 1982).

Sebaceous carcinoma is said to be the second most occurring malignant eyelid tumour (Rao et al., 1982). There are twice as many sebaceous glands in the upper lid as in the lower lid (fig. 2b). Accordingly, about twice as many sebaceous carcinomas occur in the upper lids as do in the lower lids. They may originate in Meibomian glands, which are localized in the tarsal plate, or in Zeis glands in the lid margins, or in caruncular sebaceous glands or in those localized in the eyebrows. They may originate at multiple sites. Sebaceous carcinoma is the most frequently metastasizing eyelid tumour (Rulon & Helwig, 1974; Weigent & Staley, 1976; Russell et al., 1980; Lee & Roth, 1979; Apple & Naumann, 1980). As to lethality it stands second to malignant melanoma (Rao et al., 1982). Sebaceous carcinoma elsewhere in the skin has a better prognosis (Rulon & Helwig, 1974).

Squamous cell carcinomas are rare on the eyelids. Clinically the tumour is indurated, scaly, elevated with a central ulcer with crusts (Fig. 1b). They can mimic keratoacanthoma, basal cell carcinoma and pseudo-epitheliomatous hyperplasia (Boniuk et al., 1963; Jacobiec & Zimmerman, 1982). The choice of therapy is similar as for basal cell carcinomas.

Intra-epidermal carcinoma (morbus Bowen) is characterized by a slightly red plaque of about 1 cm diameter, sometimes

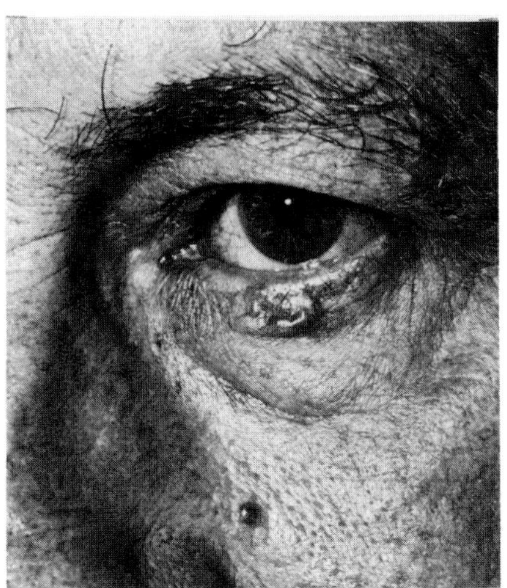

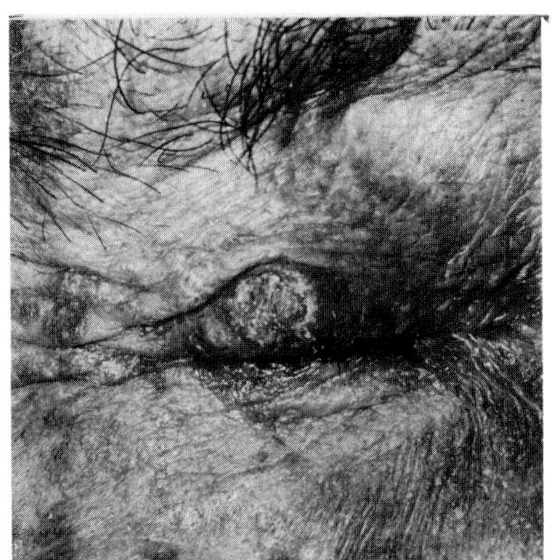

Fig. 1a. Basal cell carcinoma with raised translucent pearly borders.
1b. Squamous cell carcinoma of the upper eyelid.

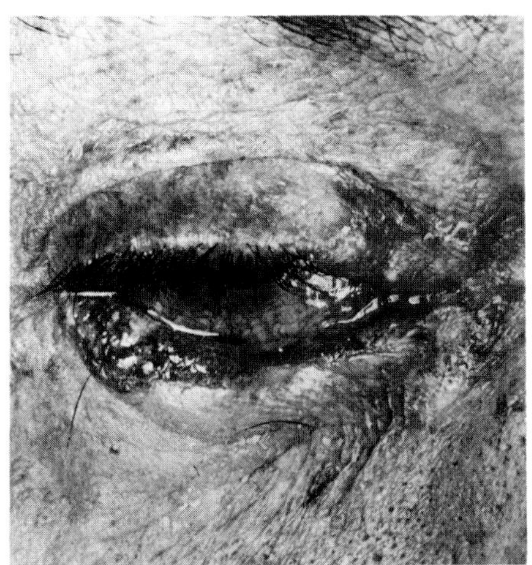

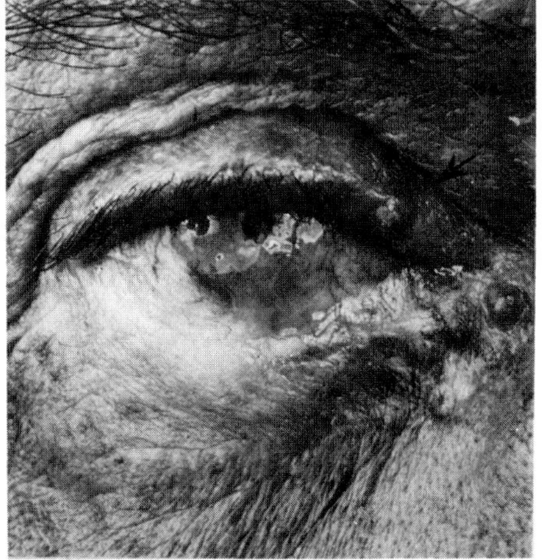

Fig. 2a. Intra-epidermal carcinoma of the lower eyelid.
2b. Same patient three years after therapy of the intra-epidermal carcinoma. Note sebaceous carcinoma in upper eyelid (arrow).

with an ulcerative surface. The lesion need not be confined to the epidermis but may extend into the palpebral and bulbar conjunctiva (Fig. 2a). Histological examination is necessary. Radiation therapy or cryosurgery will give good results.

Actinic keratoses are regarded as premalignant lesions and are characterized by small hyperkeratotic slightly infiltrated lesions of a sun-damaged skin. They always are multiple and scattered over the sun-exposed areas of the face and arms. In any doubt histological examination has to be performed. Therapy with liquid nitrogen will suffice.

Primary malignant melanomas of the eyelids are very rare (Naidoff et al., 1976). Pigmented lesions in the eyelids most frequently are extensions of a lentigo maligna or a lentigo maligna melanoma of the adjoining skin or of a conjunctival melanoma.

Malignant mesenchymal tumours of the eyelids are very rare. Localizations of a malignant lymphoma, e.g. mycosis fungoides confined to the eyelids, are occasionally seen (Knowles & Jacobiec, 1982).

Pseudomalignant tumours

Kerato-acanthoma is a benign tumour which develops rapidly in 4-6 weeks on a previously normal skin. Its characteristic features are elevated margins and a central keratin core; it may achieve a diameter of 1 cm or more (Fig. 3). Kerato-acanthoma is easily confused with squamous cell carcinoma and histological examination is mandatory. Therapy for these lesions are curettage or surgical excision.

Benign tumours

As benign epithelial eyelid tumours hyperkeratotic papillomas, seborrhoic keratoses and various adnexal tumours, a.o. trichoepithelioma, syringoma, etc., are to be mentioned. The latter are rather infrequent, however.

Seborrhoic keratoses look as typical on the eyelids as they do elsewhere on the skin. They are common in middle-aged and elderly patients. The lesions have a round or irregular

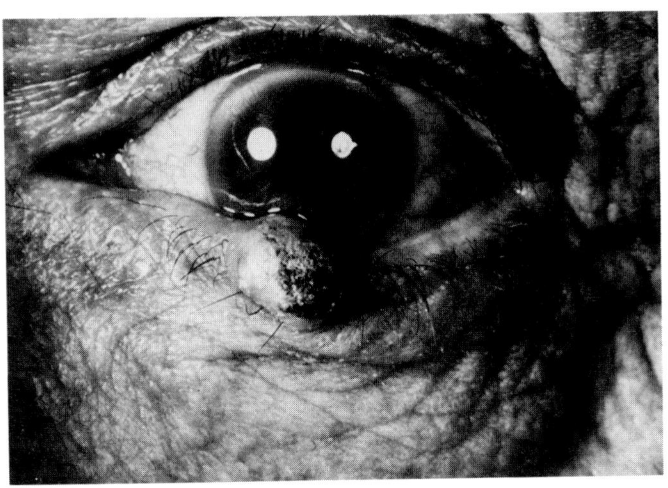

Fig. 3. Kerato-acanthoma of the lower eyelid; note the large keratin core.

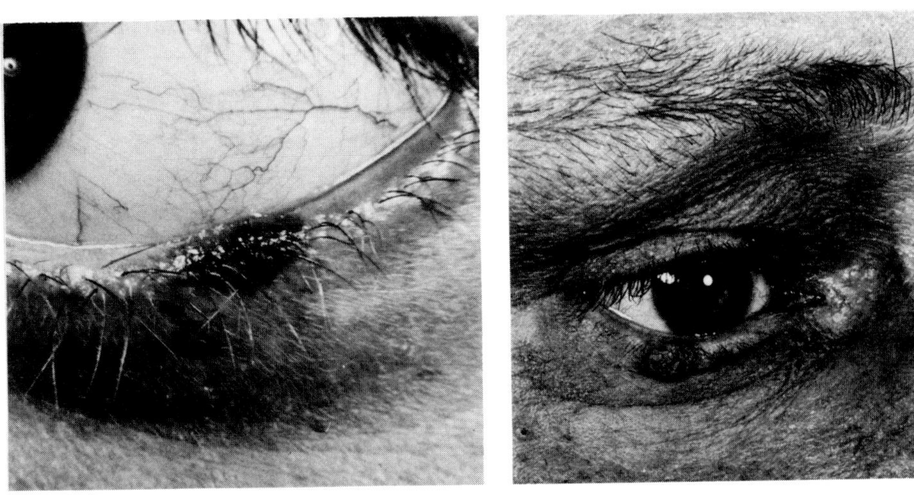

Fig. 4a. Typical naevocellular naevus of the lower eyelid.
4b. Seborrhoic keratosis of the lower eyelid.

shape with smooth borders and appear waxy and to be stuck on the skin (Fig. 4b). Seborrhoic keratosis may look like a melanoma; however, the latter can be differentiated by the more irregular shape, surface and border and a mixture of different colours in one lesion. Therapy for seborrhoic keratosis is curettage or cryotherapy.

Benign mesenchymal tumours, e.g. haemangiomas, lymphangiomas and neurofibromas, are encountered. Haemangiomas may be part of the Sturge-Weber syndrome (meningocutaneous angiomatosis).

Pigmented lesions commonly occur on the eyelids. Most of them are naevocellular naevi (Fig. 4a). A special form of pigmented naevus is the naevus of Ota, which does not only involve the eyelids but also part of the ipsilateral half of the face. Another special naevus is the "kissing naevus", consisting of 2 naevi localized opposite to each other on the upper and lower lid margins and originating from one naevocellular naevus by separation of the eyelids during the developmental period (Hamming, 1983).

Tumours of the eyelids must be differentiated from pseudotumours or reactive processes. Most frequent is the chalazion, a granulomatous inflammation of a sebaceous gland. It may, however, originate secondary to another benign or a malignant process, when a sebaceous duct is compressed or obliterated. A chalazion must be differentiated from a sebaceous carcinoma, especially if it recurs, or if the patient is elderly, or if there is a therapy-resistent blepharo-(or kerato-)conjunctivitis as well (as a result of pagetoid infiltration of the epithelium by sebaceous carcinoma cells (Rao et al., 1982). In over 28% of cases of sebaceous carcinoma there are swollen praeauricular, cervical or submandibular lymph nodes; this never occurs with a chalazion. Chalazion should, of course, also be differentiated from other forms of granulomatous inflammation.

The most frequently occurring cysts are dermoid cysts (with sweat glands and sebaceous glands in the cyst wall) and Moll cysts (with apocrine epithelium). Dermoid cysts often occur at the orbital edge. Moll cysts are localized at the lid margins.

Histological differential diagnostic clues in epithelial skin tumours

Basal cell carcinoma. Several histologic patterns and types are known:

- lobular pattern, may be adenoid or even cystic ("cysts" develop from degeneration of tumour cells) (Figs 5a, 5b); in some cases there are a certain amount of melanocytes producing melanin which gives the tumour a pigmented appearance;
- trabecular pattern, thin strands of tumour cells, lace work;
- splitting, cicatrical, morphea-like pattern (Fig. 6a), thin sheets of tumour cells with abundant stroma reaction; it may even be difficult to tell the fibroblastic response from the tumour cell strands;
- keratotic type;
- superficial (multiple) type (Fig. 6b).

Common to all basal cell carcinomas are:

- monotonous aspects of basaloid cells, in contact with the epidermis;
- palissade-like arrangement of cells on the margins of sheets, lobules or trabecular strands;
- fibroblastic stroma reaction and lymphoreticular infiltrate;
- there may be squamous differentiation centrally in sheets, even keratotic centres; however, cornification is abrupt;
- basaloid cells on the margins (DD squamous cell carcinoma).

Sebaceous carcinoma consists histologically of lobules of cells with varying sebaceous differentiation. Quite typical is pagetoid infiltrative growth into epidermis and follicular epithelium. Sebaceous differentiation is recognized by vacuolar cytoplasm reminiscent of sebaceous gland cells, staining positively with fat stains. The surrounding stroma shows proliferation of fibroblasts and lymphoreticular infiltration (Figs 7a,b,c).

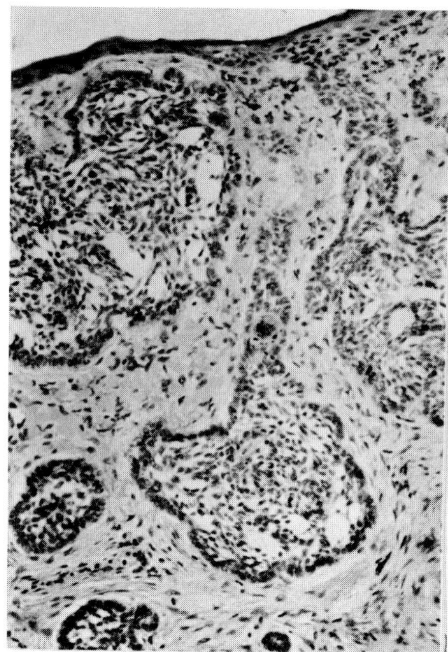

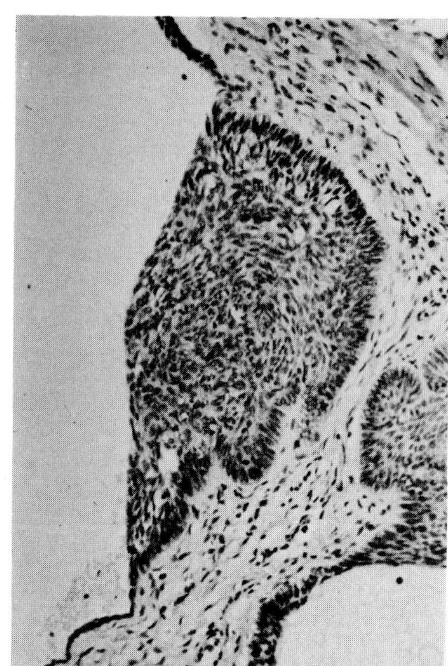

Fig. 5a. Carcinoma basocellulare; lobular pattern; centrally small area of abrupt keratinization; fibroblastic stromal reaction.

5b. Formation of cyst-like spaces in carcinoma basocellulare.

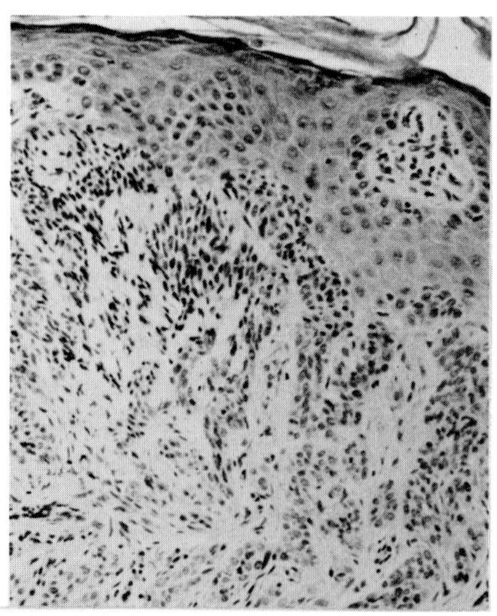

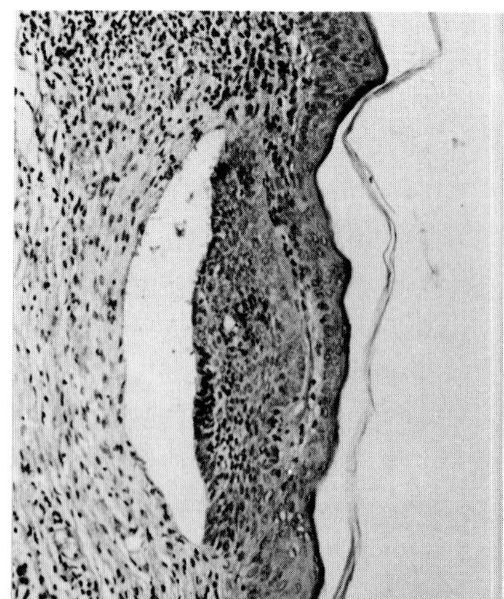

Fig. 6a. Carcinoma basocellulare; thin strands of monotonous atypical basaloid cells; abundant stromal reaction (cicatrical carcinoma basocellulare).

6b. Superficial carcinoma basocellulare; retraction artefact.

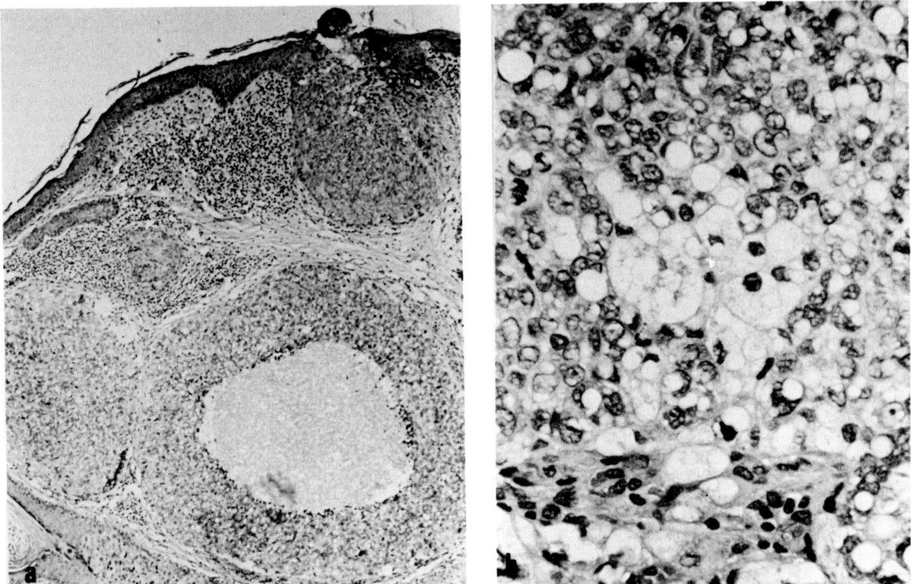

Fig. 7a. Carcinoma sebaceum, locally breaking through the epidermis. Central area of necrosis.
7b. Carcinoma sebaceum. Tumour cells are partly undifferentiated, partly show sebaceous differentiation. A few mitotic figures are seen.

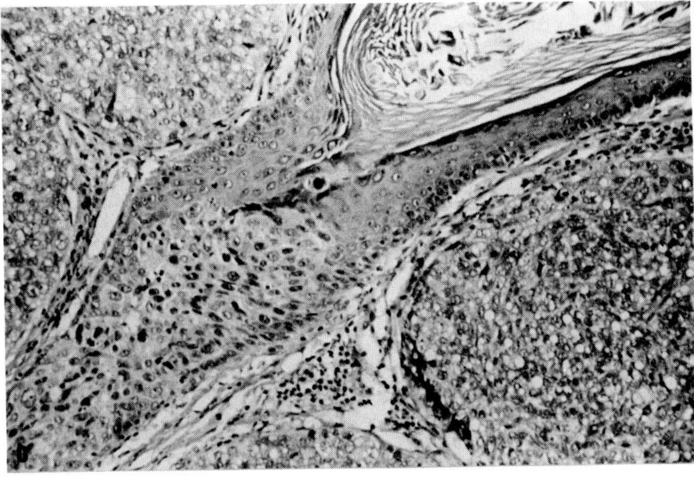

Fig. 7c. Carcinoma sebaceum. Pagetoid growth into follicular epithelium.

Squamous cell carcinoma may show varying differentiation. Well differentiated forms clearly show squamous cells with plasmodesms and keratinization of cell groups (horn pearls) and individual cells.

Differentiation from basal cell carcinoma may be difficult, as this tumour may show squamous differentiation and even, though abrupt, keratinization. However, also severely anaplastic cells are different from the basaloid cells of basal cell carcinoma. There is usually both proliferative and infiltrative stromal reaction closely associated with the tumour cell sheets and strands (Figs 8, 9).

Conditions to be differentiated from squamous cell carcinoma include kerato-acanthoma and pseudo-epitheliomatous hyperplasia. Apart from the clinical histories, important histological clues to kerato-acanthoma are:

- the presence of a central horn crater with a sharp edge;
- high squamous differentiation of the proliferated cells, also of parabasal cells, which characteristically show a glassy cytoplasm;
- moderate infiltrative growth.

It is the degree of infiltrative growth which may make differentiation from squamous cell carcinoma difficult or even impossible. Stromal reaction may be considerable, which may add to this difficulty (Fig. 11).

Pseudo-epitheliomatous hyperplasia usually forms part of a reactive pattern, together with proliferative and infiltrative stromal reactions, rather than that these reactions are obviously directed against the epithelial proliferation. The proliferated epithelium usually shows a high differentiation and no more than a slight atypia (Fig. 10).

Carcinoma in situ (m.Bowen) is characterized by an atypical epithelial cell clone proliferating through the entire thickness of the epidermis and exfoliating at the surface (atypical parakeratosis). Some cells may have large and bizarre nuclei. Mitotic figures are seen up to the uppermost epidermal cell layer. There is no infiltrative growth beyond epidermal and adnexal basal membranes. The adjoining stroma

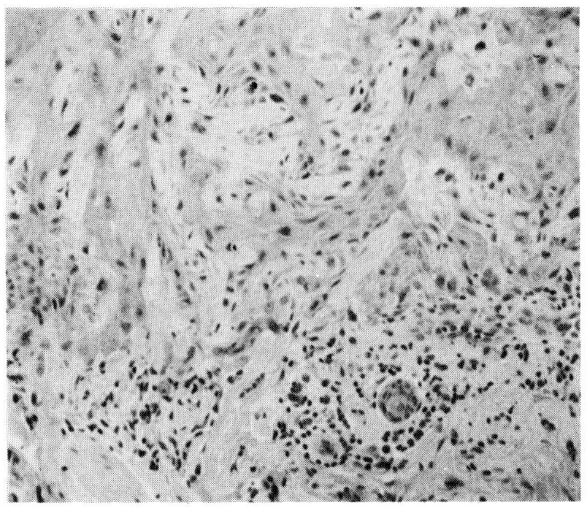

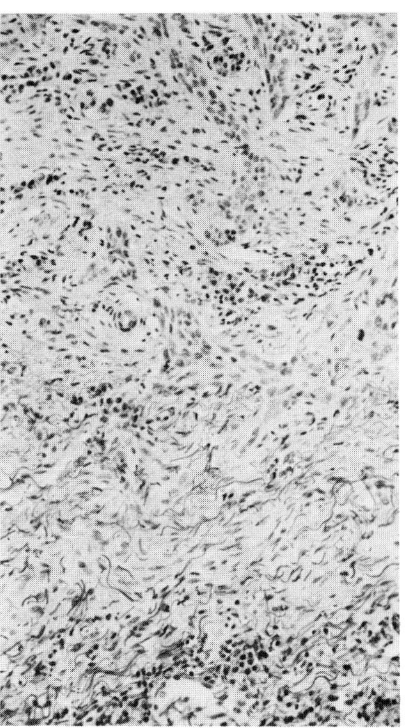

Fig. 8. Carcinoma planocellulare; the infiltrating cells show squamous differentiation. Compare Fig. 8 with Fig. 9.

Fig. 9 Carcinoma basocellulare; the infiltrating cells are monotonous basaloid cells. Same tumour as shown in Fig. 6a.

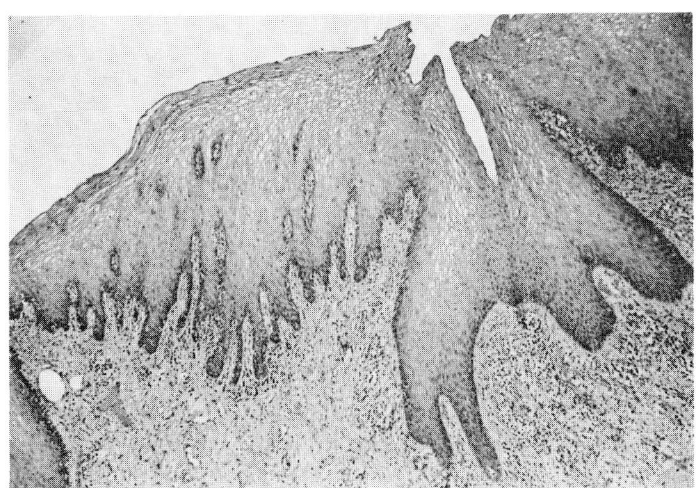

Fig. 10. Pseudo-epitheliomatous hyperplasia.

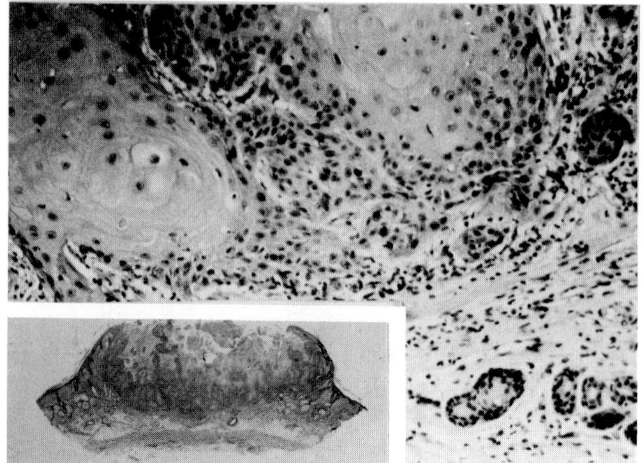

Fig. 11. Kerato-acanthoma; high squamous differentiation, also of parabasal cells: characteristically glassy cytoplasm. Inset: section of complete specimen, with central horn crater with a sharp edge.

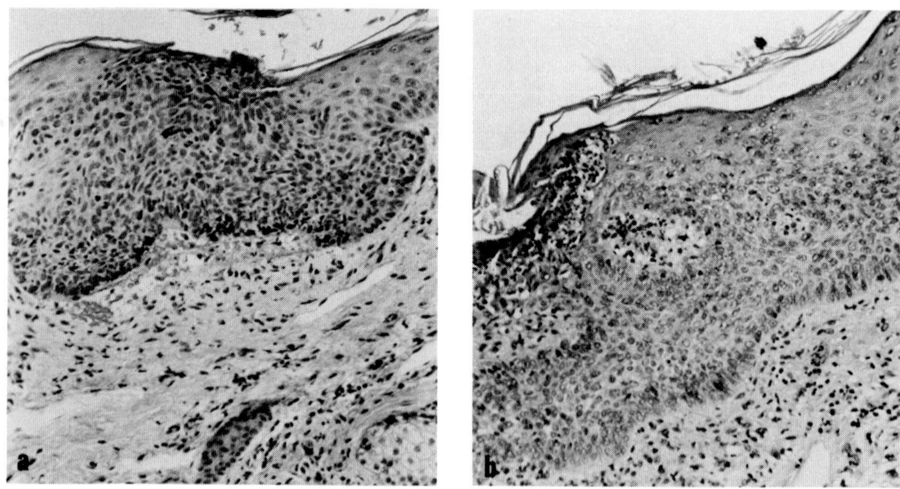

Fig. 12a. Carcinoma in situ (m.Bowen). Atypical epithelial cell clone proliferates through the entire thickness of the epidermis; sharp delineation from adjoining pre-existent keratinocytes.

12b. Idem; compare with Fig. 6b.

shows an infiltrative reaction and often elastosis. There is a sharp demarcation border between the atypical epithelial cells and the adjoining pre-existent epidermal cells. Differentiation from superficial basal epithelioma may be difficult (Figs 12a,b); this, however, "hangs on" the epidermis.

Keratosis actinica is characterized by atypia mainly of basal cells, parakeratosis confined to the areas with atypical basal cells and sharply demarcated from the adjoining normal horn layer, some proliferation of atypical basal cells, elastosis and lymphoreticular infiltration of the adjoining connective tissue. Differentiation from squamous and basal cell carcinoma is usually easy, but may sometimes pose difficulties. In so-called bowenoid actinic keratosis there are large and bizarre cells, but some differentiation in the upper epidermis is present and there are no mitotic figures in the uppermost epidermal layer.

Hyperkeratotic papillomas and seborrhoic keratoses are benign epidermal tumours. Hyperkeratotic papillomas do not show atypical epithelial cells and, unless irritated, no inflammatory response in the subepidermis tissue.

Seborrhoic keratoses may mainly consist of basaloid or of squamous cells, show so-called "pseudo-horny cysts" and no inflammatory response. There may be varying amounts of melanocytes and pigmented keratinocytes. In case of irritation there may be considerable inflammatory response and irregular differentiation patterns in the epithelium ("squamous eddies"). In rare cases, a carcinoma may develop in a seborrhoic keratosis.

References

Albright, S.D. III: Treatment of skin cancer using multiple modalities. J.Am.Acad.Dermatol. 7: 143-171, 1982.

Apple, D.J. and Naumann, G.O.H.: Okuläre Adnexe: Lider, Tränenapparat und Orbita. In: Pathologie des Auges. Ed. G.O.H. Naumann. Springer Verlag, Berlin-Heidelberg-New York, 1980, 15. Kapitel.

Aurora, A.L. and Blodi, F.C.: Lesions of the eyelids: A clinicopathologic study. Survey Ophthalmol. 15: 95, 1970.

Biro, L., Price, E. and Brand, A.: Cryosurgery for basal cell carcinoma of the eyelids and nose: five year experience. J.Am.Acad.Derm. 6: 1042-1047, 1982.
Boniuk, M., Kwitko, M.L. and Zimmerman, L.E.: Tumors of the eyelid with specific reference to lesions often confused with squamous cell carcinoma. I. Incidence and errors in diagnosis. Arch.Ophthalmol. 69: 693, 1963.
Hamming, N.: Anatomy and embryology of the eyelid. Review with special reference to the development of divided nevi. J.Paed.Dermatol. 1: 51-58, 1983.
Henkind, P. and Friedman, A.: Cancer of the lids and ocular adnexa. In: Cancer of the Skin. Eds Andrade, R., Gumport, S.L., Popkin, G.L. and Rees, T.D. Saunders Cy, Philadelphia, 1976, pp 1345-1371.
Hogan, M.J. and Zimmerman, L.E.: Ophthalmic pathology. An atlas and textbook. W.B. Saunders Cy, Philadelphia-London, 1962, chapter IV: Lids and lacrimal drainage apparatus.
Jacobiec, F.A. and Zimmerman, L.E.: Symposium on Ophthalmic Surgical Pathology, part I. Introduction. Human Pathology 13: 98, 1982.
Knowles, D.M. and Jacobiec, F.A.: Ocular adnexal lymphoid neoplasms: clinical, histopathologic, electron microscopic and immunologic characteristics. Human Pathology 13: 148, 1982.
Lee, S.C. and Roth, L.M.: Sebaceous carcinoma of the eyelid with pagetoid involvement of the bulbar and palpebral conjunctiva. J.Cutan.Pathol. 4: 134, 1977.
McMahon, R.T., Font, R.L. and McLean, I.W.: Phakomatous choristoma of eyelid. Electron microscopic confirmation of lenticular derivation. Arch.Ophthalmol. 94: 1778, 1976.
Naidoff, M.A., Bernardino, V.B., Jr. and Clark, W.H., Jr.: Melanocytic lesions of the eyelid, skin and conjunctiva. Amer.J.Ophthalmol. 82: 371, 1976.
Rao, N.A., Hidayat, A.A., McLean, I.W. and Zimmerman, L.E.: Sebaceous carcinomas of the ocular adnexa: a clinicopathologic study of 104 cases, with five-year follow-up data. Human Pathol. 13: 113, 1982.
Rulon, D.B. and Helwig, E.G.: Cutaneous sebaceous neoplasms. Cancer 33: 82, 1974.
Russell, W.G., Page, D.L., Hough, A.J. et al.: Sebaceous carcinoma of meibomian gland origin. Amer.J.Clin.Pathol. 73: 504, 1980.
Weigent, C.E. and Staley, N.A.: Meibomian gland carcinoma; report of a case with electron microscpic findings. Human Pathol. 7: 231, 1976.
Wright, J. and Font, R.L.: Mucus-secreting sweat gland carcinoma of eyelid. A clinicopathologic study of 21 cases with histochemical and electron microscopic observations. Cancer 44: 1757, 1979.
Yanoff, M. and Fine, B.S.: Ocular Pathology. A text and atlas. Harper & Row, New York-Evanston-San Francisco-London, 1975, chapter 6.
Zimmerman, L.E.: Phakomatous choristoma of the eyelid, a tumor of lenticular anlage. Amer.J.Ophthal. 71: 169, 1971.

SURGERY OF ADNEXAL TUMOURS.

J.R.O. COLLIN

The great advantage of surgery over other forms of treatment of eyelid tumours is that the excised specimen can be sent for histological confirmation of both the diagnosis and clearance. Surgery can be carried out under local or general anaesthesia. In most cases local anaesthesia is adequate and the patient can be treated as an out-patient but larger repairs may be easier under general anaesthesia as an in-patient. The tumour should be removed with approximately 4 mm. of macroscopically healthy tissue around it and if this is not possible without extending to the lid margin, a full thickness lid resection is required. It is a great comfort to surgeon and patient to know that a lesion has been completely removed before committing distant tissues to the repair since incomplete clearance has been reported in up to 50% of surgically excised specimens sent for routine histology (Rakofsky, 1973). Clearance can be confirmed with frozen section monitoring of the edges of the excised specimen at the time of surgery but if these facilities are not readily available the specimen can be sent for an urgent paraffin section and it should be possible to have the results in 24-48 hours. The wound is covered during this period and the repair can be carried out when clearance has been confirmed. A success rate of 100% has been reported with eyelid basal cell carcinomas where clearance was confirmed before the defect was repaired (Older et al., 1975).

The repair of an eyelid defect should be approached systematically (Collin, 1983). The eyelid is composed of two layers, an anterior lamella of skin and orbicularis muscle and a posterior lamella of tarsus and conjunctiva. Anterior lamellar defects can be closed directly, or with a skin-flap or skin graft (Fig. 1-3). Posterior lamellar defects can similarly be closed directly, or with a graft or tarsus, conjunctiva, buccal mucous membrane, sclera, cartilage, nasal

Oosterhuis, A. (ed.), Ophthalmic tumors.

ISBN 90-6193-528-8. Printed in the Netherlands.

septal cartilage and mucoperichondrium, or with a flap of tarso-conjunctiva (Fig. 4+5). Full-thickness defects can be closed directly, with mobilisation of the lateral lid tissues using a lateral cantholysis etc., (Fig. 6+7), or with more complicated repairs in which one of the lamellae is repaired with a flap and the other lamella is usually repaired with a graft (Fig. 8-11). In the medial canthal area defects can also be closed directly, with a skin-flap, or graft, but in addition if the defect is difficult to close and especially if there has been previous irradiation, the Laissez-Faire technique is preferred (Fox and Beard, 1964). This involves allowing the wound to granulate spontaneously (Fig. 12-14). It can be used elsewhere around the eyelids but is particularly effective for medial canthal lesions. A socket which has been exenterated to gain surgical clearance of a tumour can similarly be allowed to granulate and the cosmetic results are as acceptable as with more extensive repairs but the wound may take a long time to heal (Fig. 15-17).

Cryosurgery is relatively new in the management of eyelid and conjunctival tumours. The technique used involves a double-freeze thaw cycle using liquid nitrogen and monitoring the temperature to $-30^{o}C$. A recurrence rate for eyelid basal cell carcinomas of 6% over 5 years was reported by Fraunfelder et al. (1980). This is higher than with surgery but it is a valuable treatment in selected cases. The lacrimal drainage apparatus is relatively resistant to freezing and cryotherapy is the treatment of choice for small tumours which if treated surgically would involve damage to the lacrimal drainage apparatus and if treated with radiotherapy would involve the risk of lacrimal stenosis (Fig. 18+19). It is also the treatment of choice in situations where surgery is contraindicated on medical grounds or refused, and if radiotherapy is contraindicated such as with tumours involving the upper eyelid. Radiotherapy in this situation could lead to keratinization of the conjunctiva and symptoms or irritation of the globe. Recent work also suggests that it may be the treatment of choice for conjunctival melanoma (Jakobiec et al., 1982).

Surgical excision of eyelid tumours produces excellent cure rates of up to 100% if histological clearance is established before the defect is closed. The time taken for an operation is a disadvantage and this may be prolonged if frozen section control is used. An urgent paraffin section is an alternative. Surgery can often be performed under local anaesthesia as an out-patient limiting the use of hospital beds. If a systematic approach to surgery is adopted good cosmetic results can be achieved with relatively simple techniques. Cryosurgery is a useful adjunct to operative surgery in selected cases.

REFERENCES

1. Collin, J.R.O.: A Manual of Systematic Eyelid Surgery. Churchill Livingstone, Edinburgh. 1983.

2. Fraunfelder, F.T., Zacarian, S.A., Limmer, B.L., and Wingfield, D.: Cryosurgery for Malignancies of the Eyelid. Ophthal. 87: 461, 1980.

3. Fox, S.A., and Beard, C.: Spontaneous Lid Repair. Amer. J. Ophthal. 58: 947, 1964.

4. Jakobiec, F.A., Brownstein, S., Albert, W., Schwarg, F., and Anderson, R.: The role of cryotherapy in the management of conjunctival melanoma. Ophthal. 89: 502, 1982.

5. Older, J.J., Quickert, M.H., and Beard, C.: Surgical removal of basal cell carcinoma of the eyelids utilizing frozen section control. Trans. Amer. Acad. Ophthal. Otolaryng. 79: 658, 1975.

6. Rakofsky, S.I.: The adequacy of the surgical excision of basal cell carcinoma. Ann. Ophthal., 5: 596, 1973.

ILLUSTRATIONS

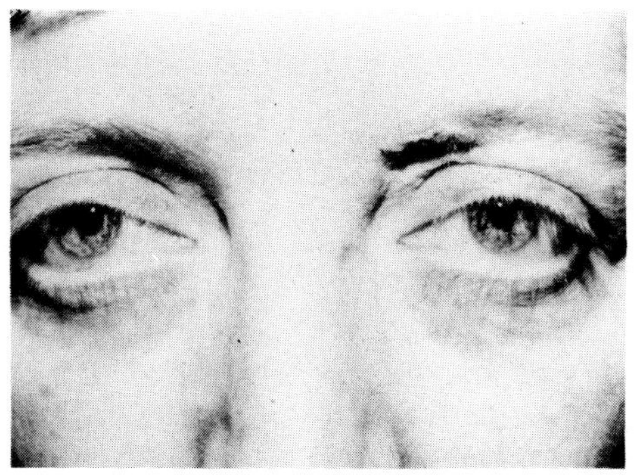

FIGURE 1. Patient with a morpheic basal cell carcinoma involving the left eyebrow and anterior lamella of the left eyelid.

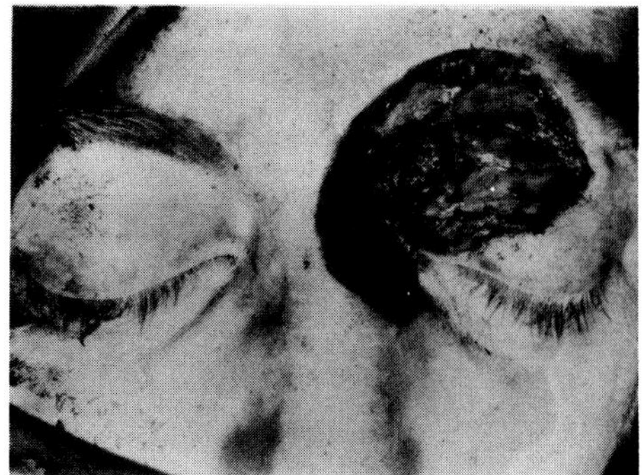

FIGURE 2a. The anterior lamella and eyebrow defect after excision of tumour.

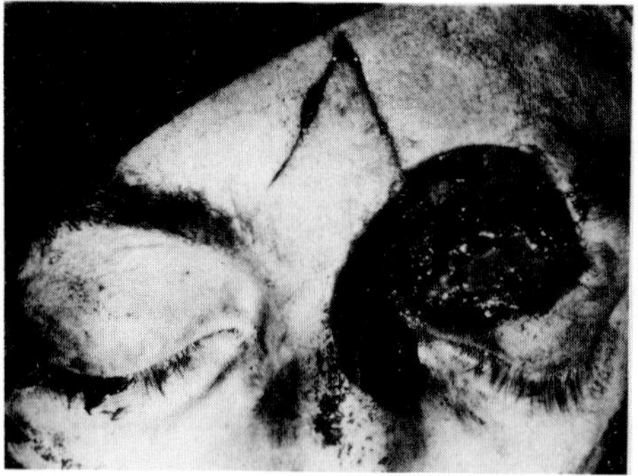

FIGURE 2b. Defect for repair with a combination of a glabellar flap and full-thickness skin graft.

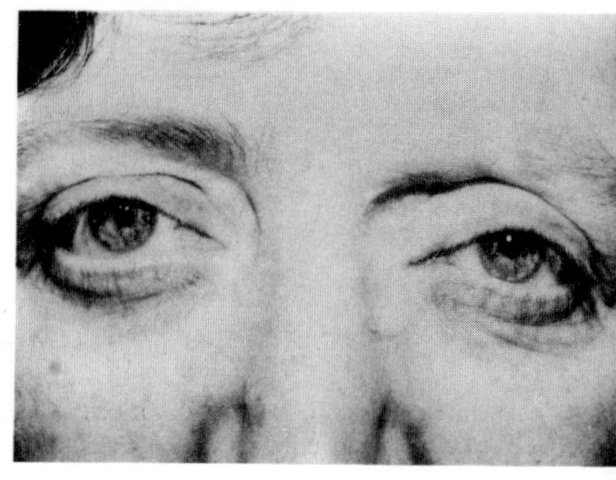

FIGURE 3. Same patient 2 years post-operatively.

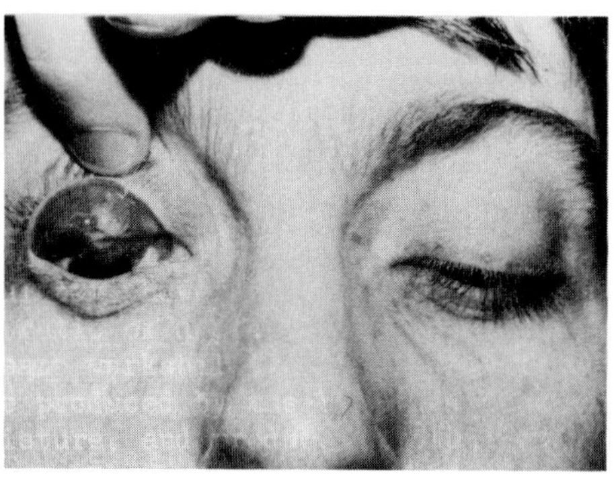

FIGURE 4. Patient with a malignant melanoma involving the posterior lamella of the eyelid.

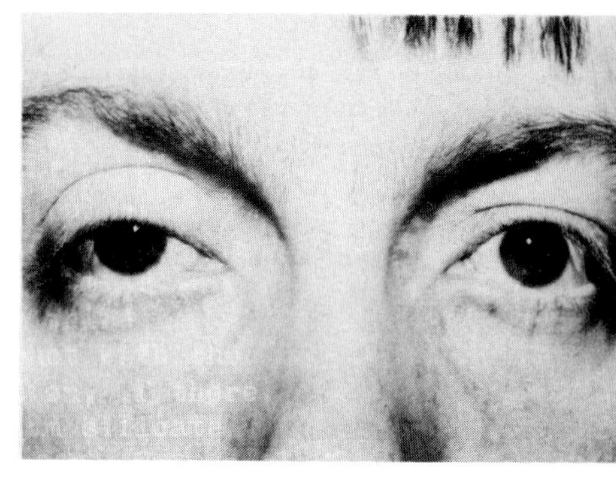

FIGURE 5. Same patient 1 year post-operatively after repair of the posterior lamella defect with a scleral graft.

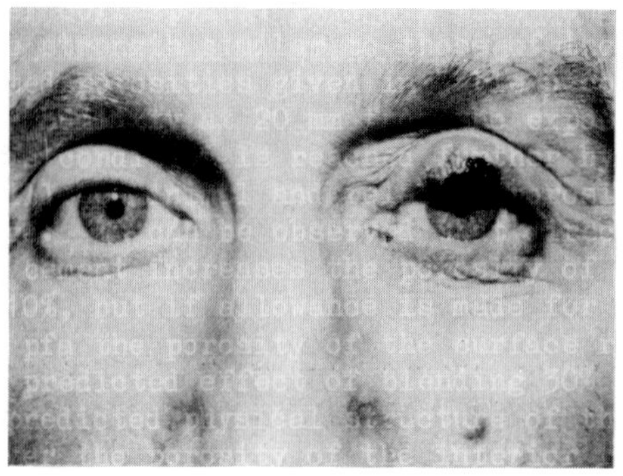

FIGURE 6. Patient with a squamous cell carcinoma of the upper eyelid.

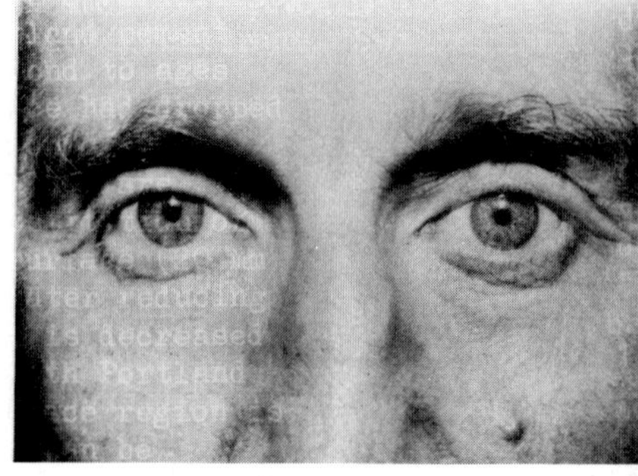

FIGURE 7. Same patient 2 years post-operatively after a full-thickness lid resection and direct closure with a lateral cantholysis and release of the orbital septum.

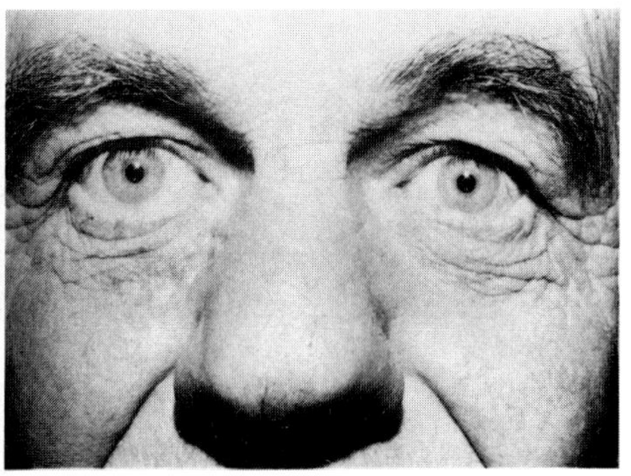

FIGURE 8. Patient with a basal cell carcinoma involving the margin of the left lower eyelid.

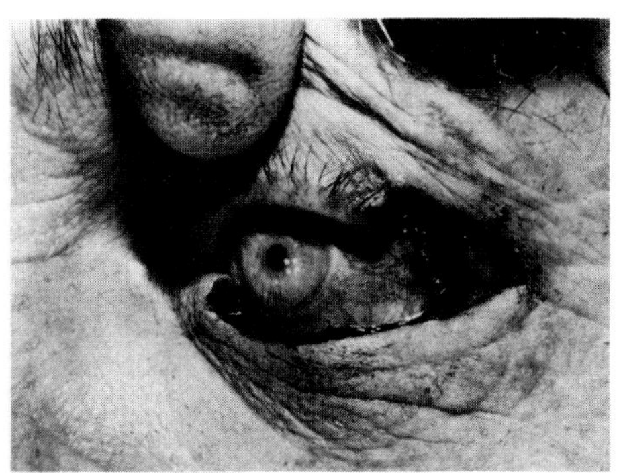

FIGURE 9. The full-thickness lid defect after excision of the tumour.

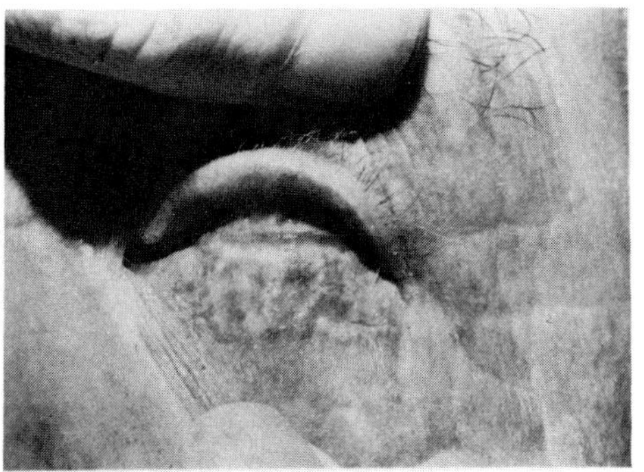

FIGURE 10. The defect repaired with a tarso-conjunctival flap from the upper lid and a full-thickness skin graft.

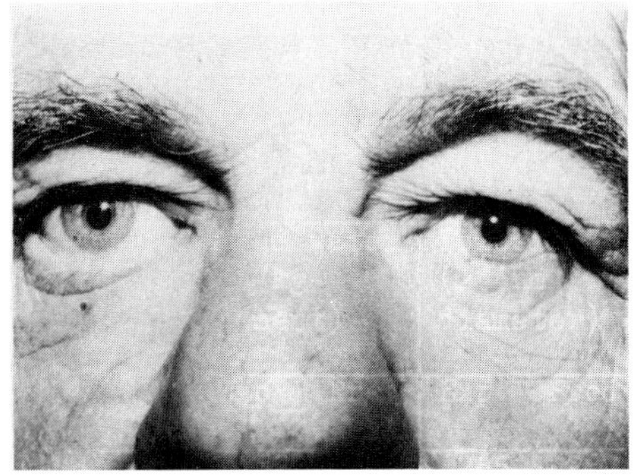

FIGURE 11. Same patient 2 years after division of the tarso-conjunctival flap.

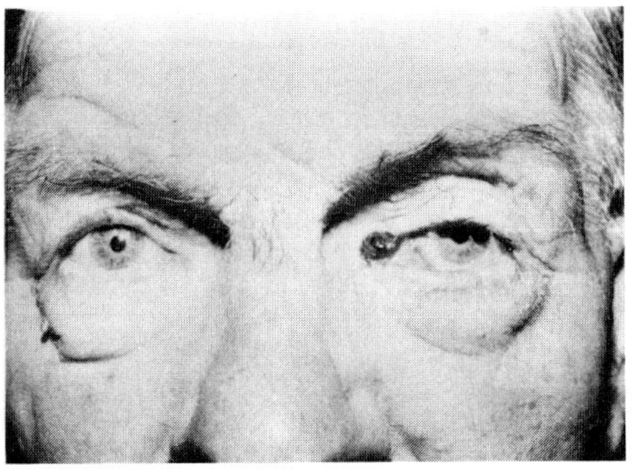

FIGURE 12. Basal cell carcinoma at the medial canthus which had recurred after irradiation.

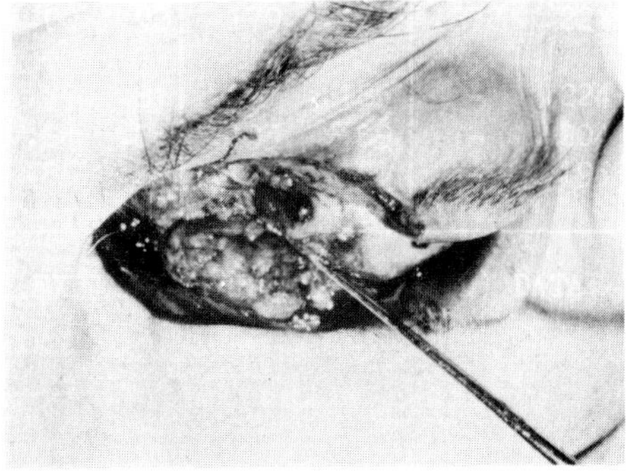

FIGURE 13. The defect after wide surgical clearance with a squint hook under the medial rectus muscle.

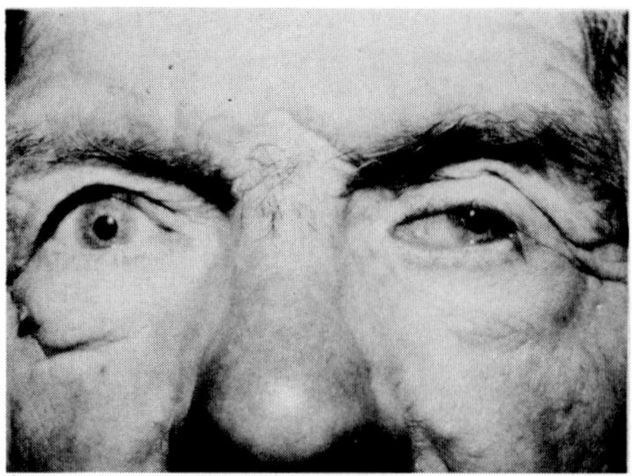

FIGURE 14. Same patient 2 years after the defect was allowed to granulate spontaneously (Laissez-Faire technique).

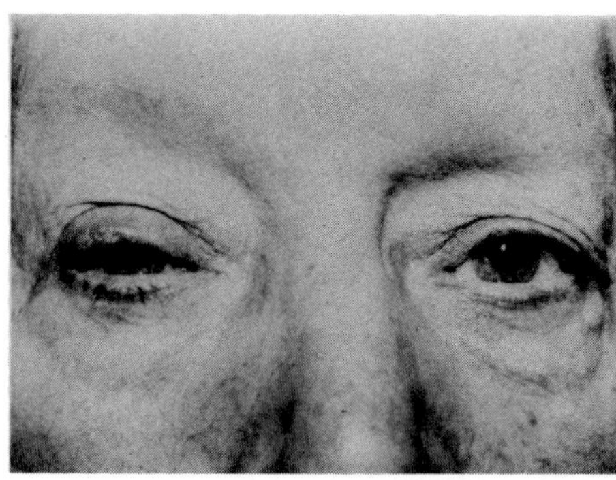

FIGURE 15. Patient with a meibomian gland carcinoma involving the upper and lower conjunctival fornix and the globe.

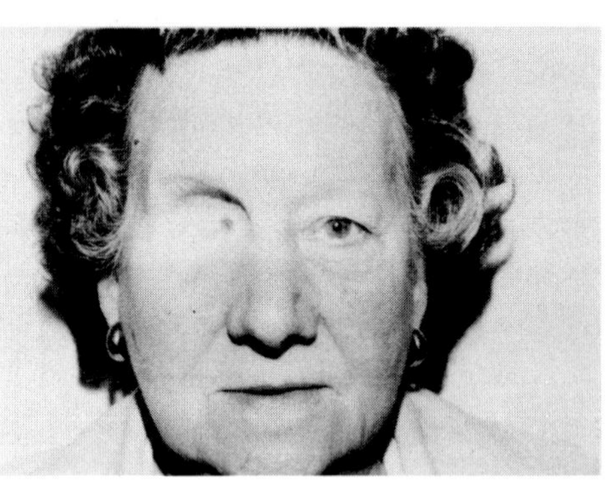

FIGURE 16. Same patient 18 months after exenteration and spontaneous granulation of the socket.

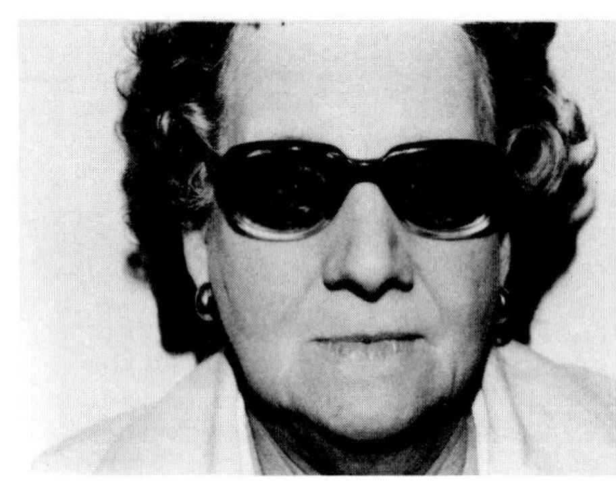

FIGURE 17. Same patient with spectacle-borne prosthesis.

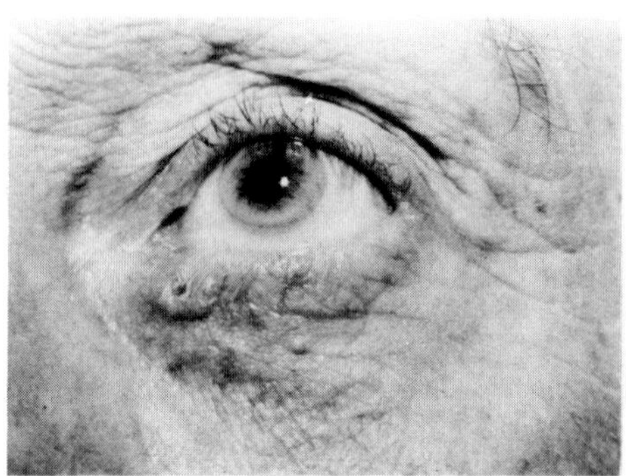

FIGURE 18. Small basal cell carcinoma involving the canaliculus.

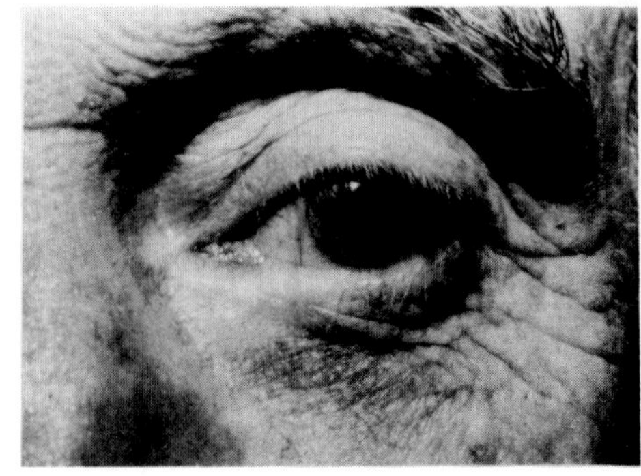

FIGURE 19. Same patient 18 months after cryosurgery with liquid nitrogen spray.

LIQUID NITROGEN CRYOSURGERY OF LID BASALIOMAS

W. BUSCHMANN

INTRODUCTION

Zacarian (1969, 1970, 1972, 1973), Matthäus (1973, 1976), Beard (1975, 1976, 1977, 1979), Fraunfelder (1977, 1980) as well as Allen (1979) and their co-workers reported on successful use of N_2-cryosurgery for treatment of lid basaliomas. The rate of recurrences was found to be as low as in surgical excision techniques (or even less). The functional and cosmetic results, however, were better. The lacrimal pathways usually remained patent, even if they had to be involved in the area of treatment; tarsus and lid margin could maintain their functions and the skin in the treated area corresponded to normal skin even in its surgical properties (elasticity, wound healing capacity). There were no visible scars except slight depigmentation, which is unimportant in a white population but is noteworthy in patients with pigmented skin.

The equipment and the application techniques used by the above mentioned authors differ to some extent. The machine developed and used by Matthäus is not available in the Western world. Therefore, we decided to evaluate the potential of N_2-cryosurgery in lid basaliomas on the basis of an equipment which is commercially available here for other applications of N_2-cryosurgery. Up to now, our material as well as the follow-up periods are too small for a final evaluation.

The potential of the method is elucidated much better by Matthäus' publications (1973, 1981), who reported on 820 basalioma cases with 5.5% recurrences within 5 years. Our material can be seen as a supplement to his work, and it may give an idea as to whether or not we have succeeded in achieving similar results with the equipment and application

Oosterhuis, A. (ed.), Ophthalmic tumors.

ISBN 90-6193-528-8. Printed in the Netherlands.

technique used by us.

METHOD

The basic principles of liquid nitrogen cryosurgery in lid basaliomas were studied thoroughly by Zacarian (1969) and Matthäus and co-workers (1973, 1976) including investigations on effectiveness of different techniques and postoperative histopathological studies.

Liquid nitrogen is used for preservation of living tissues, e.g. the cornea, with the aim to keep alive as many cells as possible. How can we expect to succeed with the same liquid nitrogen in killing all tumour cells? The point is the freezing rate (temperature decrease per second in the treated tissue), not just the temperature. Apparently, this was not fully recognized in the past, not even by all those authors who favoured N_2-cryosurgery of tumours, since some only mentioned temperature and application time in their papers but not the freezing rate.

Cornea preservation requires a well controlled low freezing rate, especially between 0° and $-30^{o}C$ of tissue temperature (2 to $5^{o}C/min$). This results in "heterogeneous nucleation" which is the term for solely extracellular ice formation with "freeze-drying" of cells. Water is moved out of the cells which thereby are protected against cryogenic destruction. Contrary to this, a very high freezing rate of about $100^{o}C/min$ in the tissues is required for cryosurgical tumour destruction. This results in "homogeneous nucleation", which means simultaneous intra- en extracellular ice formation. This, as well as the slow de-freezing, kills the cells.

Structure elements like bone, tarsus fibres, vessel walls and basal membranes of epithelium are apparently rather resistant to cryogenic destruction, so that cells can effectively regenerate along these structures. Long-term freezing of a tumour area would not enhance the cryogenic tumour cell destruction but would add ischaemic necrosis of the tumour and adjacent normal structures, which would be undesirable (scar formation); the blood supply is interrupted as long as the tissue is frozen.

The freezing rate required for tumour cryosurgery can only be achieved if - in addition to effective equipment - all other means available for enhancement of the freezing rate in the tissue are applied (e.g. local anaesthesia with vasoconstrictor, wet coupling of the probe with pressure, pre-cooling of the probe). The details are described below.

The liquid nitrogen can be applied to the tumour area either directly (spray technique) or via probes with a closed tip. Spray application can be most effective but simultaneous tissue compression (for reducing the tissue depth which must be reached with sufficient freezing rate) can not be applied, and the area of treatment, in our experience, can not be controlled with the same reliability as with closed cryo-probes. Swirling spray motions must be avoided, the nitrogen jet should be moved in a meanderlike fashion with a 45-60° angle of incidence so that the N_2-vapour is blown away and does not prevent the liquid nitrogen from reaching the tissue surface (Fraunfelder, 1977). Matthäus as well as Allen and co-workers preferred spray application in the majority of their cases, and Matthäus restricted the use of closed probes to treatment of small basaliomas. Contrary to that, we used in nearly all of our patients probes with a closed tip and restricted spray application (with regard to the above mentioned disadvantages) to basaliomas which already covered a very large area.

This difference may be explained at least partially by the equipment available. Matthäus constructed his own lab model with a very flexible, but apparently not vacuum-insulated supply line. It seems to work excellently in the spray technique but is possibly not as effective as the machine we used when probes with closed tips are applied. We have a comparatively primitive instrument for spray application (ERBOCRYO S), consisting of a thermo-flask with pressure valve and interchangeable spray tips.

The effectivity of equipment with closed tip probes (blind-ended tubes) depends very much on the equipment construction. Several primitive models were recommended and became available at low cost, but unfortunately, these are

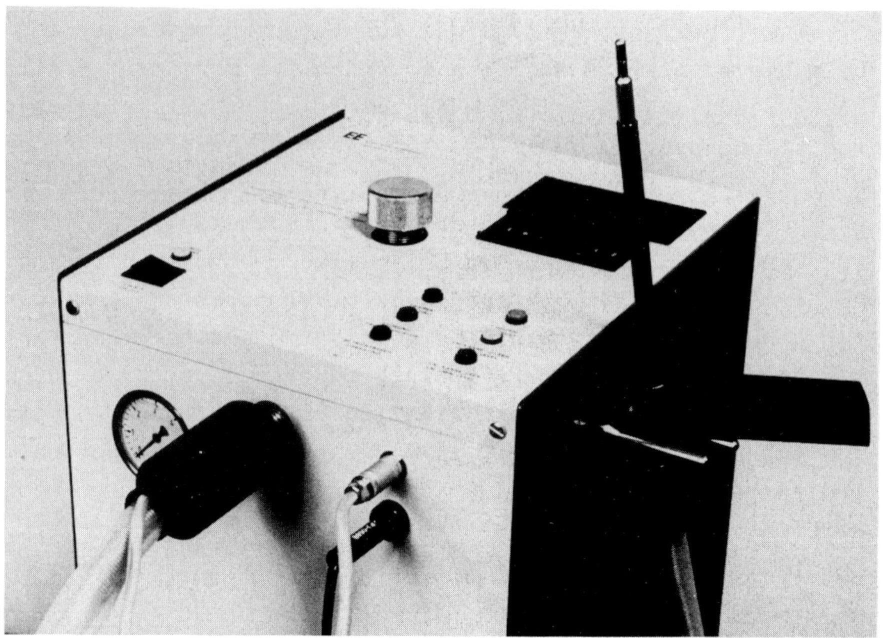

Fig. 1: Apparatus ERBOCRYO-P for liquid nitrogen cryosurgery.

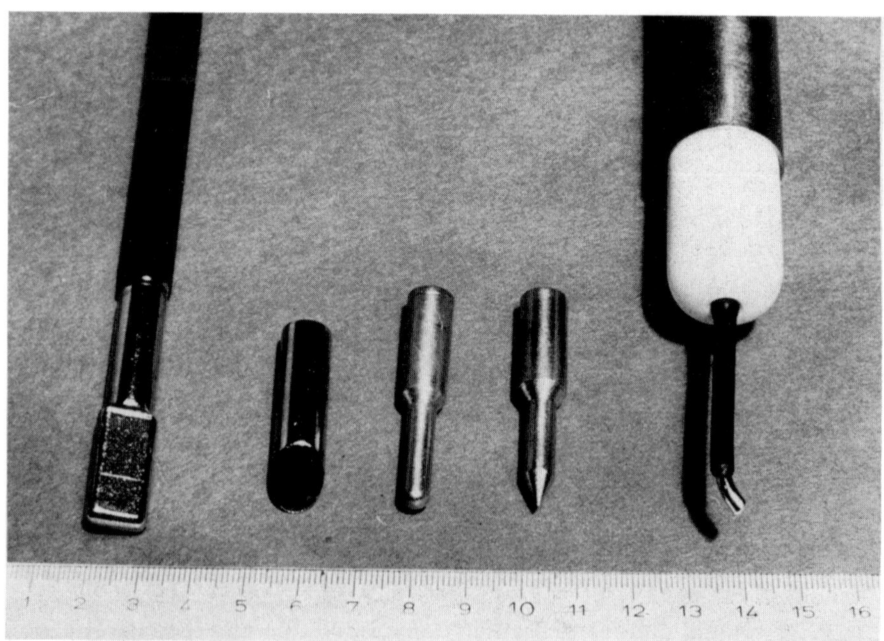

Fig. 2: Interchangeable probe tips for liquid nitrogen cryosurgery.

insufficient. Apparently, the authors were not aware of the handicaps which the vaporization of the liquid nitrogen may produce. A thermo-flask with a blind-ended tip at the bottom could never provide the necessary freezing rate in the tissue because, after contact with the tissue surface, vaporization of the liquid nitrogen in the probe's tip would prevent the inflow of a sufficient amount of further liquid nitrogen. The cooling effect would become weaker and the freezing rate in the tissue would be inadequate. The insulation effect of this vapour can be imagined by watching a water bubble on a hot stove: temperature and heat capacity of the hot plate would suffice by far for changing this drop of water into vapour within fractions of a second; nevertheless, we can see it dancing for several seconds on the hot plate. The vapour formed in the area of contact between water and hot plate lifts the water bubble, thus insulating it from further heat, until gravity presses the vapour away and the water bubble gets near enough to the plate's surface for further vaporization. With tissue temperature of $+37^{o}C$ and liquid nitrogen of $-196^{o}C$ it is just the same effect. Care must be taken, therefore, to get the nitrogen in its liquid form down to the blind end of the closed-tip probe which is in contact with the tissue, and to remove the nitrogen vapour effectively.

Therefore, we decided to use the ERBOCRYO-OP (later on the smaller ERBOCRYO-P, which is easier to handle). Both machines have a vacuum-insulated supply line and probes with closed interchangeable tips. The vacuum insulation of the supply line makes it more clumsy than that in Matthäus's apparatus but appears to contribute markedly to the effectiveness, especially in closed-tip technique. We have not yet had an opportunity to carry out comparative measurements with Matthäus's apparatus and ours, but we compared the freezing effect of spray application and that of our closed-tip technique by using a brass block with thermo-couples. In this way, it was proven that with the closed-tip probes and the ERBOCRYO-P we can get the same freezing rate as in spray application (fig. 1-3). Therefore, we preferred the closed-tip technique

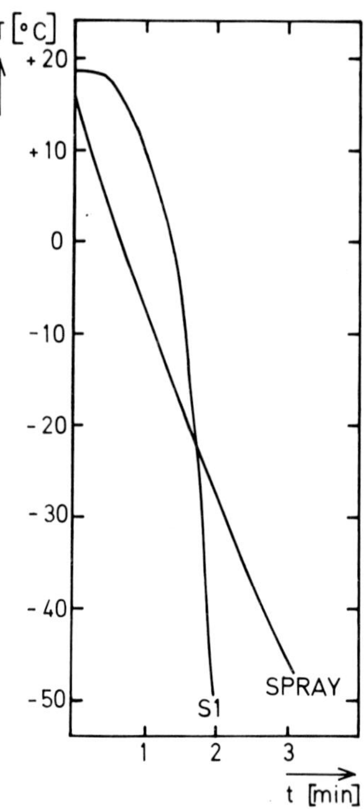

Fig. 3: Comparative measurement of the freezing rate achieved in a brass block. Thermo-couples in the brass block were used for temperature recording. Freezing started more slowly with our closed-tip probe S1 and the ERBOCRYO-P, compared with spray application (ERBOCRYO-S). However, the freezing rate in the decisive range (0°C to -40°C) was considerably higher with the closed probe (wet coupling).

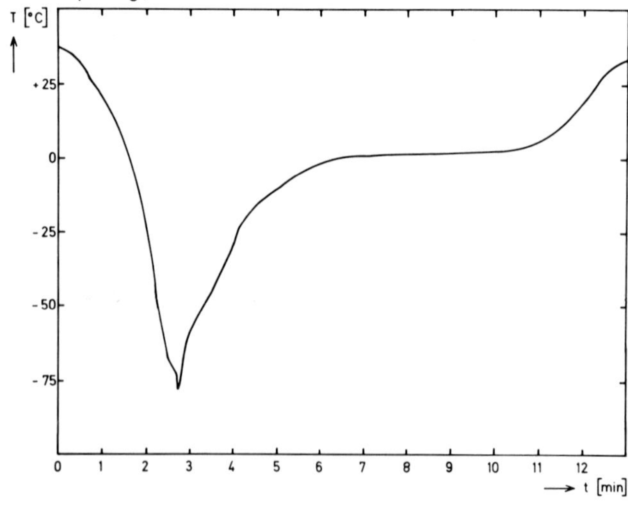

Fig. 4: Tissue temperature recorded by means of a thermo-couple needle which is placed in the tissue behind the tumor base. The freezing rate achieved between zero and -40°C is just sufficient for this thermo-couple location. The slow thawing is also demonstrated.

which allows better control of the treated area and provides the possibility to reduce the tissue thickness by applying the probe with some pressure.

Local anaesthesia and application technique

We prefer local anaesthesia (bupivacain-HCl) with epinephrine. The margin of the area to be treated is marked by using a microscope and a suitable pencil or a very superficial skin incision. Thermo-couples are placed below the tumour tissue (opposite to the side of cryo-probe application) and connected to a temperature recorder so that the drop of temperature per second can be seen from the recordings. Nowadays, we use the recording of tissue temperature preferably in tumours beyond the lids which can not be treated from skin and tarsus side. Surgeons starting to use this method, however, are well advised to use it in all cases, in spite of the fact that one can not be sure to have the thermo-couple needle placed exactly at the posterior margin of the tumour (Gill and Long, 1971). Tissue temperature recording demonstrates the effectiveness of the apparatus and the application technique used as well as the limitations of the method (fig. 4). It proves that the area of effective treatment (i.e. sufficient tissue freezing rate) is much smaller than the ice ball in the tissue!

Monitoring of the probe tip temperature would not be sufficient, because this provides by no means sufficient information on the freezing rate achieved in the tissues, where temperature decreases markedly more slowly than in the probe tip.

A biopsy is taken using an Elliot trephine either before or after the first cryo-application. This provides not only a histopathological diagnosis but also better probe-coupling and, therefore, more effective cryotherapy, especially in non-ulcerous basaliomas.

The histopathological diagnosis is not hampered by previous cryo-application. Histopathologically visible cryogenic cell alterations need some time after cryo-application to develop (Matthäus and Krantz, 1973).

The first cryo-application is started not earlier than 20 minutes after injection of the local anaesthetic. The modern local anaesthetics are effective for some hours. We have optimum conditions for cryotherapy 20 minutes after injection: the injection-induced oedema has gone and the tissue anaemia is at its maximum. Blood supply means heat supply and counteracts the cryo-effect! The lid area has a very effective blood supply and we have to reduce it during tumour cryotherapy. Therefore, the vasoconstrictor is indispensable. If general anaesthesia were to be used for any reason, local application of epinephrine might be contraindicated; then we use a prodrug, POR 8, for local vasoconstriction.

The area of probe-tissue contact should be wet and the probe be applied with some pressure to reduce tissue thickness. A plastic spatula is introduced into the conjunctival sac. We use it to protect the eyeball, to lift the lid from the bulbus and to press it against the cryo-probe. We soon noticed that probe-coupling and effectiveness are especially good in ulcerous basaliomas. Thus, we use in non-ulcerous basaliomas the biopsy site for probe-coupling.

Each area of the tumour should be frozen three times at an effective freezing rate with slow, complete defreezing in between. Defreezing must not be accelerated. Therefore, the probe (which is automatically heated after stopping the nitrogen inflow) has to be removed from the tissue as soon as it is defrozen. The tissue is then allowed to defreeze spontaneously (no application of warmed salt solution etc.!). We apply two cryo-cycles from the skin side and the third cycle from the conjunctival (tarsal) side in lid tumours. This is facilitated by the interchange of the probe-tips. The spatula-shaped probe-tip is particularly suitable for the application from the conjunctival side. All three cycles are applied from the skin side if the tumour can not be reached from the conjunctival sac. A plastic spatula protects the bulbus, if the probe is applied from the conjunctival side. The lid is lifted with the probe tip from the bulbus to protect the latter and to couple with pressure. The conjunctival sac must be kept free of fluid to avoid ice bridges to structures which should not be involved.

Skin incision and cryo-probe application from the tumour basis (after undermining of the basalioma area) were successfully used for treating a larger skin basalioma beyond the eyelids but this technique is still at a preliminary stage.

The cryo-probe is cooled once to -30°C probe temperature without tissue contact; after defreezing it is coupled to the tissue and activated again. This way, the maximum freezing rate is achieved already for the first treatment cycle.

The area of effective cryotherapy is about 2-3 mm larger in diameter than the area of probe-tissue contact; due to tissue compression, it is somewhat more in depth. We select from our probe tip collection the tip which covers best the area to be treated, and in most small and medium sized basaliomas we can cover this area with one application site. If the tumour is larger, a second or third application site can be used subsequently (overlapping). This is much better than prolongation of the cryo-application at the first application site, which would enlarge the ice ball (= area of frozen tissue), but not the area of effective tumour treatment. The freezing rate in tissue decreases markedly with the distance from the probe surface.

The duration of the cryo-applications is determined either by thermo-couple recording of tissue temperature, or by observation of the freezing effect in the tissues (experience required). A -30°C probe-tip temperature usually corresponds to the start of tissue freezing; therefore, we count the time from reaching -30°C in the probe, and then one cryo-application usually needs about 30-90 seconds. The probe temperature may go down to -196°C within this time but this must not be reached (especially not in small tumours).

Matthäus and Scholz (1981) recommend the use of the impedance measurement method (Pliquett) for evaluation of the cryosurgical effect; the recorded waveform (rectangular pulses) changes as soon as the cell membranes are destroyed. Doubtlessly, a failure of the cryo-applications to destroy the majority of cells could be detected this way. We have not yet applied this method because, in our opinion, the more important problem of detecting a few surviving cell groups could probably not be solved in this way.

MATERIAL

Indications and limitations in lid basaliomas - selection of patients

The following rules have been derived from the literature mentioned above and from our own experience.

N_2-cryosurgery should be preferred if

- the basalioma approaches or involves the lacrimal pathways (chance of postoperatively patent lacrimal passage);
- the tumour is a recurrence after previous radiation or surgical excision, and if size and location permit cryotherapy (see below);
- the tumour covers a large, flat area (e.g. of the lid margin), which would require extended plastic surgery, especially in relatively young patients;
- it is clinically uncertain whether or not the periosteum or even superficial bone layers of the nose or the orbital rim should be removed as a safety measure if surgical treatment were chosen.

In the latter case, the surgeon might sometimes hesitate to remove periosteum and bone, and this could cause recurrences (which, of course, could be prevented by using series of frozen sections!). If skin and fat are not too thick, periosteum and superficial bone layers can well be reached cryosurgically with an effective freezing rate. The structural elements remain intact and the cells and periosteum regenerate completely. There is no reason for hesitation; periosteum and bone can be subjected to cryosurgical tumour therapy without any disadvantage.

A relative indication for cryosurgery would be given in all other (especially smaller) lid basaliomas which could be removed surgically as well without need of extended plastic

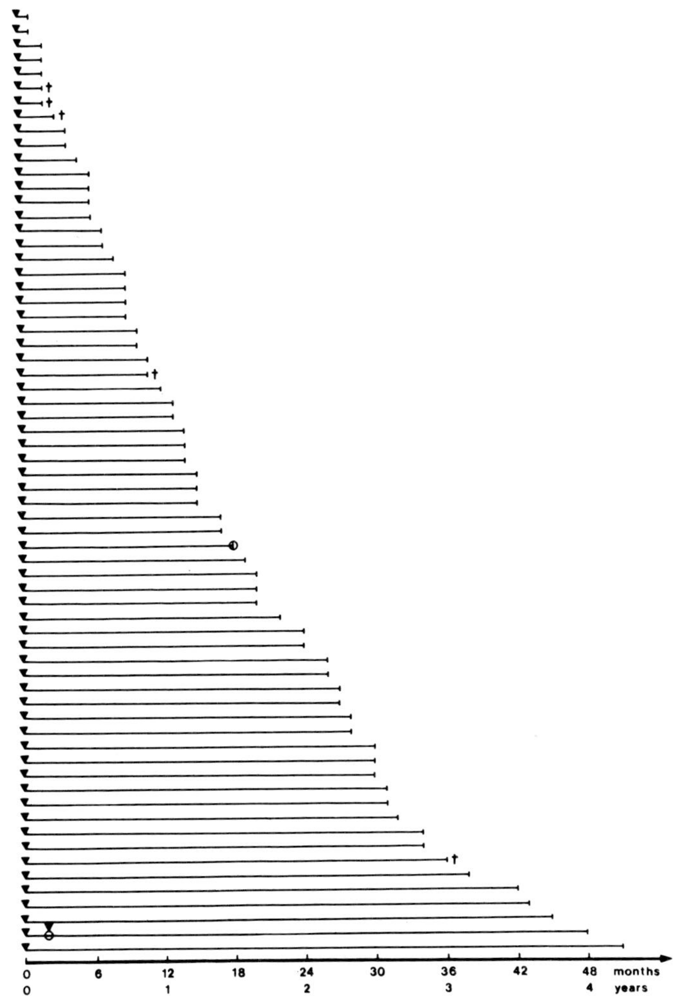

Fig. 5: Follow-up periods after cryosurgery.
▼ = cryosurgery; O = surgical excision; ϟ = radiation therapy; † = patient died from other disease.
28 cases have until now been followed up more than 2 years postoperatively (21 after primary cryosurgery and 7 after cryosurgery of recurrences).

Fig. 5a: Cryosurgery as primary treatment.
2 persisting tumours were treated subsequently by excision , or by excision and cryosurgery of tumour base.

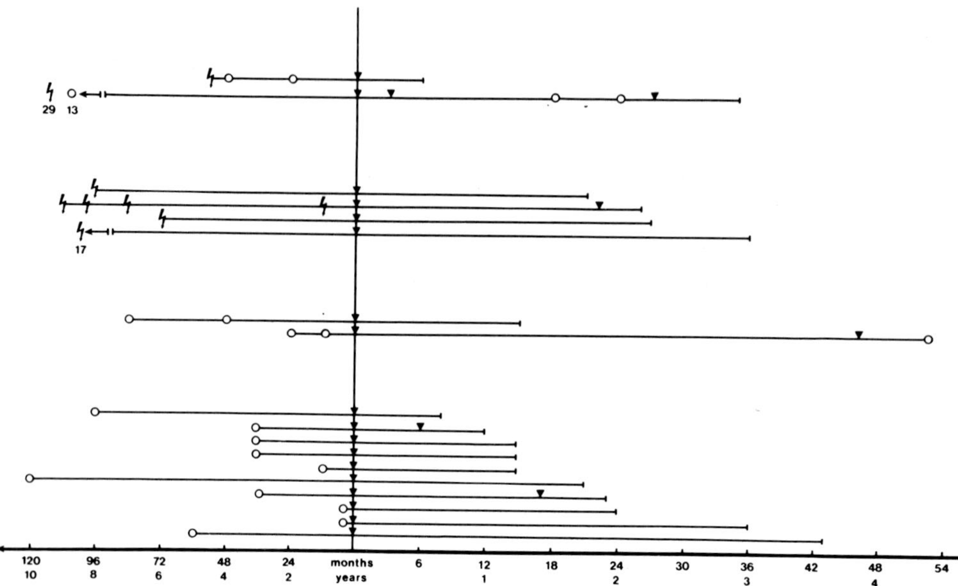

Fig. 5b: Cryosurgery for basalioma recurrences after surgical excision or radiation therapy or multiple previous approaches.
5 recurrences after cryosurgery were treated by excision or repeated cryosurgery or both.
The second case from above was Naevus flammeus, irradiated, 29 years ago; subsequently, 13 years ago, excision of a basalioma in this area, and now repeated cryosurgery and excisions for small basalioma recurrences, because larger plastic surgery would be difficult in this pretreated area.
A recently taken biopsy specimen was free of basalioma.

surgery. We preferred cryosurgery in all these cases.

Cryosurgery would be contraindicated, however, in all basaliomas in which it would not be possible to reach all areas of the tumour with a sufficient freezing rate. Figures have been given above. Basaliomas with a depth of more than 4 mm in the compressed tissue, which can not be treated additionally from behind (due to location beyond the lid), would be out of range for this kind of treatment. This applies especially to basaliomas invading the orbit, penetrating the orbital septum and/or reducing already the motility of the eyeball.

Our material consists of 84 consecutive cases with lid basaliomas, treated cryosurgically from 1979 (when we started with this method) to June 30, 1983 (see Table 1). All patients had been asked to show up for postoperative controls quarterly for at least 3 years after their operation. If they lived in distant places, they were advised to see their ophthalmologists accordingly, and we asked these colleagues to report repeatedly on the postoperative findings. Following a check-list we reminded patients and doctors, respectively, if control reports were missing.

RESULTS

The resulting control periods can be seen in Figure 5. Patient examples are shown in Figures 6 to 11.

The patients who developed tumour recurrences after surgical or radiation treatment and were treated cryosurgically later on are listed in Table 2 and Figure 5b.

Recurrences after cryosurgery were treated by a second cryosurgical approach or by excision. The kind of treatment, the subsequent follow-up period and the further results (repeated recurrence or not) are shown in Figure 5b.

Postoperative course and treatment

Following cryosurgery, a local oedema developed, which disappeared spontaneously within a few days after treatment of small and medium sized basaliomas. Its extent and duration were closely correlated with the intensity and area of cryo-

TABLE 1: Liquid nitrogen cryosurgery of lid basaliomas; 84 consecutive cases, treated from 1979 until June 1983.

	No. of patients
Lid basaliomas - cryosurgical treatment	84
1. Cryosurgery as primary treatment	66
1.1. postoperative recurrences	0
1.2. persistence of tumour	2
2. Cryosurgical treatment for lid basalioma recurrences after previous surgery or radiation therapy	18
2.1. recurrence after cryosurgery	5
2.2. slight irritation still visible	2

TABLE 2: Cryosurgical treatment of lid basalioma recurrences after surgical or radiation treatment (follow-up periods see fig. 5).

	No. of patients
Patients treated for basalioma recurrences after surgical or radiation therapy	18
1. Recurrent basalioma following surgical removal treated by cryosurgery	10
- recurrences thereafter until now	2
2. Recurrent basalioma following 2 surgical approaches treated by cryosurgery	2
- recurrence thereafter until now	1
3. Recurrent basalioma following radiation therapy treated by cryosurgery	4
- recurrence thereafter until now	1
4. Recurrent basalioma following radiation and 2 surgical excisions treated by cryosurgery	2
- recurrence thereafter until now	1

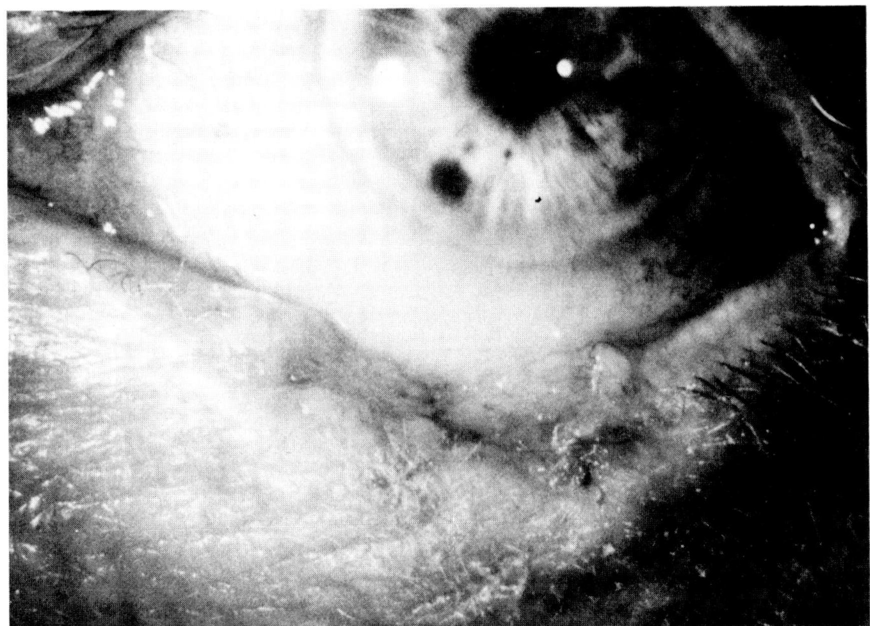

Fig. 6: Basalioma extending along lower lid margin.

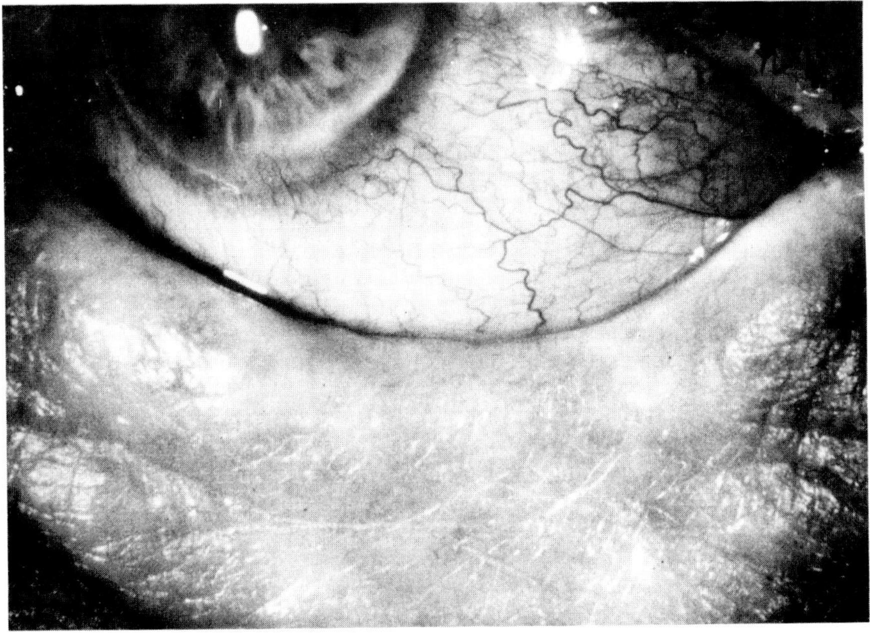

Fig. 7: Same patient as in fig. 6, 3 1/2 years after cryosurgery.

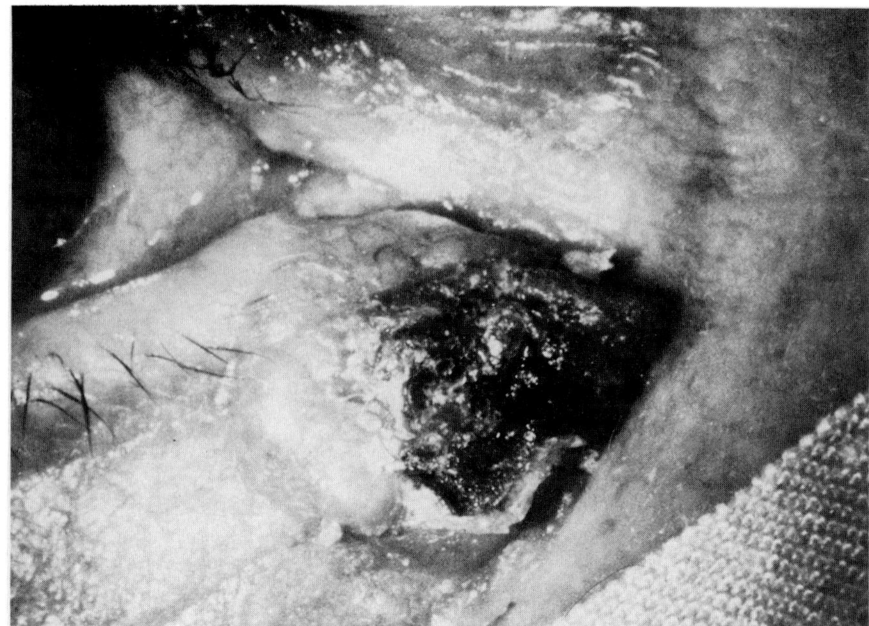

Fig. 8: Relatively large basalioma near medial canthus.

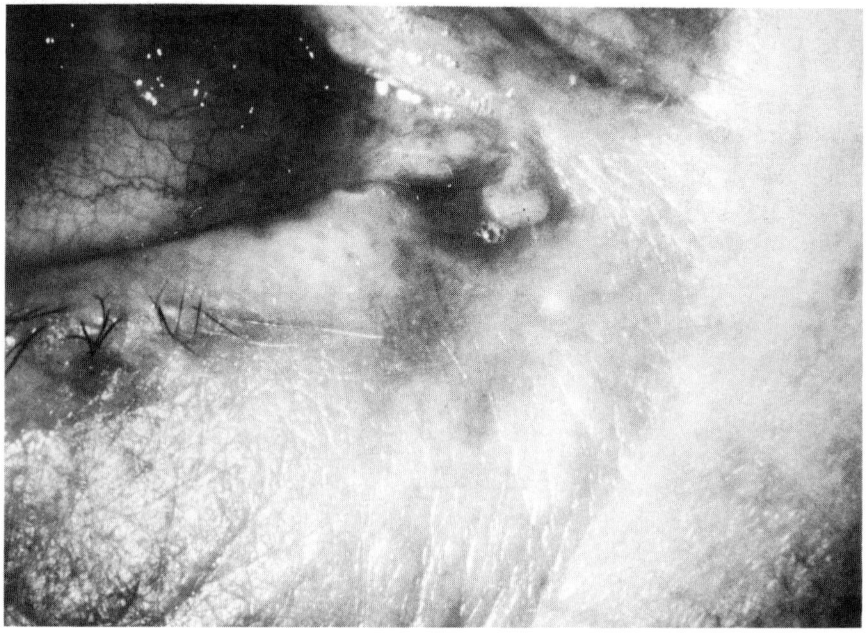

Fig. 9: Same patient as in fig. 8, 6 months after cryosurgery. Follow-up period now 2 years and 8 months. Lacrimal pathways patent.

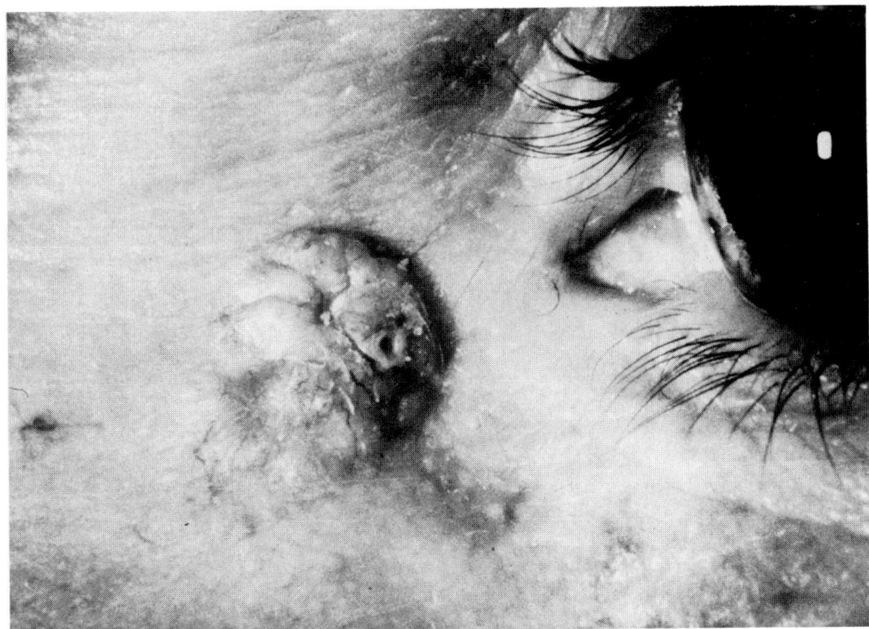

Fig. 10: Basalioma near medial canthus.

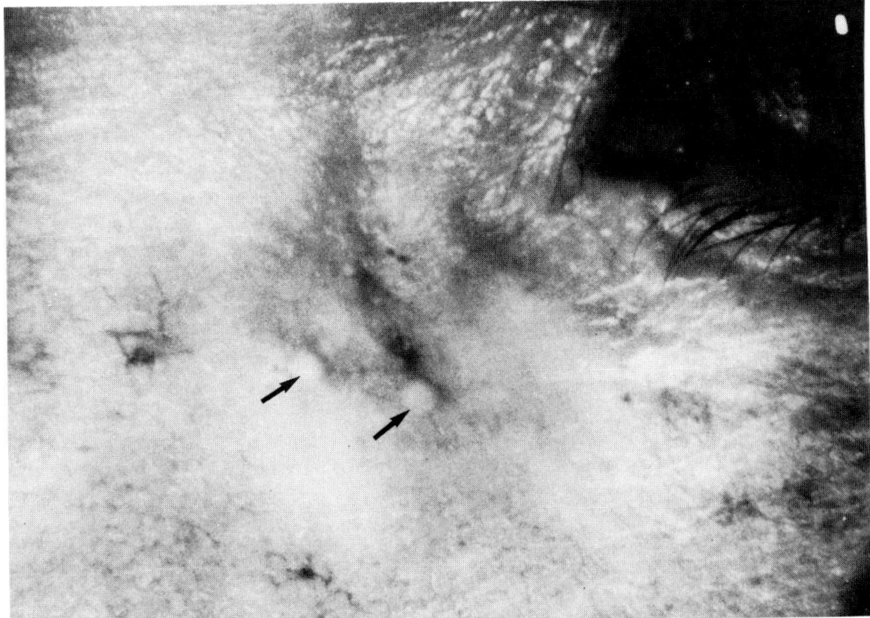

Fig. 11: Same patient as in fig. 10, 8 months postoperatively. The visible nodules are epithelial hyperplasia (pseudorecidivism, Zacarian) and disappeared spontaneously. Lacrimal pathways patent. Postoperative follow-up period 2 1/2 years.

surgical treatment. It was more pronounced in size and duration after treatment of more extended tumours, and even some orbital oedema occurred. We have seen this after particularly intensive treatment of a larger basalioma in the medial parts of the lower and upper lid and canthus. Then, systemic application of Reparil[R] or Venoruton[R] was helpful.

Nebacetin[R]-ointment was applied to the conjunctival sac after cryotherapy; we did not use bandages if the treated area could be kept dry on the skin side. A dry eschar permitted good wound healing. If, however, the tears could reach the treated skin or lid margin, a dry eschar could not develop and Nebacetin[R]-ointment with bandages was used. Wound healing was then good as well. The antibiotic ointment proved necessary to avoid superinfection.

The lacrimal pathways remained patent in nearly all of our cases where they had been patent prior to cryosurgery, as has been reported by Fraunfelder (1977) and experimentally proven by Bullock et al. (1976) as well as by Matthäus and Baerthold (1978). They obliterated, however, if very intensive cryo-treatment was necessary for a relatively large basalioma which infiltrated this area. A slight ectropion of the lower lid was seen in some patients in the early postoperative course but in general disappeared spontaneously. Cryoepilation, however, is a permanent result in the treated area. It is negligible at the lower lid (where most of the basaliomas are located) but would matter at the upper lid. Therefore, younger patients with basaliomas near the upper lid cilia may be better treated by surgical excision.

DISCUSSION

Naturally, we aimed at the use of optimum technique and method already in the first clinical case, and in the beginning all opereations of this kind were concentrated in one hand. Later on, it proved necessary to introduce other ophthalmic surgeons of our hospital to this technique and we tried hard to enable them to work at optimum conditions. Nevertheless, we must admit that the retrospective analysis

TABLE 3: Liquid nitrogen cryosurgery of lid basaliomas - recurrence rates reported in literature.

Author	No. of basaliomas treated	Follow-up period (years)	No. of recurrences after 1 cryosurgery	%
Zacarian (1975)	82	1 to 10	7	8.5
Bullock et al. (1976)	29	1.3 (mean)	2	7.0
Beard and Sullivan (1977)	49	1.1 (mean)	2	4.0
Fraunfelder et al. (1977)				
- cryo as first treatment	93	1 (mean)	2	2.0
- cryo for recurrences after surgery or radiation	8		0	
Fraunfelder et al. (1980)	310	3 (mean)	13	4.2
- long follow-up	49	5	3	6.0
- recurrences after surgery or radiation	28	3 (mean)	1	3.5
- recurrences after primary cryosurgery	11	1.3 (mean)	0	0.0
Matthäus and Scholz (1981)	820	within 5	45	5.5
Buschmann	84	0.5 - 4	5	6.0

of our material proved that we succeeded only partially regarding these two aims. This consecutive series includes all shortcomings of the time when we worked as beginners. Nevertheless, the results in our series are encouraging in those patients who received liquid nitrogen cryotherapy as primary treatment of basalioma (Tables 1 and 3). We have had no recurrence in this group up till now. Two persistent tumours must not be attributed to the method but to our failure. In one of our earliest cases, the importance of wet coupling was not yet realized. Dry coupling was used and resulted in freezing of the tumour cells at too low a freezing rate, proven by complete lack of tumour cell destruction. Postoperatively, this tumour simply showed no change at all. It was removed by surgery 6 weeks later and even histology did not reveal any cryogenic cell destruction. In addition, a technical handicap was not yet detected at the time, which may have played a role in this case. Measurements with a brass block and thermo-couples later on showed that the freezing rate in tissue provided by our equipment was considerably lower if the liquid nitrogen container of the machine was filled only half or less instead of being full. Since then, we always start with the tank filled up completely. The manufacturers have clarified the technical background in the meantime and are at present working out a constructional change to solve this problem. Microscopic marking of the tumour margin was not used in the second persistent tumour, with the result that cryosurgery was applied to part of the tumour only. It was not until 18 months later that we got the opportunity to remove this part by excision.

The results in cryosurgery of basalioma <u>recurrences after surgical or radiation therapy</u> are less favourable (Table 2). Matthäus (1976) also mentioned a higher recurrence rate in cryosurgical treatment of basalioma recurrences (after previous radiation or surgical excision) as compared with basaliomas treated primarily by cryosurgery. It is also known that the results of surgical excision or of radiation therapy are better in primary treatment than in treatment of recurrences (25% recurrences, Zacarian 1977). Nevertheless, our percentage of recurrences in this group could probably be reduced. The failures must perhaps be attributed to the surgeons rather than to the method. The method was applied by experienced surgeons only but when they were beginners in cryosurgery of tumours, they decided in all 5 cases which later on developed recurrences to apply 1 or 2 cryocycles only instead of the 3 cycles recommended; they were very much impressed by the rapid, intensive freezing. If we decided on a second cryosurgical approach, special care was taken to apply cryotherapy at optimum conditions.

Contrary to previous surgical or radiation therapy, previous cryotherapy produced no side effects which would hamper subsequent therapeutic approaches. A second cryosurgical treatment as well as plastic surgery could be done in the area of previous cryotreatment as in tissues not treated before. The follow-up periods after a second cryotherapy have been too short up till now for evaluation of results. "Pseudorecidivism" (Zacarian, 1973) was often observed in the postoperative follow-up; the small subepithelial nodules appear mostly at the margin of the treated area. They are bright nodules without vascularization and disappear spontaneously within a few months. The informed examiner would never mistake them for real recurrences but the beginner must be warned. These nodules have been observed after irradiation therapy as well. Histologically, hyperkeratosis with papillomatosis and acanthosis, consistent with epitheliomatous hyperplasia, was found (Fig. 11).

Our cosmetic results corresponded to the favourable results reported in the afore mentioned literature. Some hyperaemia remained visible for weeks or months but later on the tissue corresponded so closely to normal skin that even our experienced photographer had often difficulty in tracing the area of treatment. Survival of the tarsus fibres allowed better function of the lid and especially the lid margin than it could be achieved with qualified plastic surgery. Depigmentation was often seen after cryosurgery (Fraunfelder et al, 1980: 42.3% of the patients), but most cases returned to their normal pretreatment pigmentation within the following year. Some patients, however, still have some degree of depigmentation even after years. Usually this became visible in our patients only after light exposure in summertime and never really was a cosmetic problem; the patients had been advised anyhow to reduce exposure to sunshine.

The biochemical and especially the immunological effects of tumour cryosurgery are still under investigation: it may be that cryogenic tumour destruction stimulates the immune system against the type of tumour treated (Federman et al., 1977).

Other diseases

Jakobiec et al. and Brownstein et al. (1981, 1982) reported on successful cryosurgical treatment of conjunctival melanomas. This is a very promising approach, because pigmented cells are particularly sensitive to cryosurgery (Beard and Sullivan, 1977), and the alternative in the past was enucleation. Sofar, we have had just one patient with a growing tumour of this kind whom we treated cryosurgically (special smaller ophthalmic probe), and until now the treatment seems to have been a success.

We have tried N_2-cryosurgery also in three small intraocular melanomas the size and location of which did not allow photocoagulation or radiation treatment, in patients who had refused enucleation. It is too early to report on details but it may be mentioned that, under certain conditions, successful tumour cryosurgery is possible in intraocular melanomas; however, the size of the tumour is a limiting factor, not only with regard to sufficient freezing rate in all parts of the tumour, but also with regard to the limited tolerance of the eye in view of the amount of necrotic tumour masses. Again, it is too early to give a detailed report or recommendations.

Large cells are more sensitive to cryotherapy than smaller ones. Therefore, we decided in favour of liquid nitrogen cryosurgery (smaller probe and less intensive applications) in a case of severe bilateral conjunctival amyloidosis of both eyes. The conjunctiva was involved bilaterally down to the upper and lower fornix and the patient sought advice at several eye hospitals. In view of the extent of the disease surgical treatment (Rieger, 1981) was considered impossible and was not attempted. Cryosurgery resulted in a prompt disappearance of all granulations and up till now no recurrence has occurred, but the patient needs artificial tears for dry eye syndrome. The execretory ducts of the lacrimal glands obliterated (owing to the disease and/or cryotherapy).

Cryoepilation, an undesired side effect in tumour cryotherapy, was successfully used by us in trichiasis, as recommended by Zacarian (1977) and Matthäus (1978). The complications described by Wood and Anderson (1981) must be attributed to their indications and technique but the combination of cryosurgery and lid splitting (Anderson and Harvey, 1981) appears to be advantageous.

CONCLUSION

As far as our material permits evaluation, we can support the recommendation of the method for basalioma treatment as given by Zacarian (1969, 1973, 1977), Matthäus (1973, 1976, 1981), Beard (1977), Fraunfelder (1977) and others.

Cryosurgery in the management of most lid malignancies is superior as compared to cryosurgery of other skin tumours, because anatomic, functional and cosmetic problems of the eyelids are unique. It is ideal for patients on anticoagulants and for those who refuse conventional surgery or probably could not endure it (Fraunfelder et al., 1977).

The recurrence rate mentioned in Table 3 should be compared with the results found after application of other methods. Bart et al. (1970) reported on 7.9% recurrences following radiation therapy and 6.8% recurrences following scalpel excision (1978). Kopf et al. (1977) reported on 5.7 to 9.8% recurrences following curettage electro-desiccation. Older et al. (1975) had 0% recurrence after excision with frozen section control, and Doxanas et al. (1981) found 5.5%

recurrences subsequent to surgical excision but 0% in the cases in which frozen section controls were applied. Unfortunately, a very limited number of hospitals in the world can actually use the frozen section method owing to staff and space problems in the operation theatre and the histopathology department.

The recurrence rate does not only depend on the method and its proper use but also on location, cell type, tumour size, pattern of tumour growth, and previous treatment. Eyelid basaliomas in general have at least a twice greater recurrence rate as compared to other locations (Bart et al., 1970, 1978). Tumours of more than 10 mm diameter and poorly outlined infiltrating tumours have higher recurrence rates (Fraunfelder et al., 1980) and so have sclerotic basal cell carcinomas (Matthäus, 1981). Recurrent tumours show a higher recurrence rate with any method of treatment (25%, as mentioned before). These details are not available in comparable form in the above mentioned publications; thus, differences in the recurrence rates may also result from differences in the tumours treated.

Equipment with sufficient freezing capacity is mandatory for cryosurgery of lid basaliomas and the surgeon must be familiar with the background of the method. He should be well experienced in plastic surgery in order to be able to select the optimum way of treatment in each case. The method should not be mistaken for an "easy" way for colleagues who want to treat basalioma cases but are not trained in plastic surgery. When watched in a theatre, the method looks very easy and it does save the surgeon much time, but I hope to have shown that "to take it easy" would end up in misuse and poor results. Proper use of the method, however, appears well to be of benefit to our patients.

SUMMARY

The curative effect of liquid nitrogen cryosurgery in lid basaliomas has been shown by Zacarian, Matthäus and their co-workers. The decisive factor is the freezing rate (not just the temperature) achieved in the tissues (not merely in the probe tip). The area of effective treatment is smaller than the area of frozen tissue. Homogeneous nucleation is required for tumour cell destruction. Equipment, operation techniques, and limitations are described. Spray application or probes with closed tips may be used, but probes for retina surgery (cooled with CO_2 or NO_2) would be inadequate. Even with liquid nitrogen, every effort has to be made to enhance the freezing rate in the tissues - e.g. vacuum-insulated N_2-supply line, wet coupling, local anaesthesia with local anaemia (via vasoconstrictor). Slow defreezing and 3 freezing-defreezing cycles for each tumour part must be applied.

Why cryotherapy? The lacrimal passage often remains patent, even if it had to be involved in the treatment area. Adjacent periosteum or superficial bone layers can be included in the area of treatment without disadvantage. After treatment the regenerated skin corresponds very closely to normal skin (also in its surgical properties).

Since 1979, 84 patients have been treated. Postoperatively, we tried hard to get follow-up findings every 3 months for at least 3 years. The resulting follow-up periods are shown, as well as the findings. Pseudo-recidivism (Zacarian) was often found during the first postoperative year and disappeared spontaneously in all cases. Two tumours persisted after apparently ineffective cryo-treatment; the reasons are discussed. Otherwise, there were no recurrences in the group of patients who received N_2-cryotherapy as the first treatment of their disease. However, 5 recurrences have been observed in the group of patients who received primarily radiotherapy or surgical excision treatment and were treated afterwards for tumour recurrences with N_2-cryotherapy. Patient examples are shown.

This material, as well as the follow-up period, would not yet allow a final evaluation of this method; however, up till now we can state as good results as those reported by Matthäus or Zacarian and their co-workers, who had treated and seen a much larger number of cases over longer periods.

REFERENCES

1. Allen ED, McGill JI, Hall VL, Bodkin RE, MacDonald H, Buchanan RB, White JE, Leppard BJ, Goodwin PS, Fraser J. Cryotherapy of basal cell lesions. Trans Ophthalmol Soc UK 1979; 99:264.
2. Anderson RL, Harvey JT. Lid splitting and posterior lamella cryosurgery for congenital and acquired distichiasis. Arch Ophthalmol 1981; 99:631-34.
3. Bart RS, Kopf AW, Petratos MA. X-ray therapy of skin cancer:evaluation of a "standardized" method for treating basal cell epitheliomas. Proc Natl Cancer Conf 1970; 6:559-69.
4. Bart RS, Schrager D, Kopf AW, Bromberg J, Dubin N. Scalpel excision of basal cell carcinomas. Arch Dermatol 1978; 114:739-42.
5. Beard C, Sullivan JH. Cryosurgery of eyelid disorders including malignant tumors. In: Zacarian SA (Ed): Cryosurgical advances in dermatology and tumors of the head and neck. 1977. Springfield, Thomas.
6. Beard C. Observations on the treatment of basal cell carcinoma of the eyelids. Trans Am Acad Ophthalmol Otolaryngol 1975; 79:664.
7. Beard C. Cryosurgery in the treatment of eyelid lesions. In: Hornblass A (Ed): Tumors of the ocular adnexa and orbit. 1979. St.Louis, Toronto, London, Mosby.
8. Bellows JG. Cryosurgery in Ophthalmology. In: von Leden H, Gahan WG (Ed): Cryogenics in Surgery. 1971. New York, Medical Exam. Publishing Co..
9. Brownstein S, Jakobiec FA, Wilkinson RD, Lombardo J, Jackson WB. Cryotherapy for precancerous melanosis (atypical melanocytic hyperplasia) of the conjunctiva. Arch Ophthalmol 1981; 99:1224-31.
10. Bullock JD, Beard C, Sullivan JH. Cryotherapy of basal cell carcinoma in oculoplastic surgery. Am J Ophthalmol 1976; 82:841.
11. Buschmann W, Linnert D. Zur Kryotherapie von Tumoren. 1979. In: Ber Dtsch Ophthalmol Ges 1980; 77:305-11. Heidelberg, Bergmann.
12. Buschmann W, Linnert D. Stickstoff-Kryotherapie von Lidbasaliomen. Klin Mbl Augenheilk 1980; 177:345-53.
13. Doxanas MT, Green WR, Iliff ChE. Factors in the successful surgical management of basal cell carcinoma of the eyelids. Am J Ophthalmol 1981; 91:726-36.
14. Federman JL, Felberg NT, Shields JA. Effect of local treatment on antibody levels in malignant melanoma of the choroid. Trans Ophthalmol Soc UK 1977; 97:436.
15. Fraunfelder FT, Wallace TR, Watkins III J, Hendrickson R, Smead WJ, Limmer BL. The role of cryosurgery in external ocular and periocular disease. Trans Am Acad Ophthalmol Otolaryngol 1977; 83:713-24.

16. Fraunfelder FT, Zacarian SA, Limmer BL, Wingfield D. Cryosurgery for malignancies of the eyelid. Ophthalmology 1980; 87:461-65.
17. Gill W, Long WB. A critical look at cryosurgery. Internat Surg 1971; 56:344.
18. Jakobiec FA, Brownstein S, Albert W, Schwarz F, Anderson R. The role of cryotherapy in the management of conjunctival melanoma. Ophthalmology 1982; 89:502-15.
19. Kopf AW, Bart RS, Schrager D, Lazar M, Popkin GL. Curettage electrodesiccation treatment of basal cell carcinomas. Arch Dermatol 1977; 113:439-43.
20. Matthäus W, Krantz H. Kryotherapie in der Augenheilkunde. 1973. Dresden, Steinkopff.
21. Matthäus W, Lange G, Roitzsch E. Die Kryotherapie von Lid- und Bindehauttumoren. Ophthalmologica (Basel) 1976; 173:53.
22. Matthäus W, Sebastian G, Scholz A. Die Kryotherapie des Basalioms. Arch Geschwulstforsch 1977; 47/5:412.
23. Matthäus W, Baerthold W. Das Verhalten der Tränenwege nach Kryotherapie von Lidtumoren. Ophthalmologica (Basel) 1978; 176:150.
24. Matthäus W. Die Kryoepilation - ein neues Verfahren zur Behandlung der Trichiasis. Folia Ophthalmol 1978; 3:139-41.
25. Matthäus W, Scholz A. 9jährige Erfahrungen mit der Kryotherapie von Tumoren im Kopfbereich in 1540 Fällen. Klin Mbl Augenheilk 1981; 178:355-59.
26. Older JJ, Quickert MH, Beard C. Surgical removal of basal cell carcinomas of the eyelids utilizing frozen section control . Trans Am Acad Ophthalmol Otolaryngol 1975; 79:OP-658-OP-663.
27. Rieger G. Isolierte Amyloidose der Bindehaut. Klin Mbl Augenheilk 1981; 179:432-33.
28. Vistnes LM, Harris DR, Fajardo LF. An evaluation of cryosurgery for basal cell carcinoma. Plast & Reconstr Surg 1975; 55:71-75.
29. Wood JR, Anderson RL. Complications of cryosurgery. Arch Ophthalmol 1981; 99:460-63.
30. Zacarian SA. 1969. Cryosurgery of skin cancer and cryosurgical techniques in dermatology. Springfield, Thomas.
31. Zacarian SA. The cryogenic approach to treatment of lid tumors. Ann Ophthalmol 1970; 2:706.
32. Zacarian SA. Cancer of the eyelid - a cryosurgical approach. Ann Ophthalmol 1972; 4:473.
33. Zacarian SA. Cryosurgery of tumors of the skin and oral cavity.1973. Springfield, Thomas.
34. Zacarian SA (Ed). Cryosurgical advances in dermatology and tumors of the head and neck. 1977. Springfield, Thomas.
35. Zacarian SA. Cryosurgery of skin cancer - in proper perspective. J Dermatol Surg 1975; 1:3.

CONTRIBUTORS

G.S. Baarsma, Stichting Oogziekenhuis, Schiedamsevest 180, 3000 LM Rotterdam, The Netherlands.

N. Bornfeld, Universitätsklinikum der Gesamthochschule Essen, Augenklinik und Poliklinik, Hufelandstrasse 55, 4300 Essen 1, Federal Republic of Germany.

Dr. E.N. Brons, Academisch Ziekenhuis, Afdeling Keel-, Neus-, Oorheelkunde, Rijnsburgerweg 10, 2333 AA Leiden, The Netherlands.

Prof.Dr. W. Buschmann, Universitäts-Augenklinik, Josef-Schneider-Strasse 11, 8700 Würzburg, Federal Republic of Germany.

Prof.Dr. F.J. Cleton, Academisch Ziekenhuis, Afdeling Klinische Oncologie, Rijnsburgerweg 10, 2333 AA Leiden, The Netherlands.

J.R.O. Collin, Moorfields Eye Hospital, City Road, London EC1V 2PD, Great Britain.

M. Foerster, Universitätsklinikum der Gesamthochschule Essen, Augenklinik und Poliklinik, Hufelandstrasse 55, 4300 Essen 1, Federal Republic of Germany.

Prof. W.S. Foulds, University of Glasgow, Tennent Institute of Ophthalmology, Western Infirmary, Glasgow G11 6NT, Great Britain.

Prof. Cl. Gailloud, Hôpital Ophtalmique, Clinique Ophtalmologique Universitaire, 15, Av. de France, 1004 Lausanne, Switzerland.

Dr. J.P.A. Gillissen, Academisch Medisch Centrum, Afdeling Keel-, Neus-, Oorheelkunde, Meibergdreef 9, 1105 AZ Amsterdam, The Netherlands.

Dr. D. Hallermann, Universitäts-Augenklinik, Martinistrasse 52, 2 Hamburg 20, Federal Republic of Germany.

Prof.Dr. B.D. de Jong, Academisch Ziekenhuis, Afdeling Plastische Chirurgie, Catharijnesingel 101, 3583 CP Utrecht, The Netherlands.

Prof.Dr. P.T.V.M. de Jong, Stichting Oogziekenhuis, Schiedamsevest 180, 3000 LM Rotterdam, The Netherlands.

H.M. Kakebeeke-Kemme, Academisch Ziekenhuis, Afdeling Oogheelkunde, Rijnsburgerweg 10, 2333 AA Leiden, The Netherlands.

Dr. R.J.W. de Keizer, Afdeling Oogheelkunde, Academisch Ziekenhuis, Rijnsburgerweg 10, 2333 AA Leiden, The Netherlands.

Prof.Dr. J.A. Oosterhuis, Afdeling Oogheelkunde, Academisch Ziekenhuis, Rijnsburgerweg 10, 2333 AA Leiden, The Netherlands.

Prof.Dr. H.A. van Peperzeel, Instituut voor Radiotherapie, Academisch Ziekenhuis, Catharijnesingel 101, 3583 CP Utrecht, The Netherlands.

Dr. B.C.P. Polak, Stichting Oogziekenhuis, Schiedamsevest 180, 3000 LM Rotterdam, The Netherlands.

Dr. P.J. Ringens, Stichting Oogziekenhuis, Schiedamsevest 180, 3000 LM Rotterdam, The Netherlands.

Prof.Dr. E. Scheffer, Pathologisch Laboratorium, Rijksuniversiteit van Leiden, Wassenaarseweg 62, 2333 AL Leiden, The Netherlands.

J. Schipper, Stichting Koninklijk Nederlands Gasthuis voor Ooglijders, F.C. Dondersstraat 65, 3572 JE Utrecht, The Netherlands.

Prof.Dr. W.A. van Vloten, Afdeling Dermatologie, Academisch Ziekenhuis, Rijnsburgerweg 10, 2333 AA Leiden, The Netherlands.

Prof.Dr. A. Wessing, Universitätsklinikum der Gesamthochschule Essen, Augenklinik und Poliklinik, Hufelandstrasse 55, 4300 Essen 1, Federal Republic of Germany.

D. de Wolff-Rouendaal, Afdeling Oogheelkunde, Academisch Ziekenhuis, Rijnsburgerweg 10, 2333 AA Leiden, The Netherlands.

J.E. Wright, Moorfields Eye Hospital, City Road, London EC1V 2PD, Great Britain.

L. Zografos, Hôpital Ophtalmique, Clinique Ophtalmologique Universitaire, 15, Av. de France, 1004 Lausanne, Switzerland.